Diseases of the Nervous System

Diseases of the Nervous System

Diseases of the Nervous System

Editor: Victor Mahoney

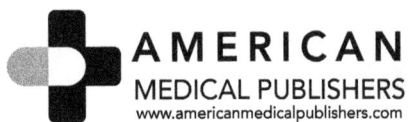

AMERICAN
MEDICAL PUBLISHERS
www.americanmedicalpublishers.com

AMERICAN
MEDICAL PUBLISHERS
www.americanmedicalpublishers.com

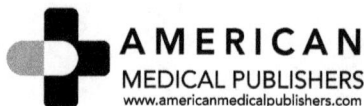

Cataloging-in-Publication Data

Diseases of the nervous system / edited by Victor Mahoney.
    p. cm.
Includes bibliographical references and index.
ISBN 978-1-63927-292-1
1. Nervous system--Diseases. 2. Neurology. 3. Neurophysiology. I. Mahoney, Victor.
RC346 .D57 2022

616.8--dc23

American Medical Publishers,
41 Flatbush Avenue,
1st Floor, New York,
NY 11217, USA

ISBN 978-1-63927-292-1 (Hardback)

Contents

Contents

Preface

Nervous system diseases are also known as neurological disorders. The nervous system consists of central and peripheral nervous systems. The brain and spinal cord together make the central nervous system. The brain is present in the skull and protected by cranium whereas the spinal cord is protected by the vertebrae. Nervous system diseases are neurological disorders that affect the functioning of the whole system. They are majorly caused by traumatic brain injury, infection in the brain or spinal cord or structural defects such as anencephaly and hypospadias. The symptoms of the nervous system diseases are pain in the face, arms, back or legs, lack of concentration, loss of feeling and constant headache. Epilepsy, spina bifida, Parkinson's disease, seizure disorders and amyotrophic lateral sclerosis are some examples of the diseases of the nervous system. This book contains some path-breaking studies related to the diseases of the nervous system. It presents researches and studies performed by experts across the globe. It is appropriate for students seeking detailed information in neurology as well as for experts.

This book is the end result of constructive efforts and intensive research done by experts in this field. The aim of this book is to enlighten the readers with recent information in this area of research. The information provided in this profound book would serve as a valuable reference to students and researchers in this field.

At the end, I would like to thank all the authors for devoting their precious time and providing their valuable contribution to this book. I would also like to express my gratitude to my fellow colleagues who encouraged me throughout the process.

Editor

Evaluation of speed-accuracy trade-off in a computer task in individuals with cerebral palsy

Deborah Cristina Gonçalves Luiz Fernani[1,2*], Maria Tereza Artero Prado[1,2], Talita Dias da Silva[3], Thais Massetti[4], Luiz Carlos de Abreu[2], Fernando Henrique Magalhães[3], Helen Dawes[5,6] and Carlos Bandeira de Mello Monteiro[2,3,4]

Abstract

Background: Individuals with Cerebral Palsy (CP) present with sensorimotor dysfunction which make the control and execution of movements difficult. This study aimed to verify the speed-accuracy trade-off in individuals with CP.

Methods: Forty eight individuals with CP and 48 with typical development (TD) were evaluated (32 females and 64 males with a mean age of 15.02 ± 6.37 years: minimum 7 and maximum 30 years). Participants performed the "Fitts' Reciprocal Aiming Task v.1.0 (Horizontal)" on a computer with different sizes and distance targets, composed by progressive indices of difficulty (IDs): ID2, ID4a and ID4b.

Results: There were no statistical differences between the groups in relation to the slope of the curve (b1) and dispersion of the movement time (r^2). However, the intercept (b0) values presented significant differences ($F(1.95) = 11.3; p = .001$), with greater movement time in the CP group compared to the TD group. It means that for individuals with CP, regardless of index difficulty, found the task more difficult than for TD participants. Considering CP and TD groups, speed-accuracy trade-off was found when using different indices of difficulty (ID2 and ID4). However, when the same index of difficulty was used with a larger target and longer distance (ID4a) or with a narrow target and shorter distance (ID4b), only individuals with CP had more difficulty performing the tasks involving smaller targets. Marginally significant inverse correlations were identified between the values of b1 and age ($r = -0.119, p = .052$) and between r^2 and Gross Motor Function Classification System ($r = -0.280, p = .054$), which did not occur with the Manual Ability Classification System.

Conclusion: We conclude that the individuals with CP presented greater difficulty when the target was smaller and demanded more accuracy, and less difficulty when the task demanded speed. It is suggested that treatments should target tasks with accuracy demands, that could help in daily life tasks, since it is an element that is generally not considered by professionals during therapy.

Keywords: Cerebral palsy, Motor activity, Disabled people, Motor skills

* Correspondence: deborah@unoeste.br
[1]University of West Paulista, Presidente Prudente, SP, Brazil
[2]Laboratory Design and Scientific Writing Department of Basic Sciences, ABC Faculty of Medicine, Av. Príncipe de Gales, 821, Vila Principe de Gales, Santo André, SP 09060-650, Brazil
Full list of author information is available at the end of the article

Background

Cerebral palsy (CP) is a common cause of motor dysfunction that affects children and adults [1], defined as a non-progressive disorder in the brain that occurs during the fetal period or early childhood [2, 3]. The motor alterations in these individuals yield varying degrees of involvement of the upper limbs [4], impairing functionality and hindering the control and execution of movements [5–8]. Due to these difficulties in motor control, several motor limitations in the upper limbs, such as longer movement durations, reduced trajectory straightness and lower peak velocities, are observed to affect daily activities and participation in several occupational tasks throughout life [9–11].

When considering optimal training programs for individuals with CP, a number of exercise interventions have been considered to be effective including: endurance, strength, speed and power interventions [12–15]. However, there is limited evidence to support the effectiveness of these training approaches for improving mobility and function.

A recent review suggests that speed rather than strength training might be effective in improving functional mobility of CP individuals [13]. However, there is limited understanding as to the relationship between speed and accuracy in individuals with CP. The speed accuracy relationship is particularly important when considering upper limb functional tasks as compared to functional mobility. In typically developed (TD) individuals, movement speed and accuracy, and their relationship, is inversely proportional except when the need for accuracy and speed coexists whereby both can be achieved [16]. For a movement to be performed accurately, muscle coordination and co-contraction need to occur [17, 18]. When a movement is performed quickly, generally a speed modulation strategy is used, whereby muscle co-contraction is reduced with a subsequent reduction in accuracy [16–18].

The mechanisms underlying the speed-accuracy trade-off are more complex than previously thought, with individuals being able to utilize a speed-energy-accuracy trade-off for goal-directed movements; whereby individuals can move faster while preserving movement accuracy by using a strategy where muscles are co-contracted around the joint but at a high energetic cost [16]. As such, a speed modulation strategy is preferred to a co-contraction strategy for faster movements, and a strategy to preserve energy economy typically prevents us from executing faster accurate movements [16].

Considering individuals with CP, changing the distance of a movement may be less taxing, as this can be controlled through a simpler model of agonist and antagonist muscle activity as compared to that required for more accurate movements [19–21]. However, Imms et al. [22] states that spasticity is the most common motor disorder in CP, characterized by a velocity-dependent increase in the tonic stretch reflex which leads to slow and effortful movement. Meskers [23] also pointed out that individuals with movement disorders caused by neurological diseases, such as CP, due to impaired muscle control have atypical force generation and inappropriate tension regulation affecting the normal movement velocity profile, which is essential to obtain fast movements, thus this characteristic could make tasks that demand speed more challenging for people with CP.

Regarding the conflicting evidence about the influence of speed or accuracy demand during a task in individuals with CP, the assessment and investigation of the speed-accuracy trade-off is essential in order to develop optimal exercise interventions that consider the speed at which movements should be performed when trying to facilitate accuracy and the components of a task (distance, size of the target). Task manipulation may for instance increase difficulty and require individuals with CP to move slower and with greater neuromuscular cost. Perhaps more importantly a better understanding will inform the design of systems and devices for individuals with CP, such as modification of computer switch systems to integrate considerations of distance and target accuracy in order to improve and ease engagement in occupational tasks.

In order to better understand the relationships between distance and accuracy, participants were engaged in a movement time task with different indices of difficulty (IDs). The same ID was performed in two ways (considering the relation between widths and distances), where tasks were performed with thicker sidebars and longer distances between them and thinner sidebars with shorter distances, in order to evaluate if the size of the target (accuracy demand) has more influence in the performance than the distance between them (speed demand).

Given this, this study aimed to verify the speed-accuracy trade-off in individuals with CP. We hypothesize that there should be an inverse relationship between task difficulty and performance (measured by means of movement time) for both TD and CP individuals, whereby the CP individuals should be generally slower than the TD controls and this effect would be more pronounced during movements with higher levels of difficulty. We further hypothesized that the greater the severity of CP, the greater should be the impairment in performance, but with no differences between tasks with same index of difficulty, i.e. tasks that demand more accuracy (size of target) or speed (distance between targets).

Methods
Study design
An observational study that analyzed the motor control system by evaluating the performance in a computer task in individuals with CP and in a control group of typically developed individuals.

Participants
In total, 96 individuals were evaluated, being 48 individuals with CP and 48 with typical development (TD), matched by age and sex. The sample was composed of 32 females and 64 males with a mean age of 15.02 ± 6.37 years (minimum 7 and maximum 30 years). The participants of the CP group comprised 25 individuals with hemiparesis, 19 with diparesis and 4 with quadriparesis. A previous statistical analysis was made to find out differences between type of CP, considering the indices of difficulty as dependent variables, with no difference found ($p > 0.05$). Thus, we include all participants in the study, wherein all individuals in the CP group showed to be able to perform the task.

In the Gross Motor Function Classification System (GMFCS) [24], 29 individuals were classified with level I, 6 with level II, 6 with level III and 7 with level IV. According to the Manual Ability Classification System (MACS) [25], 34 individuals obtained level I, 9 level II and 5 level III.

The inclusion criteria were a medical diagnosis of CP, of levels I to IV according to the GMFCS, a classification system that ranks individuals with CP from I to V, in which children in Level I present some difficulty with speed, balance, and coordination, but with ability to perform all the activities of their age-matched peers, while children in level V present difficulty in achieving any voluntary control of movement and controlling their head and trunk posture in most positions [26]. For the inclusion criteria, they should also be between levels I to III according to MACS, that similarly to GMFCS, but considers upper limb function specifically and consists of five levels, where level I represent the highest functional level and level V the lowest functional level [25]. These classification were made by two professionals specialized in CP. The last inclusion criterion was previous use of mouse in their computational activities.

The exclusion criteria were the presence of surgery or a chemical neuromuscular blockade in the upper limbs within 6 months prior to participation in the study and disorders in cognitive function that would prohibit comprehension of the experimental instructions. The comprehension ability was determined through two trials to perform the task, with lack of comprehension being determined on individuals not attempting to follow instructions and perform the task.

Material
The software used in this study was "Fitts' Reciprocal Aiming Task v.1.0 (Horizontal)" developed by Okazaki [27], in the public domain and available on the Internet, which was performed on a Toshiba notebook®, model Satellite A60-S1561, Fortrek® OM-302.

This instrument is used to verify motor control through analysis of the speed and accuracy of movement, which is determined through the log-linear relation between target size and task distance between them using a mathematical equation, and analyzed by Fitts' law, which describes the relation between movement accuracy and speed [28], resulting in the difficulty index. And, the more difficult the task, this will require greater movement time for execution [29]. Thus, the ID2 was composed by target sidebars thicker (3 cm), with little distance between them (6 cm) – ($Log2 [(2 \times 6)/3] = Log2\ 4 = 2$), the ID4a had thicker sidebars (3 cm) with a greater distance between them (24 cm) – ($Log2 [(2 \times 24)/3] = Log2\ 16 = 4$), and the ID4b had thinner target sidebars than used in ID4a (1.5 cm), however, the with less distance between them (12 cm) – ($Log2 [(2 \times 12)/1.5] = Log2\ 16 = 4$) [30, 31].

The task was composed of targets of different sizes, being that the smaller targets require more time to execute due to the necessity of increased accuracy [32, 33] and, if the distance between targets reduces, the speed of movement becomes greater and the accuracy decreases.

Therefore, to evaluate the trade-off between speed and accuracy, two different indices of difficulty were used (ID2 and ID4). The difficulty level was increased by changing the width and distance between the bars (Fig. 1). In addition, to evaluate if the size of the target (accuracy demand) requires more movement time when compared to the distance between them (speed demand), ID4 was used in two different ways (ID4a and ID4b), for which the distance between the bars and the width were different, but the ID was maintained. As the ID was maintained, should not exist difference in movement time between ID4a and ID4b.

Procedure
The experiment was composed of three trials at each of the indices of difficulty: ID2, ID4a and ID4b. The participants performed the tasks individually in a room, with only the evaluator present, seated on a chair (or their own wheelchair), which was adjusted in height according to the needs of the individual. A footrest was available, when necessary. The computer was placed on a table, and each participant was given instructions and presented with the task, in which the individual, after hearing an alarm from the computer, was required to click alternately and intermittently with an external mouse cursor on two parallel bars with three sizes of target and three distances which were used to determine different

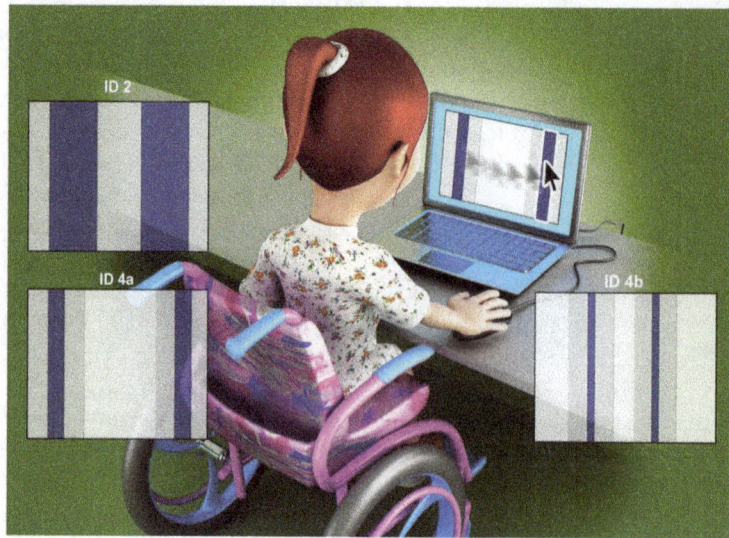

Fig. 1 Individual in a wheelchair* performing the task interfaces at different indices of difficulty *some individuals in this study were seated on a regular chair. Source: figure created by the authors

indices of difficulty, and arranged vertically. The instructions given were 'on hearing the alarm click with the greatest speed and accuracy possible, for a period of 10 seconds, until you hear a second alarm which indicates the end of your attempt'.

Directly following the attempt, the total movement time was registered by software, dividing the seconds obtained in each attempt by the number of "clicks" on targets. If more than two clicks were wrong, the individual repeated the task.

We did not assess or give instructions about the pattern of movement, so they could perform the task in the easier way for each one, i.e. movement of the upper limb in general (hand, wrist, elbow, and shoulder).

Statistical analysis

Regarding the comparisons for movement time on each index of difficulty, an ANOVA with factor 2 (groups: Cerebral Palsy - CP, Typical Development - TD) by 3 (index of difficulty - ID: ID2, ID4a, ID4b) was conducted, with repeated measures for the factor index of difficulty. Post hoc test was carried out using Tukey-HSD ($p < .05$).

In order to establish whether the groups responded to the relation between accuracy and speed, a linear regression analysis was performed on the movement time data, using the curve estimation and obtaining the values of: b0 (intercept), b1 (slope of the curve) and r^2 (movement time dispersion) of each participant; every attempt at the indices of difficulty being considered. MANOVA One way was used to compare the means of the groups in the three variables of interest (b0, b1 and r^2).

A multiple linear regression analysis considering increase in movement time (Δ between 4a and 2; and between 4b and 4a) was performed to determine which factors (age, gender, Gross Motor Function Classification System - GMFCS, Manual Ability Classification System - MACS) influenced the increase in movement time.

To verify associations between GMFCS, MACS, age, b0, b1 and r^2, the Pearson correlation coefficient was used. The software package used was SPSS, 20.0.

Results

In this study it was verified that the CP group used longer movement time to complete the task than TD group. An inverse relationship was observed between speed and accuracy of movement in individuals with TD, but not in those with CP.

The ANOVA with factors groups (CP and TD) and index of difficult (ID2, ID4a, ID4b), with repeated measures for the factor ID was performed to explore the effects of index of difficult on the movement time, determined in items below.

ID2 – ID4a

There was a statistically significant difference between the indices of difficult [F(1.94) = 69.3; $p < .001$; $\eta^2 = 0.42$]. This result demonstrates that the movement time increased significantly from ID2 (mean = 1019 ± 60 ms) to ID4a (mean = 1449 ± 60 ms). However, no interaction was found between Groups and indices of difficult.

In addition, an effect for groups [F1.94) = 33.9; $p < 0.001$; $\eta^2 = 0.27$] was found, in which the individuals with CP (mean = 1575 ± 80 ms) were 682 ms slower than those in the TD group (mean = 893 ± 80 ms).

ID4a – ID4b

There was a statistically significant difference between the indices of difficult [$F_{(1.94)}$ = 4.62; p = .034; η^2 = 0.05] and interaction between index of difficult and Groups [$F_{(1.94)}$ = 6.85; p = .010; η^2 = 0.07]. This result demonstrates that the movement time increased significantly from ID4a (mean = 1449 ± 60 ms) to ID4b (mean = 1614 ± 6 ms). However, this increase was significant in the CP group from ID4a (mean = 1791 ± 92 ms) to ID4b (mean = 2157 ± 154 ms), while in the TD group the increase was not significant (mean = 1107 ± 92 ms for mean = 1071 ± 154 ms, respectively).

The difference between groups remained [$F_{(1.94)}$ = 29.7; p < .001; η^2 = 0.24]; the individuals of the CP group (mean = 1974 ± 115 ms) were 885 ms slower than the TD group (mean = 1089 ± 115 ms).

These findings suggest that this group with CP did not total obey the relation between size and distance of targets (see Fitts' law). This observation becomes evident when comparing the results of ID4a and ID4b, which should have presented the same difficulty. However, we found that movement time increased significantly from ID4a to ID4b in individuals with CP, while in the TD group this difference did not occur, respectively). Interestingly, this result is controversial to our hypothesis that there would be no differences between ID4a and ID4b.

MANOVA was used to compare the slope of the regression line (Fig. 2) and there was no statistical difference between the groups in relation to the slope of the curve (b1) or between the dispersion of movement time (r²) data between the groups. However, the b0 (intercept), values presented statistically significant differences [$F_{(1.95)}$ = 11.3; p = .001], with a greater movement time in the CP group [mean = 1150 ± 1100 milliseconds (ms)] compared to the TD group (mean = 560 ± 70 ms).

Marginally significant inverse correlations were identified between the values of the slope of the curve and age and between the dispersion of movement time and GMFCS (Table 1) using the Pearson correlation, which did not occur with the MACS.

The linear regression analysis revealed a significant finding, $F_{(6, 41)}$ = 2.44, p = 0.041, r2 = 0.263, resulting in the following equation: increase in movement time (ID4a – ID2) = 0.045 × GMFCS. In other words, only the GMFCS influenced the increase in movement time, but age, gender and MACS did not contribute. To understand which factors influenced the increase in movement time from ID4a to ID4b, another regression analysis was performed between difference between ID4a and ID4b with age, gender, GMFCS and MACS, but there were no significant findings for the regression model.

Discussion

The majority of functional manual skills upper limb require fast and accurate performance which we observed was affected in individuals with Cerebral Palsy (CP), who demonstrated significantly greater movement time regardless of the task difficulty when compared with typically developed individuals. For individuals with CP, a typical payoff between speed and accuracy was found, except importantly that they presented with more difficulty performing tasks involving smaller targets than when moving longer distances. Our findings are important as for the first time we can specifically evidence both therapy and device us in this group.

Considering this specific motor control difficulty, and the associated higher neuromuscular cost for individuals

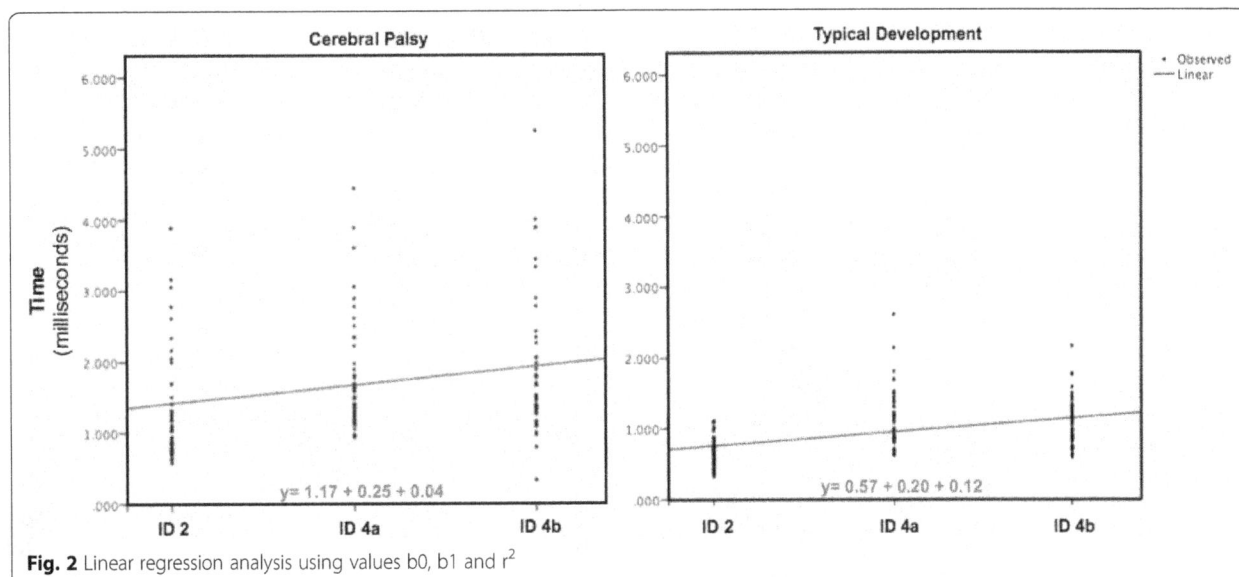

Fig. 2 Linear regression analysis using values b0, b1 and r²

Table 1 Pearson's correlation between the values of b0, b1 and r^2, age, GMFCS and MACS

Variables	Age		GMFCS		MACS	
	r	p	r	p	r	p
b0	−0.035	0.737	0.022	0.880	0.151	0.306
b1	−0.119	0.052*	0.216	0.141	0.129	0.384
r^2	0.083	0.421	−0.280	0.054*	−0.224	0.125

GMFCS, Gross Motor Function Classification System; MACS, Manual Ability Classification System; *marginally statistically significant difference

with CP, particularly those with more severe disability, we propose therapists should consider the difficulty performing dexterous tasks that involve fine control, and implement adaptations to increase target size in particular when aiming to reduce neuromuscular demand in occupational situations. Our findings inform therapeutic exercises and the design of a number of occupational tasks for example in the optimal design of communication computer switch systems.

In this study it was verified that the CP group used longer movement times to complete the tasks than did the typical developed (TD) group. An inverse relationship was observed between speed and accuracy of movement in individuals with TD but not in those with CP. These findings, as presented before, are contrary to our hypothesis and suggest that this group with CP did not obey the relation between size and distance of targets (see Fitts' law). This observation becomes evident when comparing the results of ID4a and ID4b, which should have presented the same difficulty. However, we found that movement time increased significantly from ID4a (mean = 1791 ± 92 ms) to ID4b (mean = 2157 ± 154 ms), in individuals with CP, while in the TD group this difference did not occur (mean = 1107 ± 92 ms for mean = 1071 ± 154 ms, respectively).

These results partially corroborate the findings of Smits-Elgesman [34], who affirmed that individuals with CP require more time to perform the task. The authors also reported that both CP and control groups responded similarly to increasing indices of difficulty, in agreement with the relation between speed and accuracy. This was only partially observed in our present study: in fact, based on our present findings, when observing results from ID2 compared with ID4 there is an influence between speed and accuracy. In ID2 both groups had a smaller movement time compared with ID4. However, considering ID4a versus ID4b individuals with CP had more problems with accuracy (narrow targets, ID4a) than speed (more distant targets, ID4b), this is probably due to weakness, altered reflexes and difficulties in body coordination, that lead to impaired postural control [35, 36].

Davies [4] also found evidence of individuals with CP not following the relation between speed and accuracy.

These authors stated that the International Organization for Standardization indicates that tasks requiring accuracy, such as a point-and-click task, present a low ID if less than 4 and a high ID if greater than 6. However, the study of Davies [4] showed that the ID for individuals with bilateral CP should be limited to a maximum of ID2, which could also be associated with the different performance of CP individuals between the ID4a and ID4b found in this study.

Michmizos [31] reported that the analysis of movement time is an indicator of neurological integrity. In this context, delays in movement time have been seen in studies that evaluated individuals with CP [37, 38], in agreement with that shown in the present study, in which was noted that individuals with CP began to execute the task with a movement time greater (mean = 1150 ± 1100 ms) than the TD group (mean = 560 ± 70 ms).

Considering the slope of the curve (b1), the CP group did not differ from TD group in the present study, which demonstrates that the individuals with CP evolved during the attempts, similarly to those with TD, although the group with CP maintained greater movement time for all levels of difficulty compared to the TD. This can be confirmed by the analysis of the performance differences in the indices of difficulty, in which greater time of movement was observed from ID2 to ID4a for both groups.

Both groups did not differ also regarding dispersion of movement time (r^2) in the evaluated groups; however, both groups presented r^2 values less than 1, which means that there was variation in movement time values. Although, with no significance, the CP group presented greater variation during the execution of attempts than the TD, verified by a lower value of dispersion of movement time (see Fig. 2). These findings (i.e., the lower movement speed and larger dispersion of the data of the CP group), have also been reported in several studies [4, 34, 39–41], which further suggests a decline in the motor control system associated with impairments that affect both nervous and muscular structures. Furthermore, there is evidence from previous studies that movement time is much larger in individuals with CP than in those with TD [42–45].

The correlation analyses performed to investigate the association between the task measurements and MACS, GMFCS and age (made by Pearson coefficients) showed that there was no correlation between MACS and age, intercept, slope of the curve and movement time dispersion. This finding can be explained by the sample classification (levels I, II, III), as they were able to manipulate the mouse and adequately perform the task. This was also emphasized by Davies [46], who related that individuals with levels I, II and III are able to use a mouse to access a computer, thus the MACS was not sensitive to this relation. In addition, Eliasson [25], described that approximately 65% of individuals with CP are classified as levels I to III of MACS, a fact that confirms the levels used in this study.

On the other hand, there was a significant negative correlation between slope of the curve and age, movement time dispersion and GMFCS. These findings demonstrate that the higher the age of the individual, the less the slope of the curve, i.e. the less time this individual would need to perform the task (older individuals were less sensitive to increases in indices of difficult), and the higher the level of the GMFCS, the lower the value of movement time dispersion (i.e. higher the level of the GMFCS, greater the dispersion of the movement time data). As well as the regression analysis showed that the GMFCS influenced the increase in movement time from ID2 to ID4a, i.e., the higher the GMFCS, the greater the increase in movement time.

With respect to impairment in motor function, studies such as those by Haak [47] and Hanna [48], reported that there is a decline in motor function into adulthood in individuals with severe CP, which can be explained by decreased activity, increased body size and changes in spinal alignment, therefore, it is believed that the better performance displayed by older individuals in the present study was due to higher levels of motor function, i.e. we did not evaluated severe levels, GMFCS V and MACS IV and V.

Thus, to improve the motor performance in individuals with CP which targets the performance of activities of daily living, it is necessary to construct and adapt rehabilitation therapies, including tasks that involve speed and accuracy demands [31]. Moreover, as with CP individuals had larger movement times for increased accuracy demands as compared to increased speed it is suggested that treatments should target accuracy demands, an element that is generally not considered by professionals during conventional therapy, which often emphasizes stretching and strengthening exercises.

Limitations and future studies
A limitation of this study is, that we were unable to explore the relationships of motor (spasticity and range of motion), visual or sensory functioning to speed and accuracy data; the impact of these variables should now be explored in an appropriately powered study. The variation of the topographic type, MACS and GMFCS levels can be considered vies in this study, however the sample represents the distribution of impairment in this population. In addition, we did not assess kinematic features of the movement to strength our results, as well as we did not evaluate more indices of difficulties, so we believe that further studies in CP should insert these evaluations

as additional analysis considered alongside presenting symptoms.

Conclusions
Individuals with CP presented greater difficulty when the target was smaller and demanded more accuracy, and less difficulty when the task demanded speed. It is suggested that treatments should target accuracy demands, that could help in daily life tasks and is an element that is generally not considered by professionals during therapy.

Thus, therapists should be made aware of this difficulty performing tasks that involve fine control, and consider implementing adaptations to increase target size in particular when aiming to reduce neuromuscular demand in occupational situations, with appreciation the training of functional activities that address the motor control with focus on the evolution of accuracy of movement.

Our results advise the need to implement precision training in therapies and therefore the adaptation of computer systems to integrate considerations of distance and target accuracy in order to improve and ease engagement in occupational tasks.

Abbreviations
b0: Intercept; b1: Slope of the curve; CP: Cerebral palsy; GMFCS: Gross motor function classification system; ID: Index of difficulty; ID2: Index of difficult 2; ID4a: Index of difficult 4a; ID4b: Index of difficult 4b; MACS: Manual ability classification system; r^2: Dispersion of the movement time; TD: Typical development

Acknowledgements
We thank the participants who provided their data for the study.

Funding
No funding.

Authors' contributions
DCGLF, MTAP and CBMM designed and coordinated the study. TDS performed the statistical analyses and interpreted the data. DCGLF, MTAP, TM and CBMM drafted the article and interpreted the data. DCGLF and MTAP collected the patient data. LCA, FHM and HD revised the manuscript critically for important intellectual content. All authors read and approved the final manuscript.

Competing interests
The authors declare that they do not have any competing interests.

Author details
[1]University of West Paulista, Presidente Prudente, SP, Brazil. [2]Laboratory Design and Scientific Writing Department of Basic Sciences, ABC Faculty of Medicine, Av. Príncipe de Gales, 821, Vila Principe de Gales, Santo André, SP 09060-650, Brazil. [3]School of Arts, Sciences and Humanities, University of São Paulo, São Paulo, SP, Brazil. [4]Post-graduate Program in Rehabilitation Sciences, Faculty of Medicine, University of São Paulo, São Paulo, SP, Brazil. [5]Oxford Institute of Nursing and Allied Health Research, Oxford Brookes University, Oxford, UK. [6]Department of Clinical Neurology, University of Oxford, Oxford, UK.

References

1. Yeargin-Allsopp M, Van Naarden BK, Doernberg NS, Benedict RE, Kirby RS, Durkin MS. Prevalence of cerebral palsy in 8-year-old children in three areas of the United States in 2002: a multisite collaboration. Pediatrics. 2008; doi: 10.1542/peds.2007-1270.
2. Bax M, Goldstein M, Rosenbaum P, Leviton A, Paneth N. Proposed definition and classification of cerebral palsy. Dev Med Child Neurol. 2005;47:571–6.
3. Rosenbaum P, Paneth N, Leviton A. Goldstein M; Bax M. A report: the definition and classification of cerebral palsy April 2006. Dev Med Child Neurol 2007; 109:8-14.
4. Davies TC, Almanji A, Stott NS. A cross-sectional study examining computer task completion by adolescents with cerebral palsy across the manual ability classification system levels. Dev Med Child Neurol. 2014; doi:10.1111/dmcn.12521.
5. Thiel EV, Steenbergen B. Shoulder and hand displacements during hitting, reaching, and grasping movements in hemiparetic cerebral palsy. Mot Control. 2001;5:166–82.
6. Law K, Lee EY, Fung BK, Yan LS, Gudushauri P, Wang KW, et al. Evaluation of deformity and hand function in cerebral palsy patients. J Orthop Surg Res. 2008; doi:10.1186/1749-799X-3-52.
7. Sorsdahl AB, Moe-Nilssen R, Kaale HK, Rieber J, Strand LI. Change in basic motor abilities, quality of movement and everyday activities following intensive, goal-directed, activity-focused physiotherapy in a group setting for children with cerebral palsy. BMC Pediatr. 2010; doi: 10.1186/1471-2431-10-26.
8. Park ES, Sim EG, Rha DW. Effect of upper limb deformities on gross motor and upper limb functions in children with spastic cerebral palsy. Res Dev Disabil. 2011; doi:10.1016/j.ridd.2011.07.021.
9. Arnould C, Penta M, Thonnard JL. Hand impairments and their relationship with manual ability in children with cerebral palsy. J Rehabil Med. 2007;39:708–14.
10. Öhrvall AM, Eliasson AC, Löwing K, Ödman P, KrumlindeSundholm L. Self-care and mobility skills in children with cerebral palsy, related to their manual ability and gross motor function classifications. Dev Med Child Neurol. 2010;52:1048–55.
11. Figueiredo PR, Silva PL, Avelar BS, da Fonseca ST, Bootsma RJ, Mancini MC. Upper limb performance and the structuring of joint movement in teenagers with cerebral palsy: the reciprocal role of task demands and action capabilities. Exp Brain Res. 2015;233(4):1155–64. doi:10.1007/s00221-014-4195-3.
12. Ross SM, MacDonald M, Bigouette JP. Effects of strength training on mobility in adults with cerebral palsy: a systematic review. Disabil Health J. 2016; doi:10.1016/j.dhjo.2016.04.005.
13. Moreau NG, Bodkin AW, Bjornson K, Hobbs A, Soileau M, Lahasky K. Effectiveness of rehabilitation interventions to improve gait speed in children with cerebral palsy: systematic review and meta-analysis. Phys Ther. 2016; doi:10.2522/ptj.20150401.
14. Dewar R, Love S, Johnston LM. Exercise interventions improve postural control in children with cerebral palsy: a systematic review. Dev Med Child Neurol. 2015; doi:10.1111/dmcn.12660.
15. Novak I, McIntyre S, Morgan C, Campbell L, Dark L, Morton N, Stumbles E, Wilson SA, Goldsmith S. A systematic review of interventions for children with cerebral palsy: state of the evidence. Dev Med Child Neurol. 2013; doi:10.1111/dmcn.12246.
16. Missenard O, Fernandez L. Moving faster while preserving accuracy. Neuroscience. 2011; doi:10.1016/j.neuroscience.2011.09.020.
17. Gribble PL, Mullin LI, Cothros N, Mattar A. Role of Cocontraction in arm movement accuracy. J Neurophysiol. 2003; doi:10.1152/jn.01020.2002.
18. Popescu F, Hidler JM, Rymer WZ. Elbow impedance during goal-directed movements. Exp Brain Res. 2003;152:17–28.
19. Selen LP, Beek PJ, van Dieën JH. Impedance is modulated to meet accuracy demands during goal-directed arm movements. Exp Brain Res. 2006;172:129–38.
20. Selen LP, Franklin DW, Wolpert DM. Impedance control reduces instability that arises from motor noise. J Neurosci. 2009; doi:10.1523/JNEUROSCI.2826-09.2009.
21. Wong J, Wilson ET, Malfait N, Gribble PL. Limb stiffness is modulated with spatial accuracy requirements during movement in the absence of destabilizing forces. J Neurophysiol. 2009; doi:10.1152/jn.91188.2008.
22. Imms C, Wallen M, Elliott C, Hoare B, Randall M, Greaves S, Adair B, Bradshaw E, Carter R, Orsini F, Shih ST, Reddihough D. Minimising impairment: protocol for multicentre randomised controlled trial of upper limborthoses for children with cerebral palsy. BMC Pediatr. 2016;16:70. doi:10.1186/s12887-016-0608-8.
23. Meskers CGM, de Groot JH, de Vlugt E, Schouten AC. NeuroControl of movement: system identification approach for clinical benefit. Front Integr Neurosci. 2015; doi:10.3389/fnint.2015.00048.
24. Palisano RJ, Cameron D, Rosenbaum PL, Walter SD, Russell D. Stability of the gross motor function classification system. Dev Med Child Neurol. 2006; doi:10.1111/j.1469-8749.2006.tb01290.x.
25. Eliasson AC, Krumlinde Sundholm L, Rösblad B, Beckung E, Arner M, Öhrvall AM, Rosenbaum P. The manual ability classification system (MACS) for children with cerebral palsy: scale development and evidence of validity and reliability. Dev Med Child Neurol. 2006; doi:10.1111/j.1469-8749.2006.tb01313.x.
26. Morris C, Bartlett D. Gross motor function classification system: impact and utility. Dev Med Child Neurol. 2004;46(1):60–5.
27. Okazaki VHA. Discrete Aiming Task (v.2.0). 2007. http://okazaki.webs.com/softwaresdownloads.htm#297051518. Accessed 4 July 2011.
28. Ifft PJ, Lebedev MA, Nicolelis MAL. Cortical correlates of Fitts' law. Front Integr Neurosci. 2011; doi:10.3389/fnint.2011.00085.
29. Fitts PM. The information capacity of the human motor system in controlling the amplitude of movement. J Exp Psychol. 1954;47:381–91.
30. Schmidt RA, Zelaznik H, Hawkins B, Frank JS, Quinn JT. Motor-output variability: a theory for the accuracy of rapid motor acts. Psychol Rev. 1979;47(5):415–51.
31. Michmizos KP, Krebs HI. Reaction time in ankle movements: a diffusion model analysis. Exp Brain Res. 2014; doi:10.1007/s00221-014-4032-8.
32. Boyd LA, Vidoni ED, Siengsukon CF, Wessel BD. Manipulating time-to-plan alters patterns of brain activation during the Fitts' task. Exp Brain Res. 2009;194:527–39.
33. Lam MY, Hodges NJ, Virji-Babul N, Latash ML. Evidence for slowing as a function of index of difficulty in young adults with down syndrome. Am J Intellect Dev Disabil. 2009;114:411–26.
34. Smits-Engelsman BCM, Rameckers EAA, Duysens J. Children with congenital spastic hemiplegia obey Fitts' law in a visually guided tapping task. Exp Brain Res. 2007; doi:10.1007/s00221-006-0698-x.
35. Do JH, Yoo EY, Jung MY, Park HY. The effects of virtual reality-based bilateral arm training on hemiplegic children's upper limb motor skills. Neuro Rehabilitation. 2016; doi:10.3233/NRE-161302.
36. Seruya M, Johnson JD. Surgical treatment of pediatric upper limb spasticity: the shoulder. Semin Plast Surg. 2016; doi:10.1055/s-0035-1571253.
37. Horgan JS. Reaction-time and movement-time of children with cerebral palsy: under motivational reinforcement conditions. Am J Phys Med. 1980;59:22–9.
38. Chang JJ, Wu TI, Wu WL, Su FC. Kinematical measure for spastic reaching in children with cerebral palsy. Clin Biomech. 2005; doi:10.1016/j.clinbiomech.2004.11.015.
39. Bravo PE, Legare M, Cook AM, Hussey S. A study of the application of Fitts' law to selected cerebral palsied adults. Percept Mot Skills. 1993;77:1107–17.
40. Legare M, Wolak C, Doyle B. Stimulus-response compatibility in a small sample of cerebral palsied adults. Percept Mot Skills. 1994;79:1459–74.
41. Gump A, Legare M, Hunt DL. Application of Fitts' law to individuals with cerebral palsy. Percept Mot Skills. 2002;94:883–95.
42. Keates S, Hwang F, Langdon P, Clarkson PJ, Robinson P. Cursor measures for motion-impaired computer users. Proceedings of the fifth international ACM conference on assistive technologies. ACM: Edinburgh; 2002. doi:10.1145/638249.638274.
43. Hwang F, Keates S, Langdon P, Clarkson J. Mouse movements of motion-impaired users: a submovement analysis. J SIGACCESS Access Comput. 2003; doi:10.1145/1028630.1028649.
44. Hwang F, Keates S, Langdon P, Clarkson J. A submovement analysis of cursor trajectories. Behav Inf Technol. 2005; doi:10.1080/01449290412331327474.
45. Wobbrock JO, Fogarty J, Liu S, Kimuro S, Harada S. The angle mouse: target-agnostic dynamic gain adjustment based on angular deviation. Proceedings of the 27th international conference on human factors in computing systems; Boston, MA: ACM, 2009:1401–10.

46. Davies TC, Chau T, Fehlings DL, Ameratunga S, Stott NS. Youth with cerebral palsy with differing upper limb abilities: how do they access computers? Arch Phys Med Rehabil. 2010;91:1952–6.

47. Haak P, Lenski M, Hidecker MJC, Li M. Paneth N. Dev Med Child Neurol. 2009; doi:10.1111/j.1469-8749.2009.03428.x.

48. Hanna SE, Rosenbaum PL, Bartlett DJ, Palisano RJ, Walter SD, Avery L, Russell DJ. Stability and decline in gross motor function among children and youth with cerebral palsy aged 2 to 21 years. Dev Med Child Neurol. 2009;51(4):295–302.

2

A comparison of central nervous system involvement in patients with classical Fabry disease or the later-onset subtype with the IVS4 +919G>A mutation

Han-Jui Lee[1,2†], Ting-Rong Hsu[3,4†], Sheng-Che Hung[1,2,5*] ⓘ, Wen-Chung Yu[2,6], Tzu-Hung Chu[2,4], Chia-Feng Yang[2,4], Svetlana Bizjajeva[7], Chui-Mei Tiu[1,2] and Dau-Ming Niu[3,4*]

Abstract

Background: Patients with the later-onset IVS4+919G>A (IVS4) Fabry mutation are known to have positive central nervous system involvement compared with age- and sex-matched controls. This study compares central nervous system manifestations in patients with the IVS4 mutation or classical Fabry mutations.

Methods: This was a retrospective analysis of magnetic resonance imaging (MRI) data from Taiwanese patients enrolled in the Fabry Outcome Survey (sponsored by Shire; data extracted March 2015).

Results: Twenty-five IVS4 (19 males) and 12 (four males) classical Fabry patients underwent MRI at a median (range) age of 60.7 (45.0–70.4) and 43.0 (18.0–61.4) years, respectively. All patients received agalsidase alfa enzyme replacement therapy; two (16.7%) classical Fabry patients underwent MRI before treatment start. The pulvinar sign occurred in eight (32.0%; seven males) IVS4 and six (50.0%; three males) classical Fabry patients. Infarction occurred in eight (32.0%) IVS4 and four (33.3%) classical Fabry patients. Fazekas scores of 0, 1, 2, and 3 were found for 15 (60.0%), seven (28.0%), two (8.0%), and one (4.0%) of the IVS4 patients and for six (50.0%), four (33.3%), two (16.7%), and 0 classical Fabry patients, respectively. Abnormal height bifurcation of the basilar artery was observed in 40.0% of IVS4 and 58.3% of classical Fabry patients; abnormal laterality was observed in 4.0% of IVS4 and 16.7% of classical Fabry patients. Median (range) basilar artery diameter was 2.7 (1.4–4.0) mm in IVS4 and 3.2 (2.3–4.7) mm in classical Fabry patients ($P = 0.0293$); vascular stenosis was noted in 8.3% of IVS4 patients but in no classical Fabry patients.

Conclusions: A similar range of MRI findings was found for both IVS4 and classical Fabry patients. Notably, basilar artery diameter was larger in classical Fabry patients than IVS4 patients.

Keywords: Agalsidase alfa, Central nervous system manifestations, Fabry Outcome Survey, Later-onset Fabry disease, Magnetic resonance imaging

Background

Fabry disease (FD, MIM 301500) is an X-linked lysosomal disorder resulting from lysosomal α-galactosidase A deficiency, which subsequently leads to the accumulation of glycosphingolipids, primarily globotriaosylceramide, throughout the body [1]. This multisystemic disorder commonly manifests in childhood or adolescence with symptoms including acroparesthesia, cornea verticillata, and gastrointestinal complaints [2]. Progression to renal failure, hypertrophic cardiomyopathy, and cerebrovascular complications occurs in later life; these comprise the leading causes of premature death in FD [3]. Organ failure attributed to FD can reduce life expectancy by approximately 25 years in males [4] and 15 years in females [5]. Enzyme replacement therapy (ERT) can slow disease progression [6] and, if started early

* Correspondence: hsz829@gmail.com; dmniu1111@yahoo.com.tw
†Equal contributors
[1]Department of Radiology, Taipei Veterans General Hospital, Taipei, Taiwan
[3]Institute of Clinical Medicine, National Yang-Ming University, Taipei, Taiwan
Full list of author information is available at the end of the article

enough, may even be able to prevent irreversible organ damage.

Neurological signs and symptoms are commonly reported in FD and can start during childhood or adolescence [7]. Neuropathic pain, vertigo, tinnitus, stroke, and transient ischemic attack are some of the commonly reported neurological features of FD [8, 9]. White matter lesions and infarction, increased signal intensity in the lateral pulvinar (known as the pulvinar sign), and increased diameter and tortuosity of the basilar artery [8, 10–12] are some of the abnormalities that have been observed upon brain magnetic resonance imaging (MRI) in patients with FD. Increased diameter of the basilar artery and presence of the pulvinar sign are reportedly useful in FD diagnosis, particularly when found alongside other, less specific, neurological findings that are also known to occur in FD [10–12].

The incidence of FD ranges from 1 in 40,000 to 1 in 117,000 live births in the general population [1, 13]. There are 2 major phenotypes of FD, "classical" (type 1) and "later-onset" (type 2) subtypes [14]. In Taiwan, the Chinese hotspot IVS4+919G>A (IVS4) mutation occurs at a high frequency [15, 16] and is reported to be a pathogenic, later-onset, cardiac-specific Fabry mutation [17]. Despite its high frequency, the pathology and neurological complications of FD in individuals with the later-onset IVS4 mutation currently are not well understood. In our previous comparison of patients carrying the IVS4 mutation with healthy age- and sex-matched controls, we found a greater frequency of infarctions (35% vs 0%; $P = 0.001$) and the pulvinar sign (30% vs 0%; $P = 0.002$), and a greater volume of white matter hyperintensities (1.1583 cm^3 vs 0.1354 cm^3; $P = 0.004$) in patients with IVS4-type FD [18]. The objective of the current study is to retrospectively review and compare the severity of central nervous system manifestations in Taiwanese patients with the later-onset IVS4 mutation or classical Fabry mutations.

Methods

Study design

This was a retrospective analysis of MRI data from Taiwanese patients enrolled in the Fabry Outcome Survey (FOS; sponsored by Shire Human Genetic Therapies, Inc). At the Taipei Veterans General Hospital (TVGH), brain imaging is routinely performed for patients with FD. The protocol for white matter (fluid-attenuated inversion recovery [FLAIR]) and cerebral artery (MR angiography) imaging has been optimized but not restricted to the same machine; thus, patients receive similar imaging protocols but can be randomly assigned to different scanners. This study analysed MRI and neurological signs and symptoms data gathered at the TVGH along with demographics and baseline data collected in

FOS for the same patients. The FOS registry collates outcomes data from patients with confirmed FD who are receiving, or are eligible for, ERT with agalsidase alfa. Treated patients receive agalsidase alfa 0.2 mg/kg body weight every other week. Inclusion criteria for this analysis were being Taiwanese, presence of the Chinese hotspot IVS4 mutation or classical Fabry mutations, as confirmed by molecular analysis, and having undergone brain MRI at any point after FD diagnosis. The data for this analysis were extracted from the FOS database in March 2015.

The Institutional Review Board of TVGH approved participation in FOS and the MRI analysis, and all patients gave written informed consent before their data were entered into the FOS database. Two board certified neuroradiologists, who were blinded to the type of disease, reviewed the brain MRIs from all patients by consensus.

Brain imaging

Non-contrast MRIs were obtained on one of three 1.5-tesla or 3-tesla scanners (Signa Excite 1.5T, GE Healthcare, Milwaukee, WI, USA; SignaHDxt 1.5T, GE Healthcare; Discovery MR750 3.0T, GE Healthcare). Axial spin-echo T1-weighted imaging parameters were 1.5T, 600–700/8–11/2 (TR/TE/NEX) and 3T, 360/9/1 (TR/TE/NEX). Axial FLAIR imaging parameters were 1.5T, 9000/92/2250 ms (TR/TE/TI) and 3T, 9000/145/2250 ms (TR/TE/TI). Time-of-flight angiography parameters were 1.5T, 26–28/6.8 ms (TR/TE) and 3T, 25/2.8 ms (TR/TE); flip angle 20°, voxel size 0.4 x 0.4 x 0.5 mm.

Qualitative assessment

The methods used for image analysis are described in our previous study [18]. The presence and location of infarction was categorized as none, anterior circulation alone, posterior circulation alone, or both anterior and posterior circulation. Furthermore, high signal changes on T1-weighted images bilaterally at the lateral pulvinar were considered as the pulvinar sign [11].

Semi-quantitative assessment

Deep white matter hyperintensities on T2-weighted images or FLAIR sequences were graded according to the Fazekas scale, which classifies white matter hyperintensities according to the following scoring system: 0, absent; 1, punctate foci; 2, beginning of confluence of foci; and 3, large confluent areas [19].

The degree of elongation and tortuosity of the basilar artery were evaluated using Smoker's criteria [20] according to the height of basilar artery bifurcation and its most lateral position. The scale used to categorize the height of basilar artery bifurcation was as follows: 0, at or below the dorsum sellae; 1, within the suprasellar cistern; 2, at the level of the floor of the third ventricle; and 3, indenting and elevating the floor of the third ventricle. The most lateral position of the basilar artery was graded as follows: 0, midline throughout; 1, medial to lateral margins of the clivus or dorsum sellae; 2, lateral to lateral margins of the clivus or dorsum sellae; and 3, situated in the cerebellopontine angle cistern.

Quantitative assessment

The diameter of the basilar artery was measured on a workstation (AZE Virtual Place Plus, AZE Ltd., Tokyo, Japan) by an observer who was blinded to all clinical information. A line was drawn perpendicular to the middle portion of the basilar artery on the sagittal view of a three-dimensional time-of-flight magnetic resonance angiogram at the maximum intensity projection. The observer then recorded the diameter as the full width at half maximum of this middle segment. Vascular stenosis was identified when the diameter of the basilar artery was less than 2 mm or appeared hypoplastic.

Neurological signs and symptoms

The prevalence of neurological signs and symptoms was obtained from the FOS database and compared between patients with IVS4 or classical Fabry mutations and MRI data. The neurological signs and symptoms analysed include stroke, sudden onset of numbness or weakness in the extremities, asymmetric facial expression, dysarthria, sudden onset of blurred vision or diplopia, depression, emotional or personality changes, forgetfulness, tinnitus, and vertigo.

Statistical analysis

The statistical analysis was performed using SAS software, version 9.2 (SAS Institute Inc., Cary, NC, USA). Descriptive statistics were calculated for demographic, MRI, and signs and symptoms data. For continuous variables, 95% confidence intervals for means were calculated using t-distribution, and for binary variables exact (Clopper-Pearson) 95% confidence intervals were computed. Differences between IVS4 versus classical Fabry mutations in binary outcome variables were assessed using Fisher's exact test. Differences in continuous variables between patients with IVS4 versus classical Fabry mutations were evaluated using the Wilcoxon rank-sum test, either exact (when computationally feasible) or normal approximation. Potential associations between mutation type and presence of neurological signs and symptoms were examined using Fisher's exact test; estimated odds ratios together with 95% exact confidence limits are reported. All statistical analyses are exploratory and the results of the statistical tests (p-values) are interpreted descriptively, as hypothesis

generation rather than hypothesis testing. The level of significance was set to 5% without any multiplicity adjustment. P-values above the significance level of 5% are not considered as confirmation of no difference between the groups, and p-values below 5% are not considered as confirmation of a difference between the groups.

Results

A total of 37 Taiwanese patients registered in FOS had brain MRI data; of these, twice as many had the IVS4 mutation (67.6%) than classical Fabry mutations (32.4%). The majority of IVS4 patients were male (76.0%) whereas females comprised the majority of classical Fabry patients (67.0%; Table 1). Median age at symptom onset, diagnosis, FOS entry, and MRI assessment was greater for IVS4 patients than classical Fabry patients (Table 1). All patients received ERT with agalsidase alfa; all IVS4 patients and 83.3% of classical Fabry patients underwent brain MRI after ERT initiation (Table 1).

Brain MRI in both IVS4 and classical Fabry patients revealed infarction, deep matter hyperintensities (Fig. 1, Fig. 2), and the pulvinar sign (Fig. 1, Fig. 3). Overall, infarcts were observed in similar proportions of IVS4 and classical Fabry patients (32.0% and 33.3%, respectively; Table 2), although with some differences in the site of occurrence. Anterior circulation stroke alone and posterior circulation stroke alone each occurred in 8.0% of IVS4 patients, and both anterior and posterior circulation stroke occurred in 16.0% of IVS4 patients. Posterior circulation stroke alone was not observed in classical Fabry patients; instead, anterior circulation stroke alone and both anterior and posterior circulation stroke each occurred in 16.7% of classical Fabry patients (Table 2). Hemorrhage was noted in MRIs from 16.7% of classical Fabry patients, but not in any MRIs from IVS4 patients (Table 2).

Fazekas scores for deep white matter hyperintensities were assigned for 100.0% of both IVS4 and classical Fabry patients. In each group, the largest proportion of patients was assigned a Fazekas score of 0 (60.0% for IVS4 and 50.0% for classical Fabry patients), followed by scores of 1 (28.0% and 33.3%), 2 (8.0% and 16.7%), and 3 (4.0% IVS4 patients only; Table 2). The pulvinar sign was observed in a greater proportion of classical Fabry patients (50.0%) than IVS4 patients (32.0%; Table 2).

Abnormal height bifurcation of the basilar artery was observed in 40.0% of IVS4 and 58.3% of classical Fabry patients (at the third ventricular floor in all IVS4 and 50.0% of classical Fabry patients, and indenting and elevating the third ventricular floor in 8.3% of classical Fabry patients; Table 2). Abnormal laterality of the basilar artery was observed in 4.0% of IVS4 and 16.7% of classical Fabry patients (lateral to lateral margins of the

Table 1 Demographic characteristics of Taiwanese patients with MRI data registered in FOS as of March 2014

Characteristic	IVS4 mutation $n = 25$	Classical Fabry mutations $n = 12$	P-value
Sex, n (%)			
Male	19 (76.0)	4 (33.0)	0.0274[a]
95% CI	0.55-0.91	0.10-0.65	
Female	6 (24.0)	8 (67.0)	
Age at symptom onset, years[c]			
Mean (SD)	50.3 (7.8)	9.5 (2.0)	
95% CI	46.2-54.5	8.1-10.9	
Median (range)	48.0 (38.0-65.0)	10.0 (6.0-12.0)	<0.0001[b]
Age at diagnosis, years			
Mean (SD)	57.6 (6.9)	39.8 (14.5)	
95% CI	54.7-60.4	30.6-49.1	
Median (range)	59.0 (42.0-67.0)	40.0 14.0-60.0)	0.0001[b]
Age at FOS entry, years			
Mean (SD)	59.7 (6.7)	42.4 (14.1)	
95% CI	56.9-62.5	33.4-51.4	
Median (range)	60.3 (44.8-69.7)	43.3 (17.4-61.2)	<0.0001[b]
Received ERT, n			
Yes	25	12	NA
95% CI	0.86-1.00	0.74-1.00	
Age at treatment start, years			
Mean (SD)	58.6 (6.8)	40.9 (14.5)	
95% CI	55.8-61.5	31.7-50.1	
Median (range)	59.7 (44.1-68.3)	40.9 (14.9-61.3)	0.0001[b]
MRI after treatment initiation, n (%)			
Yes	25 (100.0)	10 (83.3)	0.0991[a]
95% CI	0.86-1.00	0.52-0.98	
Age at MRI assessment, years			
Mean (SD)	60.0 (6.8)	42.6 (14.3)	
95% CI	57.2-62.8	33.6-51.7	
Median (range)	60.7 (45.0-70.4)	43.0 (18.0-61.4)	0.0001[b]

ERT, enzyme replacement therapy; *FOS*, Fabry Outcome Survey; *IVS4*, IVS4+ 919G>A; *MRI*, magnetic resonance imaging; *NA*, not available
[a]Fisher's exact test
[b]Wilcoxon rank-sum test
[c]Data missing from 9 IVS4 ($n = 16$) and 2 classical FD ($n = 10$) patients

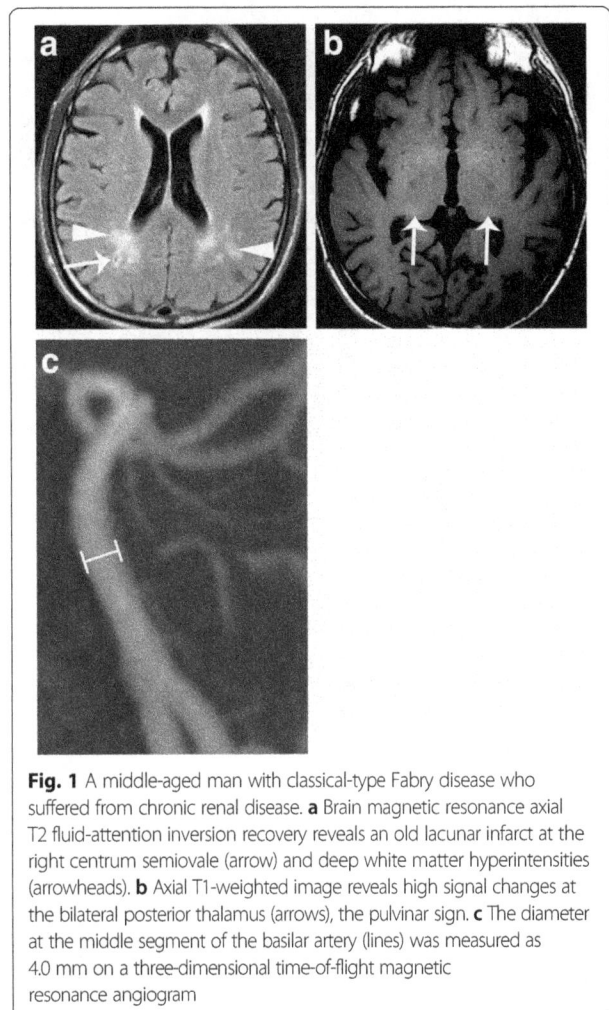

Fig. 1 A middle-aged man with classical-type Fabry disease who suffered from chronic renal disease. **a** Brain magnetic resonance axial T2 fluid-attention inversion recovery reveals an old lacunar infarct at the right centrum semiovale (arrow) and deep white matter hyperintensities (arrowheads). **b** Axial T1-weighted image reveals high signal changes at the bilateral posterior thalamus (arrows), the pulvinar sign. **c** The diameter at the middle segment of the basilar artery (lines) was measured as 4.0 mm on a three-dimensional time-of-flight magnetic resonance angiogram

clivus or dorsum sellae in all patients with abnormal laterality; Table 2).

The median diameter of the middle segment of the basilar artery was larger in classical Fabry patients than it was in IVS4 patients (3.2 mm vs 2.7 mm; $P = 0.0293$; Table 2). Vascular stenosis of the basilar artery was noted in 8.3% of IVS4 patients but in none of the classical Fabry patients (Table 2).

Of the IVS4 patients who did not demonstrate MRI evidence of infarction, eight of 17 (47.1%) presented with one or more non-specific neurological symptoms, including numbness/weakness ($n = 1$), depression ($n = 1$), forgetfulness ($n = 2$), tinnitus ($n = 2$), vertigo ($n = 4$; Table 3). For IVS4 patients with MRI evidence of infarction, six of eight (75.0%) presented with one or more non-specific neurological symptoms, including numbness/weakness ($n = 2$), asymmetric face ($n = 1$), blurred vision/diplopia ($n = 1$), emotional change ($n = 2$), personality change ($n = 1$), forgetfulness ($n = 4$), tinnitus ($n = 1$), and vertigo ($n = 1$), and two patients were clinically silent. Of the classical Fabry patients who showed no MRI evidence of infarction, four of eight (50.0%) reported neurological complaints, including numbness/weakness ($n = 1$), emotional change ($n = 3$), forgetfulness ($n = 1$), and tinnitus ($n = 1$). Of the four classical Fabry patients with MRI evidence of infarction, two reported symptoms of numbness/weakness, one of whom also reported

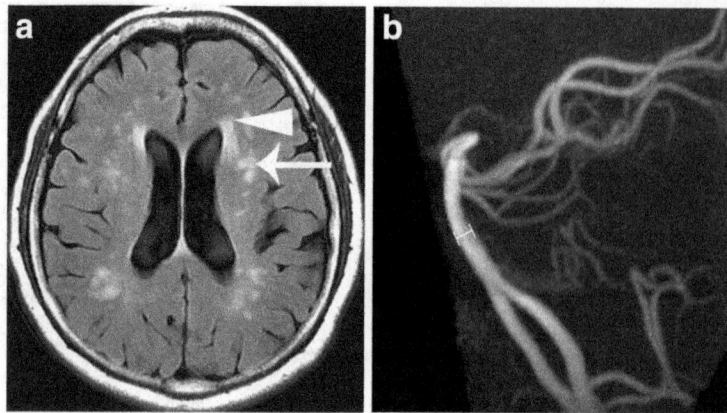

Fig. 2 A middle-aged female patient with IVS4+919G>A-type Fabry disease who suffered from hypertrophic cardiomyopathy and sudden onset of limb weakness. **a** Brain magnetic resonance axial T2 fluid-attention inversion recovery shows old lacunar infarct at the left corona radiata (arrow) and increased deep white matter hyperintensities (arrowhead). **b** The diameter at the middle segment of the basilar artery was measured as 3.3 mm on a three-dimensional time-of-flight magnetic resonance angiogram

stroke/minor stroke and dysarthria, and the other two were clinically silent. No statistically significant associations were found between the type of mutation (IVS4 or classical Fabry) and any neurological sign or symptom.

Discussion

Fabry disease is classified as the classical phenotype (type 1) or the later-onset phenotype (type 2), which tends to have

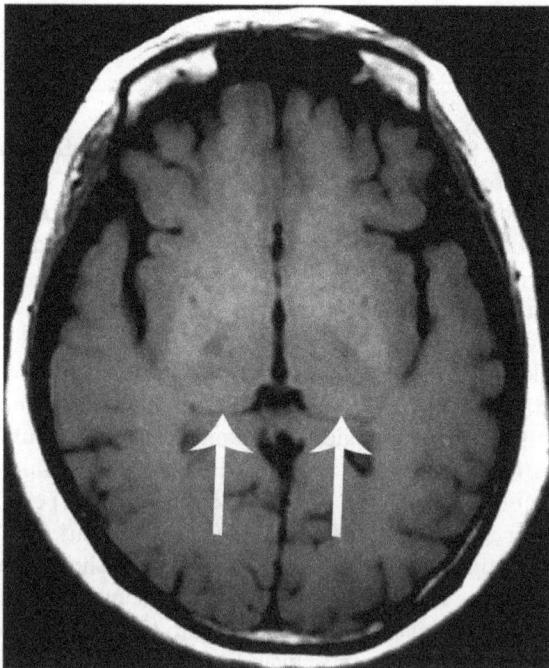

Fig. 3 A middle-aged female patient with IVS4+919G>A-type Fabry disease with hypertrophic cardiomyopathy. Brain magnetic resonance axial T1-weighted image reveals the pulvinar sign with high signal changes at the bilateral posterior thalamus (arrows)

mutation-specific renal or cardiac damage. Classical FD is characterized by frequent central nervous system involvement, which may be caused by the deposition of glycosphingolipids in cerebrovascular endothelial cells, a consequence of cardiogenic embolism from cardiomyopathy, valvular heart disease, ischemic heart disease, and/or arrhythmias [21–24]. Cardiac involvement is already acknowledged in later-onset IVS4 FD, but the degree of extra-cardiac involvement is still not well known. Brain MRI findings in our previous study demonstrated a greater degree of neurological involvement in patients with IVS4 FD compared with age- and sex-matched healthy controls [18]. In this study, we showed that patients carrying the later-onset IVS4 mutation had similar central nervous system involvement to that of classical Fabry patients, but with a lower degree of basilar artery dilatation.

In this comparison between patients with IVS4 and classical FD, the prevalence of infarction was similar in each group (32.0% for IVS4 patients and 33.3% for classical Fabry patients). The incidence of stroke found in our patients is much higher than in the general population [25], but similar to the results of other studies on FD [21, 22].

Vertebrobasilar dolichoectasia is thought to be an early and frequent sign of classical FD [26], and tends to be more frequently observed in elderly or male FD patients [18, 26]. In our study, median basilar artery diameter was larger in classical Fabry patients than IVS4 patients, despite the IVS4 group containing more males and having an older median age than the classical Fabry group. This may reflect less basilar artery involvement in IVS4 patients than classical Fabry patients. The mechanism of dolichoectasia is still not completely understood. In contrast with the histology of classical FD vasculopathy, and despite significant globotriaosylceramide accumulation in cardiomyocytes, no endothelial deposition

Table 2 MRI and MRA findings in patients with IVS4 versus classical Fabry mutations

Parameters	IVS4 mutation n = 25	Classical Fabry mutations n = 12	P-value
MRI findings			
Pulvinar sign, n (%)	8 (32.0)	6 (50.0)	0.4701[a]
95% CI	0.15-0.54	0.21-0.79	
Infarct, n (%)	8 (32.0)	4 (33.3)	0.6759[b]
95% CI	0.15-0.54	0.10-0.65	
Anterior circulation stroke	2 (8.0)	2 (16.7)	
Posterior circulation stroke	2 (8.0)	0	
Both anterior and posterior circulation stroke	4 (16.0)	2 (16.7)	
None of them	17 (68.0)	8 (66.7)	
Hemorrhage (microbleeds), n (%)	0	2 (16.7)	0.0991[a]
Fazekas score, n	25	12	0.7378[a]
0: No or a single punctate WM lesion	15 (60.0)	6 (50.0)	
1: Multiple punctate WM lesions	7 (28.0)	4 (33.3)	
2: Beginning of lesion confluence	2 (8.0)	2 (16.7)	
3: Large confluent lesion	1 (4.0)	0	
Height bifurcation of the BA, n	25	12	0.4276*
0: At or below the dorsum sellae	6 (24.0)	2 (16.7)	
1: Within the suprasellar cistern	9 (36.0)	3 (25.0)	
2: At the third ventricle floor	10 (40.0)	6 (50.0)	
3: Indenting and elevating the third ventricle floor	0	1 (8.3)	
Abnormal height bifurcation	10 (40.0)	7 (58.3)	
Laterality of the BA, n	25	12	0.3652[a]
0: Midline throughout	12 (48.0)	4 (33.3)	
1: Medial to lateral margins of clivus or dorsum sellae	12 (48.0)	6 (50.0)	
2: Lateral to lateral margins of clivus or dorsum sellae	1 (4.0)	2 (16.7)	
3: In the cerebellopontine angle cistern	0	0	
Abnormal laterality	1 (4.0)	2 (16.7)	0.2407[a]
95% CI	0.00-0.20	0.02-0.48	

Table 2 MRI and MRA findings in patients with IVS4 versus classical Fabry mutations (Continued)

MRA findings			
BA diameter, mm			
Mean (SD)	2.7 (0.6)	3.3 (0.7)	
95% CI	2.5-3.0	2.9-3.8	
Median (range)	2.7 (1.4-4.0)	3.2 (2.3-4.7)	0.0293[b]
Vascular stenosis/BA hypoplasia, n[c] (%)	2 (8.3)	0	0.5429[a]
95% CI	0.01-0.27	0.74-1.00	

BA, basilar artery; IVS4, IVS4+919G>A; MRA, magnetic resonance angiography; MRI, magnetic resonance imaging; WM, white matter
[a]Fisher's exact test
[b]Wilcoxon rank-sum test
[c]Data missing from one IVS4 patient, thus n = 24

of globotriaosylceramide was noted in our previous myocardial biopsy study [17], or in other reports on later-onset, cardiac-specific variants [27–29]. These findings support the theory that later-onset FD should be considered a unique entity that is different from classical FD, owing to the primary involvement of cardiomyocytes instead of endothelial cells. Furthermore, later-onset FD presentation and course might not be the same as typically observed in classical FD. Thus, long-term follow-up studies of IVS4 FD are needed for a more thorough understanding of the progression of this disease.

White matter hyperintensities, which are thought to be related to small vessel disease and secondary to the severity of perfusion dysfunction in FD cerebral vasculopathy, were quite similar in frequency between the two groups [30]. Furthermore, the pulvinar sign, which may be caused by regional hyperperfusion and reflect associated subtle dystrophic calcifications and end-organ damage [10, 11], was found in 32% and 50% of patients in the IVS4 and classical FD groups. This might provide supportive evidence of CNS involvement in IVS4 FD. However, the median age of the IVS4 group is higher than the classical Fabry group and patient numbers are too small to provide a solid conclusion; thus, further investigation with a larger population is necessary.

In addition to cerebrovascular events, cognitive dysfunction, although mild in nature, and depression are already known in FD patients [31]. In the current analysis, in terms of neurological presentations, IVS4 and classical Fabry patients shared several similarities. First, as previously mentioned, the observed incidence of infarction was similar in the two groups. Silent infarcts are commonly noted events in FD, but the frequency of silent brain infarcts in FD is still not yet known [32]. Second, there was a high prevalence of non-specific signs and symptoms or silent infarcts in both groups (62.5% in IVS4 patients and 50.0% in classical Fabry

Table 3 Neurological signs and symptoms in patients with IVS4 or classical Fabry mutations

Neurological sign or symptom, n (%)	IVS4 mutation n = 25	Classical Fabry mutations n = 12	Odds ratio (exact 95% CI); P-value	No MRI evidence of infarction		MRI evidence of infarction	
				IVS4 mutation n = 17	Classical Fabry mutations n = 8	IVS4 mutation n = 8	Classical Fabry mutations n = 4
Any neurological manifestation	14 (56.0)	6 (50.0)	1.27 (0.26-6.28); 1.0000	8 (47.1)	4 (50.0)	6 (75.0)	2 (50.0)
Stroke/minor stroke	1 (4.0)	1 (8.3)	0.46 (0.01-39.22); 1.0000	0	0	1 (12.5)	1 (25.0)
Numbness/weakness	3 (12.0)	3 (25.0)	0.41 (0.05-3.74); 0.3666	1 (5.9)	1 (12.5)	2 (25.0)	2 (50.0)
Asymmetric face	1 (4.0)	0	(0.03-NA); 1.0000	0	0	1 (12.5)	0
Dysarthria	0	1 (8.3)	(0.03-NA); 0.3243	0	0	0	1 (25.0)
Blurred vision/diplopia	1 (4.0)	0	(0.03-NA); 1.0000	0	0	1 (12.5)	0
Depression	1 (4.0)	0	(0.03-NA); 1.0000	1 (5.9)	0	0	0
Emotional change	2 (8.0)	3 (25.0)	0.26 (0.02-2.79); 0.3035	0	3 (37.5)	2 (25.0)	0
Personality change	1 (4.0)	0	(0.03-NA); 1.0000	0	0	1 (12.5)	0
Forgetfulness	6 (24.0)	1 (8.3)	3.47 (0.34-174.06); 0.3891	2 (11.8)	1 (12.5)	4 (50.0)	0
Tinnitus	3 (12.0)	1 (8.3)	1.50 (0.10-85.80); 1.0000	2 (11.8)	1 (12.5)	1 (12.5)	0
Vertigo	5 (20.0)	0	(0.62-NA); 0.1521	4 (23.5)	0	1 (12.5)	0

IVS4, IVS4+919G>A; *MRI*, magnetic resonance imaging; *NA*, not available

patients). These findings indicate that regular neurological and neuroimaging assessments are important and should be recommended for patients with the cardiac IVS4 mutation.

This study had some limitations that should be addressed. First, the FOS registry is not designed to confirm differences between groups of patients and because of the small group sizes the statistical tests lacked power and robustness, restricting the analyses to the descriptive level. Second, differences were observed in age at MRI assessment and in the proportion of females in each group; thus, as the incidence of stroke among patients with FD increases with age [21], the results herein must be interpreted with caution. A large longitudinal cohort comparison is needed to effectively evaluate neurological differences between patients with IVS4 and classical Fabry mutations.

Conclusions

In conclusion, the range of abnormalities found on brain MRI for classical Fabry patients is consistent with previous observations and also is similar in patients with the IVS4 mutation. Patients with the IVS4 mutation experience similar neurological signs and symptoms to patients with classical Fabry mutations.

Abbreviations

BA: Basilar artery; ERT: Enzyme replacement therapy; FD: Fabry disease; FLAIR: Fluid-attention inversion recovery; FOS: Fabry Outcome Survey; IVS4: IVS4+919G>A; MRA: Magnetic resonance angiography; MRI: Magnetic resonance imaging; WM: White matter

Acknowledgements

Under the direction of the authors, Tina Rose, an employee of Excel Scientific Solutions, provided writing assistance for this publication. Editorial assistance in formatting, proofreading, copy editing, and fact checking was also provided by Excel Scientific Solutions. SB from Shire International GmbH also reviewed and edited the manuscript for scientific accuracy.

Funding

This research was funded by Shire International GmbH.

Authors' contributions

H-JL, T-RH, S-CH, and D-MN designed the study. S-CH developed the initial draft of the manuscript. SB conducted the statistical analyses. H-JL, T-RH, S-CH, W-CY, T-HC, C-FY, SB, C-MT, and D-MN interpreted the data, revised the manuscript critically for important intellectual content, and read and approved the final manuscript.

Competing interests

T-RH and W-CY have received travel support from Genzyme and Shire. SB is an employee of, and holds stocks in, Shire. D-MN has received research and travel support from Genzyme and Shire. S-CH, H-JL, T-HC, C-FY, and C-MT declare no competing interests.

Author details

[1]Department of Radiology, Taipei Veterans General Hospital, Taipei, Taiwan. [2]School of Medicine, National Yang-Ming University, Taipei, Taiwan. [3]Institute of Clinical Medicine, National Yang-Ming University, Taipei, Taiwan. [4]Department of Pediatrics, Taipei Veterans General Hospital, Taipei, Taiwan. [5]Department of Biomedical Imaging and Radiological Sciences, National Yang-Ming University, Taipei, Taiwan. [6]Division of Cardiology, Department of Medicine, Taipei Veterans General Hospital, Taipei, Taiwan. [7]Shire, Zug, Switzerland.

References

1. Desnick RJ, Ioannou YA, Eng CM. α-Galactosidase a deficiency: Fabry disease. In: Scriver CR, Beaudet AL, Sly WS, Valle D, editors. The metabolic and molecular basis of inherited disease. 8th ed. New York: McGraw-Hill; 2001. p. 3733–74.
2. Ramaswami U, Wendt S, Pintos-Morell G, Parini R, Whybra C, Leon Leal JA, Santus F, Beck M. Enzyme replacement therapy with agalsidase alfa in

children with Fabry disease. Acta Paediatr. 2007;96:122–7.

3. Mehta A, Widmer U. Natural history of Fabry disease. In: Mehta A, Beck M, Sunder-Plassmann G, editors. Fabry disease: perspectives from 5 years of FOS. Oxford: Oxford PharmaGenesis; 2006.

4. Schiffmann R, Warnock DG, Banikazemi M, Bultas J, Linthorst GE, Packman S, Sorensen SA, Wilcox WR, Desnick RJ. Fabry disease: progression of nephropathy, and prevalence of cardiac and cerebrovascular events before enzyme replacement therapy. Nephrol Dial Transplant. 2009;24:2102–11.

5. MacDermot KD, Holmes A, Miners AH. Anderson-Fabry disease: clinical manifestations and impact of disease in a cohort of 60 obligate carrier females. J Med Genet. 2001;38:769–75.

6. Mehta A, Beck M, Elliott P, Giugliani R, Linhart A, Sunder-Plassmann G, Schiffmann R, Barbey F, Ries M, Clarke JT. Fabry Outcome Survey investigators. Enzyme replacement therapy with agalsidase alfa in patients with Fabry's disease: an analysis of registry data. Lancet. 2009;374:1986–96.

7. Mehta A, Ricci R, Widmer U, Dehout F, Garcia de Lorenzo A, Kampmann C, Linhart A, Sunder-Plassmann G, Ries M, Beck M. FOS investigators. Fabry disease defined: baseline clinical manifestations of 366 patients in the Fabry Outcome Survey. Eur J Clin Invest. 2004;34:236–42.

8. Mehta A, Ginsberg L. Natural history of the cerebrovascular complications of Fabry disease. Acta Paediatr Suppl. 2005;94:24–7.

9. Ramaswami U, Parini R, Pintos-Morell G, Kalkum G, Kampmann C. Beck M; FOS Investigators. Fabry disease in children and response to enzyme replacement therapy: results from the Fabry Outcome Survey. Clin Genet. 2012;81:485–90.

10. Moore DF, Ye F, Schiffmann R, Butman JA. Increased signal intensity in the pulvinar on T1-weighted images: a pathognomonic MR imaging sign of Fabry disease. AJNR Am J Neuroradiol. 2003;24:1096–101.

11. Takanashi J, Barkovich AJ, Dillon WP, Sherr EH, Hart KA, Packman S. T1 hyperintensity in the pulvinar: key imaging feature for diagnosis of Fabry disease. AJNR Am J Neuroradiol. 2003;24:916–21.

12. Fellgiebel A, Keller I, Martus P, Ropele S, Yakushev I, Bottcher T, Fazekas F, Rolfs A. Basilar artery diameter is a potential screening tool for Fabry disease in young stroke patients. Cerebrovasc Dis. 2011;31:294–9.

13. Meikle PJ, Hopwood JJ, Clague AE, Carey WF. Prevalence of lysosomal storage disorders. JAMA. 1999;281:249–54.

14. Bangari DS, Ashe KM, Desnick RJ, Maloney C, Lydon J, Piepenhagen P, Budman E, Leonard JP, Cheng SH, Marshall J, Thurberg BL. Alpha-galactosidase A knockout mice: progressive organ pathology resembles the type 2 later-onset phenotype of Fabry disease. Am J Pathol. 2015;185:651–65.

15. Lin HY, Chong KW, Hsu JH, Yu HC, Shih CC, Huang CH, Lin SJ, Chen CH, Chiang CC, Ho HJ, Lee PC, Kao CH, Cheng KH, Hsueh C, Niu DM. High incidence of the cardiac variant of Fabry disease revealed by newborn screening in the Taiwan Chinese population. Circ Cardiovasc Genet. 2009;2:450–6.

16. Hwu WL, Chien YH, Lee NC, Chiang SC, Dobrovolny R, Huang AC, Yeh HY, Chao MC, Lin SJ, Kitagawa T, Desnick RJ, Hsu LW. Newborn screening for Fabry disease in Taiwan reveals a high incidence of the later-onset GLA mutation c.936+919G>A (IVS4+919G>A). Hum Mutat. 2009;30:1397–405.

17. Hsu TR, Sung SH, Chang FP, Yang CF, Liu HC, Lin HY, Huang CK, Gao HJ, Huang YH, Liao HC, Lee PC, Yang AH, Chiang CC, Lin CY, Yu WC, Niu DM. Endomyocardial biopsies in patients with left ventricular hypertrophy and a common Chinese later-onset Fabry mutation (IVS4+919G>A). Orphanet J Rare Dis. 2014;9:96.

18. Lee HJ, Hung SC, Hsu TR, Ko SC, Chui-Mei T, Huang CC, Niu DM, Lin CP. Brain MR imaging findings of cardiac-type Fabry disease with an IVS4 +919G>A mutation. AJNR Am J Neuroradiol. 2016. doi:10.3174/ajnr.A4677.

19. Fazekas F, Chawluk JB, Alavi A, Hurtig HI, Zimmerman RA. MR signal abnormalities at 1.5 T in Alzheimer's dementia and normal aging. AJR Am J Roentgenol. 1987;149:351–6.

20. Smoker WR, Corbett JJ, Gentry LR, Keyes WD, Price MJ, McKusker S. High-resolution computed tomography of the basilar artery: 2. Vertebrobasilar dolichoectasia: clinical-pathologic correlation and review. AJNR Am J Neuroradiol. 1986;7:61–72.

21. Sims K, Politei J, Banikazemi M, Lee P. Stroke in Fabry disease frequently occurs before diagnosis and in the absence of other clinical events: natural history data from the Fabry Registry. Stroke. 2009;40:788–94.

22. Buechner S, Moretti M, Burlina AP, Cei G, Manara R, Ricci R, Mignani R, Parini R, Di Vito R, Giordano GP, Simonelli P, Siciliano G, Borsini W. Central nervous system involvement in Anderson-Fabry disease: a clinical and MRI retrospective study. J Neurol Neurosurg Psychiatry. 2008;79:1249–54.

23. Rolfs A, Böttcher T, Zschiesche M, Morris P, Winchester B, Bauer P, Walter U, Mix E, Löhr M, Harzer K, Strauss U, Pahnke J, Grossmann A, Benecke R. Prevalence of Fabry disease in patients with cryptogenic stroke: a prospective study. Lancet. 2005;366:1794–6.

24. Fellgiebel A, Müller MJ, Ginsberg L. CNS manifestations of Fabry's disease. Lancet Neurol. 2006;5:791–5.

25. Feigin VL, Lawes CM, Bennett DA, Anderson CS. Stroke epidemiology: a review of population-based studies of incidence, prevalence, and case-fatality in the late 20th century. Lancet Neurol. 2003;2:43–53.

26. Politei J, Schenone AB, Burlina A, Blanco M, Lescano S, Szlago M, Cabrera G. Vertebrobasilar dolichoectasia in Fabry disease: the earliest marker of neurovascular involvement? J Inborn Errors Metab Screen. 2014;2:1–6.

27. von Scheidt W, Eng CM, Fitzmaurice TF, Erdmann E, Hubner G, Olsen EG, Christomanou H, Kandolf R, Bishop DF, Desnick RJ. An atypical variant of Fabry's disease with manifestations confined to the myocardium. N Engl J Med. 1991;324:395–9.

28. Takenaka T, Teraguchi H, Yoshida A, Taguchi S, Ninomiya K, Umekita Y, Yoshida H, Horinouchi M, Tabata K, Yonezawa S, Yoshimitsu M, Higuchi K, Nakao S, Anan R, Minagoe S, Tei C. Terminal stage cardiac findings in patients with cardiac Fabry disease: an electrocardiographic, echocardiographic, and autopsy study. J Cardiol. 2008;51:50–9.

29. Germain DP. A new phenotype of Fabry disease with intermediate severity between the classical form and the cardiac variant. Contrib Nephrol. 2001;136:234–40.

30. DeVeber GA, Schwarting GA, Kolodny EH, Kowall NW. Fabry disease: immunocytochemical characterization of neuronal involvement. Ann Neurol. 1992;31:409–15.

31. Bolsover FE, Murphy E, Cipolotti L, Werring DJ, Lachmann RH. Cognitive dysfunction and depression in Fabry disease: a systematic review. J Inherit Metab Dis. 2014;37:177–87.

32. Kolodny E, Fellgiebel A, Hilz MJ, Sims K, Caruso P, Phan TG, Politei J, Manara R, Burlina A. Cerebrovascular involvement in Fabry disease: current status of knowledge. Stroke. 2015;46:302–13.

3

Ipsiversive ictal eye deviation in inferioposterior temporal lobe epilepsy

Wei Zhang[1,2], Xingzhou Liu[2], Lijun Zuo[1], Qiang Guo[2], Qi chen[3] and Yongjun Wang[1,4,5,6*]

Abstract

Background: Versive seizure characterized by conjugate eye movement during epileptic seizure has been considered commonly as one of the most valuable semiological signs for epilepsy localization, especially for frontal lobe epilepsy. However, the lateralizing and localizing significance of ictal eye deviation has been questioned by clinical observation of a series of focal epilepsy studies, including frontal, central, temporal, parietal and occipital epilepsy.

Case presentation: Two epileptic cases characterized by ipsiversive eye deviation as initial clinical sign during the habitual epileptic seizures are presented in this paper. The localization of the epileptogenic zone of both of the cases has been confirmed as inferioposterior temporal region by the findings of ictal stereoelectroencephalography (SEEG) and a good result after epileptic surgery. Detailed analysis of the exact position of the key contacts of the SEEG electrodes identified the overlap between the location of the epileptogenic zone and human MT/MST complex, which play a crucial role in the control of smooth pursuit eye movement.

Conclusion: Ipsiversive eye deviation could be the initial clinical sign of inferioposterior temporal lobe epilepsy and attribute to the involvement of human MT/MST complex, especially human MST which was located on the anterior/dorsal bank of the anterior occipital sulcus (AOS).

Keywords: Ipsiversive eye deviation, Inferioposterior temporal epilepsy, MT/MST complex, Anterior occipital sulcus

Background

Epileptic version or versive seizure, which has been defined as sustained and extreme conjugate eye movements with lateral head and body movements [1, 2], can occur during partial epileptic seizures. Contraversive epileptic eye deviation, often termed as "versive seizure", is one of the most common types of frontal lobe seizure in which frontal eye field is involved by epileptic stimulation [3, 4]. Moreover, it is considered as one of the most valuable semiological signs for lateralization of epileptogenic zone [5–7].

However, the lateralizing and localizing significance of ictal eye deviation, even the versive type, during partial epileptic seizures has been questioned by clinical observations froma series of focal epilepsy studies focusing on the

lateralization, particularly because of that the epileptic eye deviation may be ipsilateral or contralateral to the electroencephalography (EEG) focus, and has been associated with focal manifestations of EEG or neuroimaging evidence from frontal, central, temporal, parietal and occipital areas [8–22]. Although the fundamental reasons for these differences may be much more complicated than people originally understood, variations of eye movement induced by different pathophysiology during seizures must be considered.

So far, five categories of eye movements have been observed in human or non-human primates: pursuit, saccadic, vergence, vestibulo-ocular and optokinetictypes [23]. Among them, smooth pursuit is the most common type of eye movement guided by retinal imaging which mediates eye deviation to the visual stimuli [23, 24]. Although epileptic ipsiversion occurs incidentally and has been discussed curtly, it has been attributed to activation of the smooth pursuit eye movements mediated by the temporo-occipital cortex [8, 9]. By contrast, epileptic

* Correspondence: yongjunwang1962@gmail.com
[1]Department of Neurology, Beijing Tiantan Hospital, Capital Medical University, Beijing, China
[4]China National Clinical Research Center for Neurological Diseases, Beijing, China
Full list of author information is available at the end of the article

contraversion was assumed to occur as a result of the stimulation of the saccadic system by the cortico-superior collicular pathway [8, 9].

In macaque monkeys, the middle temporal (MT) and medial superior temporal (MST) areas, which play an indispensable role in normal smooth pursuit movement, locate in the inferior posterior and medial superior temporal lobe, respectively [25–27]. It has been also observed that lesions of MT produce retinotopic deficits in the initiation of pursuit eye movement [28], and lesions of MST also produce directional deficits that are especially pronounced during maintained pursuit [29]. These results highlight a general distinction between the two areas: MT is largely involved in pursuit initiation, whereas MST is important for pursuit maintenance [24].

Only a few comparative studies hitherto investigated human homology of MT/MST functional organization, and the results indicated that the vicinity of posterior branch of the inferior temporal sulcus is motion-sensitive area and direct stimulation to this area induces constant ipsilateral eye deviation [25, 30, 31]. Anatomical correlation of the eye movement disorders during epileptic seizures generated in human MT (or MST), however, has been scarcely discussed [8, 13, 32]. We present here two cases whose epileptogenic zones have been confirmed by ictal stereoelectroencephalography (SEEG) and freedom from seizures during the long term follow-up after surgery.

Cases presentation

Case-1 was a 24-year old and right-handed man with no personal or family risk factors of epilepsy and febrile seizures. The initial epileptic seizures occurred at the age of 18, which were described as generalized tonic-clonic type (GTCS), at a frequency of three or four times a year. He was treated with oxcarbazepine and levetiracetam with no response. After his age of 22, he experienced "minor seizures" which were characterized by eyes and head deviation to his right followed by bilateral asymmetric tonic posturing lasting about thirty seconds. The seizure frequency increased progressively from once a week to several tens a day without any triggering factor.

Paroxysmal delta activity followed by spike and waves activity had been detected on right temporo-occipital region in the interictal scalp EEG. During the 3 days of scalp VEEG monitoring, a total of 32 habitual seizures were recorded, each of them lasted for 10 to 30 s and two of them were followed by secondary GTCS. The semiological chronology of the seizures can be summarized as forced eye deviation to the right followed by right side turning of the head, left leg tonic posturing, left version and GTCS. The ictal EEG showed rhythmic theta-delta discharges followed by spike and waves activity over the right temporo-occipital region (Fig. 1). For presurgical evaluation, he underwent two MRI scans, 1.5

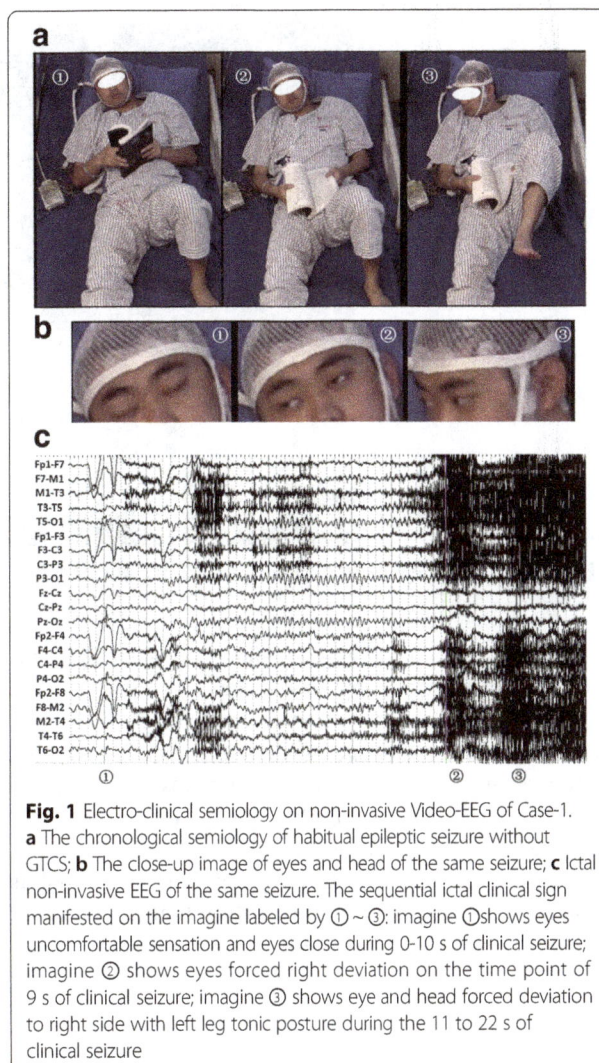

Fig. 1 Electro-clinical semiology on non-invasive Video-EEG of Case-1. **a** The chronological semiology of habitual epileptic seizure without GTCS; **b** The close-up image of eyes and head of the same seizure; **c** Ictal non-invasive EEG of the same seizure. The sequential ictal clinical sign manifested on the imagine labeled by ① ~ ③: imagine ①shows eyes uncomfortable sensation and eyes close during 0-10 s of clinical seizure; imagine ② shows eyes forced right deviation on the time point of 9 s of clinical seizure; imagine ③ shows eye and head forced deviation to right side with left leg tonic posture during the 11 to 22 s of clinical seizure

and 3.0 tesla respectively, which were performed with 3 mm thickness with no interval, and a positron emission tomography with neurotracer of fluorodeoxyglucose 18 F (FDG-PET). Both of the MRI and FDG-PET scans were unremarkable (Fig. 2).

All the SEEG electrodes with multiple contacts (10 to 15 contacts, length: 2 mm, diameter: 0.8 mm, 1.5 mm apart) were implanted with assistance of ROSA robot (Medtech, Montpellier, France). This procedure was preceded by a 3 tesla MRI scan performed with 1 mm thickness without interval for the implantation planning. A postoperative computed tomography (CT) scan without contrast was then used to verify both the absence of bleeding and the precise location of each contact. Finally, image reconstructionwas made in ROSA operating system to locate each contact anatomically along each electrode trajectory.

The patient underwent two different surgeries for SEEG implantation over his right hemisphere, and the second one, being performed 4 months after the first

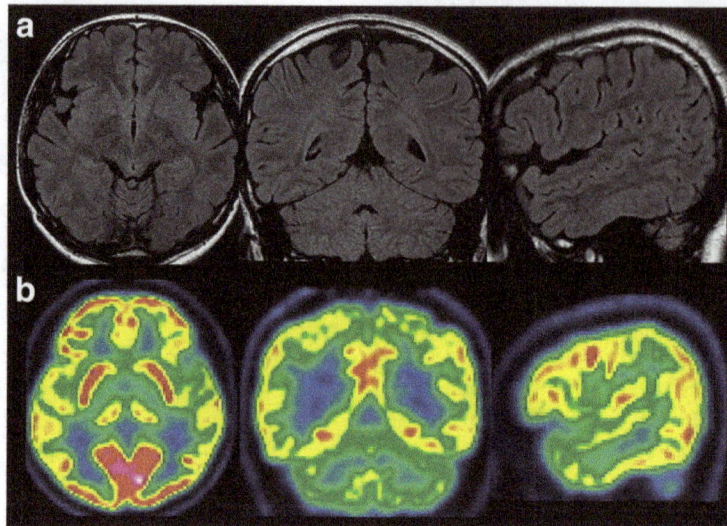

Fig. 2 a and **b** showed the Brain MRI and FDG-PET of Case-1. No evaluable changes were identified for localization of epileptogenic lesion

procedure, was in order to define the electrophysiological boundary of epileptogenic zone.

The first implantation covered extensive cortical areas related to eye movements as shown in Fig. 3, including intraparietal sulcus (IPS, anterior and posterior respectively), lateral (superior and inferior respectively) and medial parietal regions, lateral and medial occipital regions, occipito-parietaland occipito-temporal junction as well as posterior part of medial and neocortical temporal regions. According to the findings of the first SEEG recording, the second implantation focused on the cortical areas of early spreading and surrounding areas as shown in Fig. 4 including limbic and neocortical temporal areas, temporo-occipital areas, lateral and medial occipital areas.

Resembling interictal pattern was obtained from both of SEEG recordings. Continuous or subcontinuous delta activities and 1.5-2Hz spike-waves were recorded from the inferoposterior temporal neocortex adjacent to the posterior segment of right inferior temporal sulcus (ITS) during interictal SEEG recording. Both of the SEEG

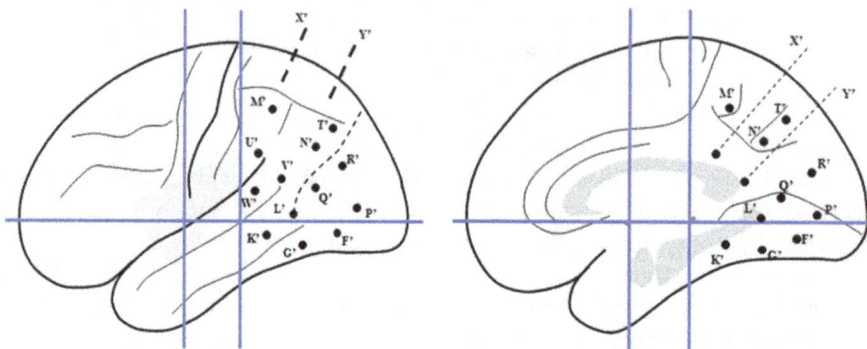

Fig. 3 Sechematic diagram of the first SEEG electrode implantation of Case-1 on lateral and medial view of the Talairach's basic referential system. X': electrode exploring the dorsal part of posterior cingulate gyrus (PCC) (medial contacts) and the anterior superior parietal lobule (SPL) (lateral contacts); Y': electrode exploring the ventral part of PCC (medial contacts) and posterior SPL (lateral contacts); M': electrode exploring anterior precuneus (medial contacts) and supramarginal gyrus (lateral contacts); T': electrode exploring posterior precuneus (medial contacts) and angular gyrus (AG) (lateral contacts); N': electrode exploring posterior precuneus on anterior bank of parieto-occipital fissure (medial contacts) and AG (lateral contacts); U': electrode exploring SMG with lateral contacts; W' and V': electrodes exploring posterior part of superior temporal gyrus (STG) adjacent to superior temporal sulcus (STS) with lateral contacts; L': electrode exploring the anterior part of lingual gyrus (LG) (medial contacts) and posterior segment of inferior temporal sulcus (ITS) (lateral contacts); K': electrode exploring posterior parahippocampal gyrus (medial contacts) and middle temporal gyrus (MTG) (lateral contacts); G': electrode exploring posterior fusiform gyrus (FG) (medial contacts) and posterior inferior temporal gyrus (ITG); Q': electrode exploring LG (medial contacts) and anterior bank of ascending limb of ITS (lateral contacts); F': electrode exploring LG (medial contacts) and posterior bank of ascending limb of ITS (lateral contacts); P': electrode exploring LG (medial contacts) and convexity of occipital lobe (lateral contacts); R': electrode exploring cuneus (medial contacts) and convexity of occipital lobe (lateral contacts)

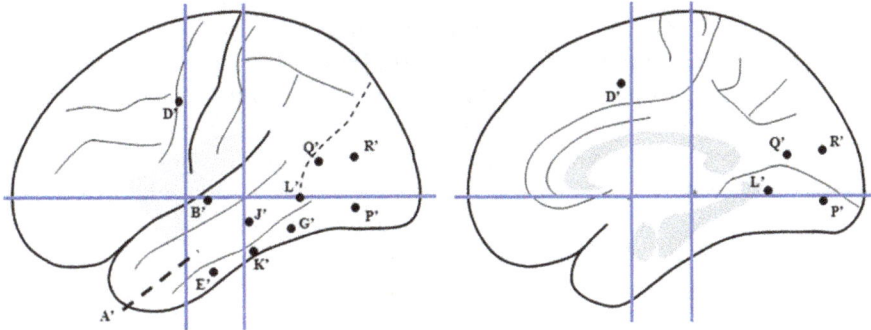

Fig. 4 Sechematic diagram of the second SEEG electrode implantation of Case-1 on lateral and medial view of the Talairach's basic referential system. G': electrode exploring the posterior part of ITG with lateral contacts and fusiform gyrus with medial contacts; L': electrode exploring the posterior segment of ITS with lateral contacts and anterior LG with medial contacts; Q': electrode exploring the anterior bank of the anterior occipital sulcus (AOS) with lateral contacts and anterior bank of parieto-occipital fissure (POF) with medial contacts; P' and R': electrodes exploring the posterior bank of AOS with lateral contacts and cuneus and LG with medial contacts; K': electrode exploring the middle part of ITG with lateral contacts and collateral sulcus with medial contacts; E': electrode exploring the anterior ITG with lateral contactsandentorhinal cortex with medial contacts; J': electrode exploring MTG with lateral contacts and hippocampus with medial contacts; A': electrode exploring the temporal pole with lateral contacts and amygdale with medial contacts; B': electrode exploring STG with lateral contacts and anterior insular long gyrus with medial contacts; D': electrode exploring the frontal eye field (FEF) with lateral contacts and cingulate cortex with medial contacts

recording showed similar initial epileptic discharges characterized as polyspikes followed by high frequency oscillations on the inferoposterior temporal regions. On the first ictal SEEG recording in which more extensive cortical areas were explored, the high frequency oscillations propagated to wide cortical areas including the temporo-occipital area, supramarginal and angular gyri, intraparietal sulcus within 600 ms (Fig. 5). The ictal SEEG of the second SEEG recording demonstrated the initial discharge originating from posterior inferior temporal gyrus (ITG) (contacts of G'8-9 and G'12), and the propagations of the high frequency oscillation involved

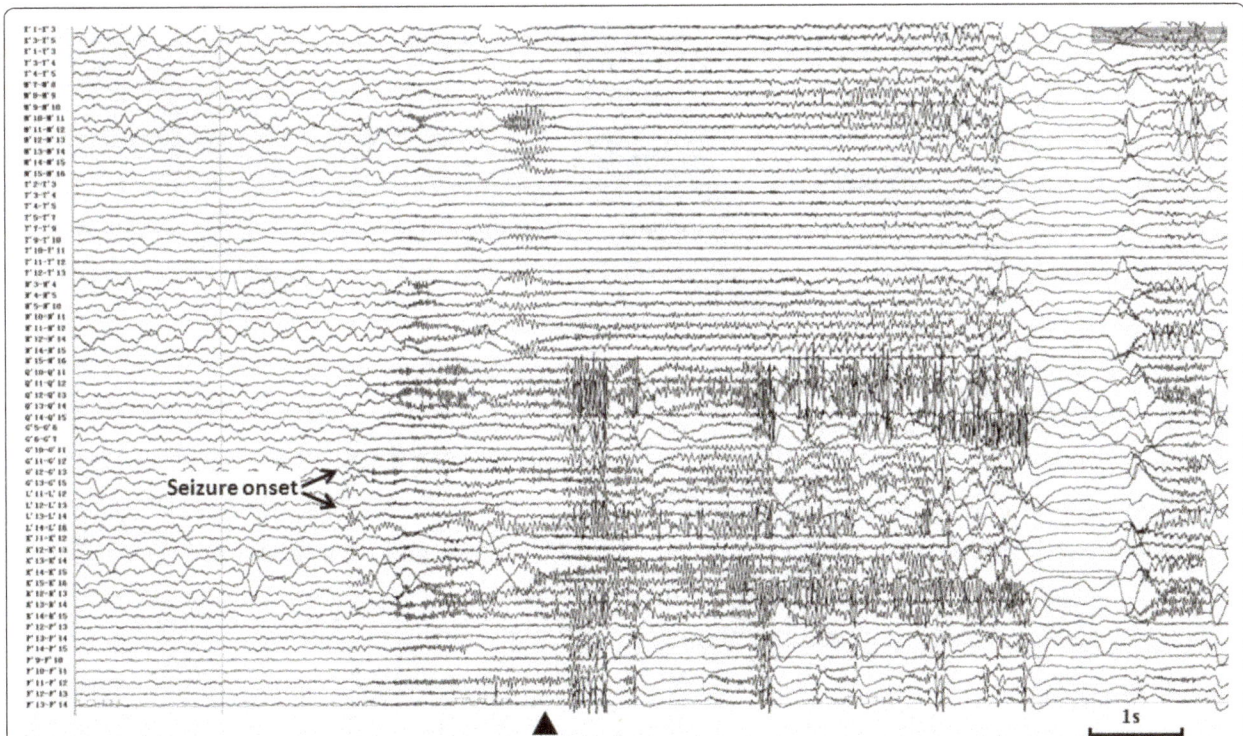

Fig. 5 Ictal SEEG after the first electrodes implantation of Case-1. Seizure-onset was on G'12-13 and L'12-13 exploring the posterior part of inferior temporal area. The initial eyes left version appeared at the time point labeled by ▲

the posterior segment of the ITS, anterior and posterior banks of anterior occipital sulcus (AOS), and lateral occipital sulcus (LOS), and even the location of frontal eyes field (FEF) within 400 ms (Fig. 6). The exact location of the key electrodes of the second SEEG electrodes implantation, obtained from postoperative CT and preoperative MRI data fusion, has been shown on Fig. 7.

The location of the seizure onset zone was confirmed over the inferotemporal region through both of the SEEG recordings, and particularly during the second SEEG. The early spreading areas of electrical seizure were located over the posterior segment of ITS, anterior and posterior bank of AOS, and extended to cortical area adjacent to the posterior segment of superior temporal sulcus (STS). The cortical resection (Fig. 8) was done and include the posterior part of the ITG and middle temporal gyrus (MTG), anterior and posterior banks of the AOS, and posterior segment of the STS. Seizure-freedom lasted 17 months since epileptic surgery.

Case-2 was a 19-year old right-handed man with normal psychomotor development. When he was 3 years old, his parents observed several episodes of abnormal behaviors during sleep, which manifested as eyes open and staring for several seconds. The treatment of Phenobarbital led to a period of seizure-freedom for 1.5 years.

Seizure recurred at the age of five after Phenobarbital withdrawn, and manifested as eyes staring and making fist of right hand lasting for 1 min with frequency of 1–2 times per day. Intentional response with external stimuli was lost during the episodes of seizures and recovered immediately after seizures. The patient reported his habitual epileptic aura as a kind of visual illusion "mimicking watching 3D movie".

Interictal scalp-EEG showed numerous spike-waves on right temporal region with the highest amplitude of single spike over the middle temporal region. Video EEG captured three habitual seizures. The typical chronological semiology could be concluded was eyes open and staring followed by forced deviation to right side, left arm tonic posturing proximally with left fist clenched, and then left facial clonia only in one seizure. Each seizure lasted for about tens of seconds and no more than 1 min with loss of consciousness. EEG onset characterized by rhythmic spikes on right middle-posterior temporal region showed by ictal scalp-EEG (Fig. 9). Brain MRI scanning demonstrated high abnormal signals involving right middle-posterior part of ITG, lateral occipito-temporal sulcus and fusiform gyrus on T2 and T2flair slices (Fig. 10), which was presumed as the epileptogenic lesion by us. Hypometabolism on brain FDG-

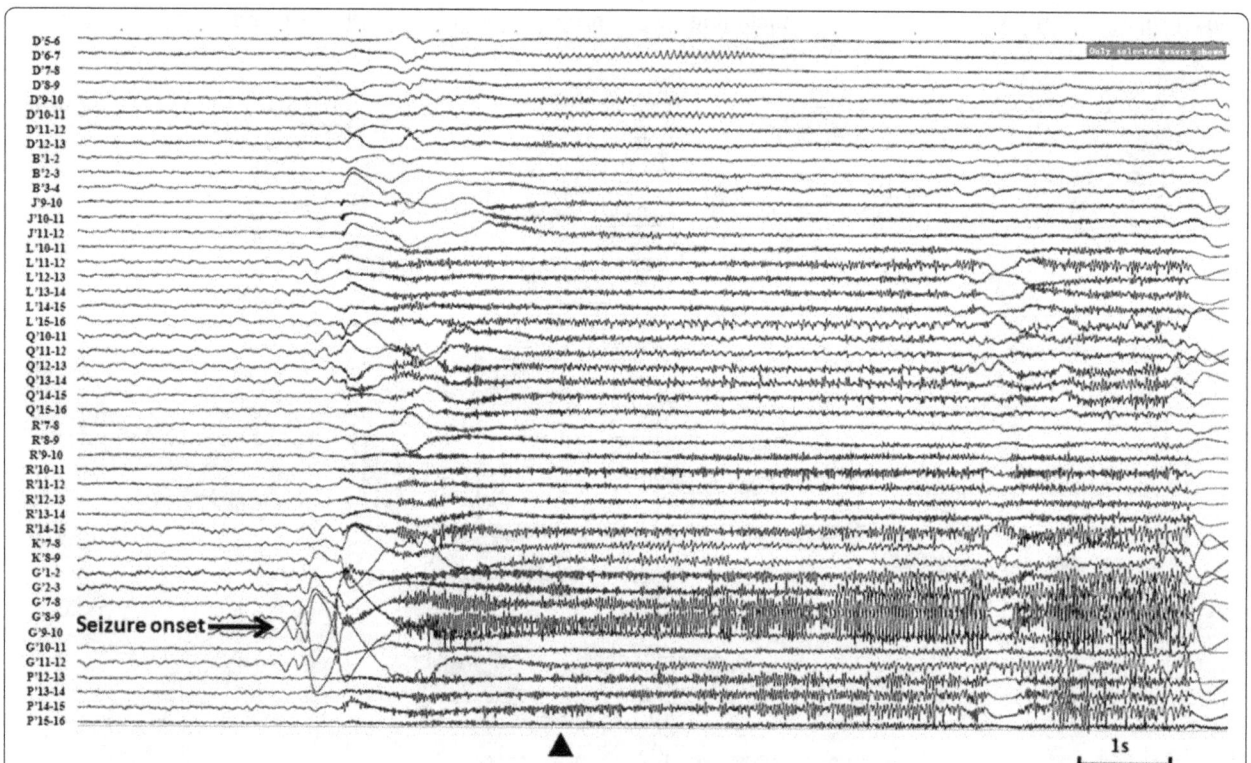

Fig. 6 Ictal SEEG after the second electrodes implantation of Case-1. EEG seizure onset characteristic as initial slow followed by high frequency oscillations (HFO) was over lateral contacts of electrode G' (G'9 and 12), which exploring the posterior ITG. The wide propagation of HFO involved multiple cortical areas, including posterior segment of ITS (L'13-16), anterior and posterior bank of AOS (Q'10-16, P'12-16), LOS (R'10-15), and even the location of FEF (D'5-12), within 400 ms

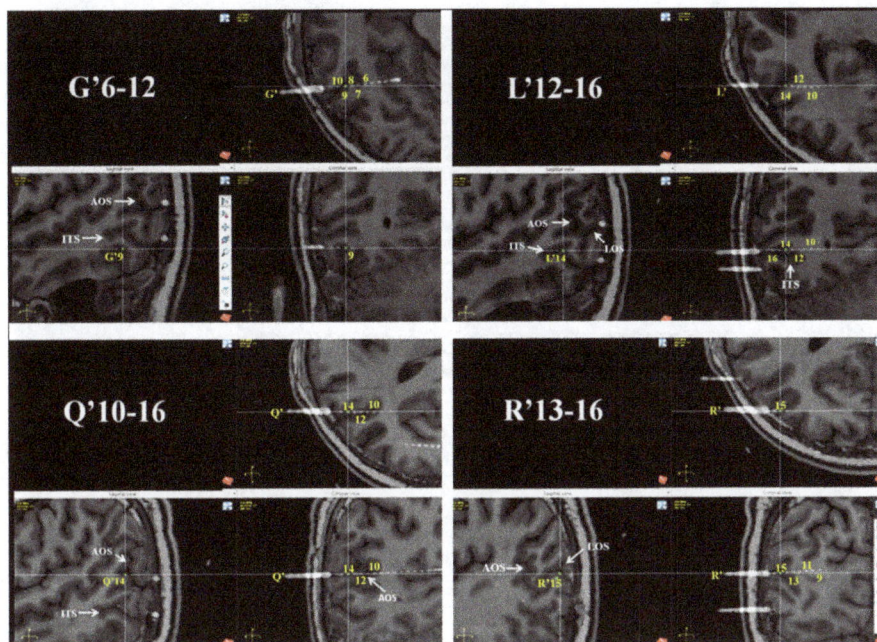

Fig. 7 The reconstruction of the exact location of key electrodes through the fusion of postoperative CT and preoperative MRI data. AOS: anterior occipital sulcus; ITS: inferior temporal sulcus; LOS: lateral occipital sulcus

PET scanning pointed to the same region and supported our hypothesis (Fig. 10).

According to our consideration, the SEEG should have been performed in order to ascertain the causal relationship between the epileptic seizure and the putative epileptogenic lesion, and confirm the involvement of MT+ during the episodes of epileptic eye movements. The electrodes were placed to explore the following cortical foci: the right middle and posterior neocortical temporal cortex, temporal pole and medial structure (Fig. 11).

Constant polyspikes and ripple were identified over the fusiform gyrus (L'1-3, H'1-3, K'1-2) and posterior ITG (S'7-9) in interictal, as well as preictal phase of SEEG. The electro-clinical semiology obtained from SEEG was stereotyped and identical with that recorded by scalp-EEG. The putative lesion had been confirmed by ictal SEEG as epileptogenic lesion and the most posterior cortical part of

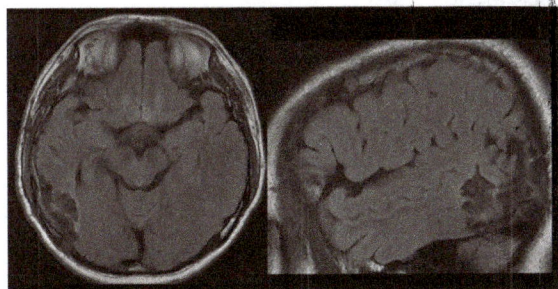

Fig. 8 Postsurgical MRI of Case 1 and seizure freedom has lasted for 17 months since cortical resection

ITG, which occupied the anterior bank of the AOS, was involved by ictal discharges within 5 s before the appearance of initial clinical sign—the ipsilateral eye deviation. The cortical resection had been guided by the neuroimaging and clinical neurophysiologic data, which had been described above in detailed. The core of the resection is the lesion identified by MRI, and the anterior border was determined by the lateral contacts of electrode O', posterior border was anterior bank of AOS, the superior border-reach the cortical areas explored by lateral contacts of the electrodes H' and R', and medial border is the collateral sulcus. The patient has been seizure-free for 25 months since the epileptic surgery without any remarkable neurological and neuropsychological deficit.

Discussion

Epileptic eye deviation in seizure originated from the parieto-temporo-occipital region had been reported previously [8–16]. The underlying mechanisms of lateralized eye deviation during epileptic stimulation had been presumed as below: contralateral eye deviation is attributed to the involvement of cortical saccadic areas, and the stimulation of smooth pursuit cortical areas during epileptic seizures causes ipsilateral ocular deviation [8, 9, 14, 33]. However, actual case of epileptic ipsiversion, manifesting as eyes conjugate deviation to the ipsilateral side of the epileptic focus, was rarely reported [33], and empirical evidence on the presumed mechanisms underlying the ipsilateral eye deviation has not been documented in details.

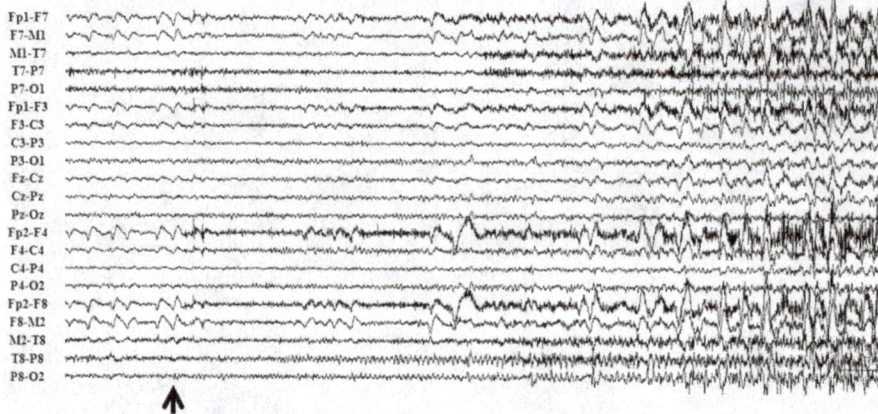

Fig. 9 Ictal scalp-EEG of Case 2 showed rhythmic spikes on right middle-posterior temporal region at EEC onset (labeled by *black arrow*)

Eyes pursuits are smooth tracking movements which maintain foveal fixation when viewing a moving object and hence stabilize the retinal image, and the stimulus for pursuit is motion of an object. In macaque cerebral cortex, area MT complex (MT+), which includes the middle temporal (MT) and medial superior temporal (MST) areas, has been considered strongly direction-selective, and important in processing neuronal signals related to visual motion [34–36]. According to the neurophysiologic data from macaque, the neural pathway of pursuits originates in the primary visual cortex, and the projections are then sent to the extrastriate V5 which includes the areas of MT and MST [37–39]. The receptive field of area MT primarily includes the contralateral visual field, while area MSTd (dorsal MST) has receptive field that extends well into the ipsilateral visual field [26, 40]. Area MT neurons respond only when retinal motion is present [41, 42], and lesions of MT produce retinotopic deficits in the initiation of pursuit eye movement [28]. In contrast, MST neurons maintain their responses to object motion even when there is no retinal counterpart [41, 42], and lesions of MST produce directional deficits that are especially pronounced during maintained pursuit [29], also known as an ipsilateral pursuit deficit [29, 43].

The existence of area V5/MT+ has been demonstrated in healthy and dyslexic human subjects in electrophysiological and functional imaging studies using PET, functional MRI (fMRI), transcranial magnetic stimulation (TMS), and magnetoencephalography (MEG) [25, 44–46]. In general, the human MT+ has been assumed to be correlated with the borders of Brodmann areas 19 and 37 or with von Economo and Kostinas' area OA and PH [47], and is typically found within a dorsal/posterior limb of the ITS, or the junction

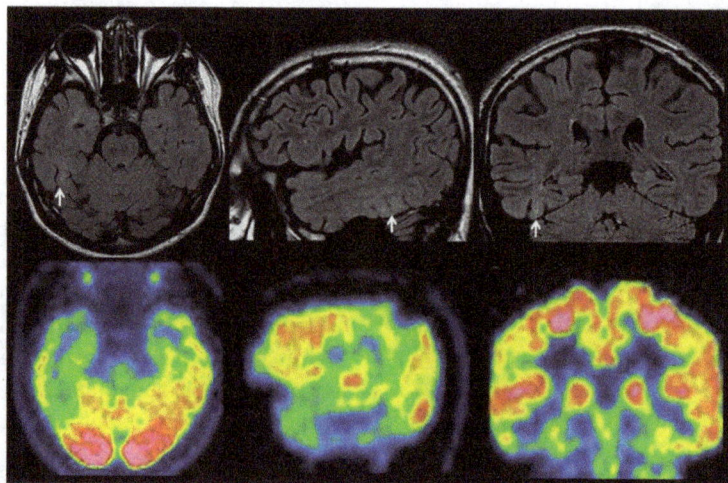

Fig. 10 Brain MRI and PET scans of Case 2. T2flair imagins of brain MRI showed the high abnormal signals involving right middle-posterior part of ITG, lateral occipito-temporal sulcus and fusiform gyrus. PET scan demonstrated the hypometabolism regions over inferior and basal aspects of right temporal lobe, as well as the medial temporal structure

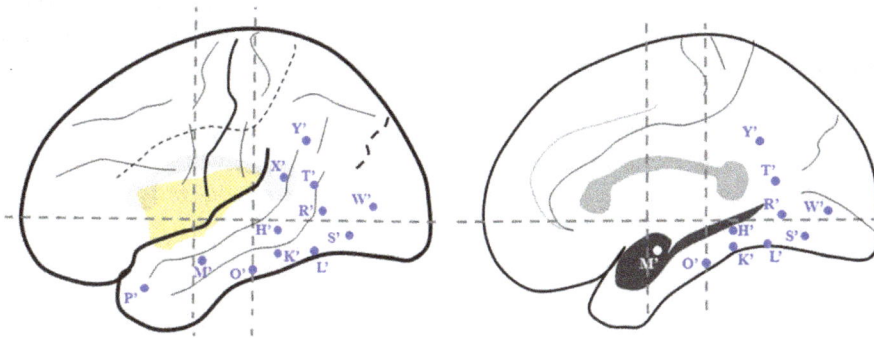

Fig. 11 Sechematic diagram of the second SEEG electrode implantation of Case-2 on lateral and medial view of the Talairach's basic referential system. K' and L': electrodes exploring the lesion on the middle and posterior part of ITG with lateral contacts and fusiform gyrus with medial contacts; O' and S': electrodes exploring the anterior and posterior border of the lesion identified by the MRI with lateral contacts and parahippocampal gyrus with medial contacts; H' and R': electrodes covered the middle and posterior MTG with lateral contacts and fusiform gyrus with medial contacts; T': electrode covered the angular gyrus with lateral contacts and ventral part of posterior cingulate gyrus with medial contacts in oblique orientation; Y': electrode exploring the supramarginal gyrus with lateral contacts and dorsal part of posterior cingulate gyrus with medial contacts; X': electrode covered the angular gyrus with lateral contacts; W': electrode exploring the most posterior part of ITG just anterior to the AOS with lateral contacts and lingual gyrus with medial contacts; M': electrode exploring the anterior part of MTG with lateral contacts and amygdala with medial contacts; P: electrode covered the temporal pole with lateral and medial contacts

between this sulcus and lateral/inferior occipital sulcus according to the fMRI results [25, 30, 48, 49]. Human fMRI studies have revealed two distinct subregions, i.e., MT and MST, which are not homogeneous and are arranged in a similar manner as that in the macaque brain [44]. Receptive field and retinotopic studies showed that MT receptive field constrained mostly to the contralateral visual field [26, 44] and exhibited retinotopic organization [25, 49], whereas MST did not demonstrate retinotopic organization but did respond to peripheral stimuli in both the contralateral and ipsilateral visual hemifields, indicating large receptive fields [25, 44]. The significant characteristics making MST different from MT are the strong responses to ipsilateral stimulation, and have no clear and orderly retinotopic map that MT did contain [25, 50]. The human MST strongly responds to peripheral stimuli with large (contralateral and ipsilateral) receptive fields [25, 50], and also receives vestibular information [51–53]. The physiological properties suggest that human MST is strongly specialized for encoding global flow properties and plays a critical role in the maintenance of smooth pursuit [50, 53, 54].

The arrangement of the two subregions of human MT+ is similar to that in the macaque brain, that is, MT is located at the posterior part of MT+ and MST borders MT area anteriorly [25, 44, 49, 50]. Huk and others located human MST on the anterior/dorsal bank of AOS (also known as the ascending limb of the inferior temporal sulcus), while area MT typically located on the posterior/ventral bank of AOS [25]. The precise position of area MT has been confirmed by cytoarchitectonic study from the Jüelich group [31], but area MST has not been well defined cytoarchitectonically.

Evidence from recent studies on eye movements revealed several features of the pursuit system as functional homologies with saccades [24], and that the overlapping networks between smooth pursuit and saccades include the typical cortical eye fields including the frontal eye field (FEF), supplementary eye field (SEF), dorsolateral prefrontal cortex (DLPFC), parietal eye field (PEF), precuneus and even MT/MST fields [55]. In fact, each of the cortical eye fields is composed of two distinct subregions which are devoted to the control of both saccadic and smooth pursuit eye movements, and has direct projections to neural centers in the brain stem which are involved in eye movement control [23]. Different from the traditional view of pursuit and saccades as distinct oculomotor subsystems, the control of pursuit and saccades might be viewed as different outcomes resulting from a single cascade of sensory-motor functions [24].

Inspired by the physiological and functional evidence from macaque and the human brain, and the precise anatomical localization of the human MST and MT based on the data from neurophysiologic and functional neuroimaging studies, we hypothesized that the mechanisms of epileptic semiology of ipsiversive eye deviation in the two cases, whose epileptogenic zone has been confirmed to be located in the inferoposterior temporal region, can be explained by involvement of the cortical network of eye movement control, specifically in terms of the smooth pursuit movement.

The two cases we reported here had both similar epileptic semiology and anatomical localization of the epileptogenic zone as ascertained by SEEG. The initial clinical sign of both cases was characterized by forced ipsilateral eye deviation with homodromous head turning, which is similar to the semiology of the case reported by Kaplan [33]. In the present Case1, the epileptogenic zone is located on the posterior ITG and extended to the anterior bank of AOS, which is the precise anatomical location of human MST. In the present Case2, the epileptogenic zone is located on the fusiform and posterior ITG, and the epileptic discharges spread to anterior bank of AOS immediately before the appearance of initial clinical sign. Therefore, the localization of epileptogenic zone in the two cases was of great similarity to the conclusion of Kaplan's case, whose epileptic seizure originated from right temporo-occiptial cortex [33]. As mentioned above, since area MST strongly responds to visual stimuli in the ipsilateral visual field, epileptic stimulation of MST has the probability to induce ipsilateral conjugate eye deviation, as that manifested by our two cases.

Case1 had two times of SEEG recordings to determine the exact location of epileptogenic zone and the boundary of cortical resection. Taking all the cortical areas covered in both SEEG recordings into consideration, we had got adequate coverage on cortical eye fields, striate and multiple extra-striate visual cortices. Meta-analysis on all the ictal SEEG of Case1 indicated that the rapid synchronization of high frequency oscillations happened within 400–600 ms among the multiple cortical eyes fields, striate and extra-striate visual cortices including MT+, inferior parietal lobule (IPL), IPS, parieto-occipital sulcus (POS), FEF, and so on. The wide and rapid synchronized ictal epileptic discharges among multiple cortical eye fields are consistent with the viewpoint that the pursuit system has a functional architecture similar to that of the saccadic system [24].

The resemblances of the two cases include ipsiversive eye deviation and the location of epileptogenic zones which were localized in the posterior part of ITG adjacent to AOS—the accurate cortical localization of human MST. According to the characteristics of retinotopic organization in the subregions of MT+ and its functional roles in smooth pursuit eye movements, we hypothesize that the lateralization of eye deviation during temporo-occipital epileptic seizures depended on whether MST is involved initially or primarily during the epileptic seizure. Epileptic seizure originated from/primarily involvedthe posterior ITG or anterior bank of AOS (human MST) would probably induce ipsilateral conjugate eye deviation initially.

Conclusion

To our knowledge, these are the first cases reports focusing on the epileptic ipsiversive eye deviation by using SEEG recordings. The advantages of SEEG include its accurate cortical mapping and electrode implantation with high spatial resolution on 3D level, and the capacity

to sample the cortical activity in the depth of cerebral sulcus. According to the neurophysiologic and functional neuroimaging evidence mentioned above, the core anatomical marker and probable boundary of the cortical location of human MST/MT is the AOS (the ascending limb of the ITS), which had been explored adequately with the exploration of its adjacent and related cortical areas in the two cases. The relationship of exact location of epileptogenic zones of the two cases and AOS convinces us that the manifestation of epileptic ipsiversive eye deviation should be attributed to the neurophysiologic and neuropsychological characteristics of MT+, especially area MST, and its functional role in cortical control of smooth pursuit eye movements.

Abbreviations
AOS: Anterior occipital sulcus; CT: Computed tomography; DLPFC: Dorsolateral prefrontal cortex; FDG-PET: Positron emission tomography with neurotracer of fluorodeoxyglucose 18 F; FEF: Frontal eyes field; GTCS: Generalized tonic-clonic seizure; IPS: Intraparietal sulcus; ITG: Inferior temporal gyrus; ITS: Inferior temporal sulcus; LOS: Lateral occipital sulcus; MEG: Magnetoencephalography; MRI: Magnetic resonance imaging; MST: Medial superior temporal area; MT: Middle temporal area; MTG: Middle temporal gyrus; PEF: Parietal eye field; POS: Parieto-occipital sulcus; SEEG: Stereoelectroencephalography; SEF: Supplementary eye field; STS: Superior temporal sulcus; TMS: Transcranial magnetic stimulation

Acknowledgements
We thank Dr Junxi Chen from the epilepsy center of Guangdong Sanjiu Brain Hospital for his help of data acquisition.

Funding
Not applicable.

Authors' contributions
WZ contributed to the data acquisition and analysis of the manuscript. XL and YW contributed to the data acquisition, analysis and redaction of the manuscript, and also the interpretation of the data. QG contributed the data acquisition. LZ and QC contributed to redaction of the manuscript. All authors read and approved the final manuscript.

Competing interests
The authors declare that they have no competing interests.

Author details
[1]Department of Neurology, Beijing Tiantan Hospital, Capital Medical University, Beijing, China. [2]Epilepsy Center, Guangdong Sanjiu Brain Hospital, Jinan University, No. 578, Sha Tai Nan Lu, Guangzhou 510510, China. [3]School of Psychology, South China Normal University, Guangzhou, China. [4]China National Clinical Research Center for Neurological Diseases, Beijing, China. [5]Department of Neurology, Tiantan Clinical Trial and Research Center for Stroke, Beijing Tiantan Hospital, Capital Medical University, Beijing, China. [6]Vascular Neurology, Department of Neurology, Beijing Tiantan Hospital, Capital Medical University, Beijing, China.

References
1. Wyllie E, Luders HO, Morris HH, Lesser RP, Dinner DS. The lateralizing significance of versive head and eye movements during epileptic seizures. Neurology. 1986;36(5):606.
2. Lüders HO, Acharya J, Baumgartner C, Benbadis S, Bleasel A, Burgess R, Dinner DS, Ebner A, Foldvary N, Geller E, Hamer H, Holthausen H, Kotagal P, Morris H, Meencke HJ, Noachtar S, Rosenow F, Sakamoto A, Steinhoff BJ,

Tuxhorn I, Wyllie E. Semiological seizure classification. Epilepsia. 1998;29(9): 1006–13.

3. Kellinghaus C, Lüders HO. Frontal lobe epilepsy. Epileptic Disord. 2004;6:223–39.

4. Bonelli SB, Lurger S, Zimprich F, Stogmann E, Assem-Hilger E, Baumgartner C. Clinical seizure lateralization in frontal lobe epilepsy. Epilepsia. 2007;48(3):517–23.

5. Loddenkemper T, Kotagal P. Lateralizing signs during seizures in focal epilepsy. Epilepsy Behav. 2005;7:1–17.

6. Olbrich A, Urak L, Gröppel G, Serles W, Novak K, Porsche B, Benninger F, Czech T, Baumgartner C, Feucht M. Seimology of temporal lobe epilepsy in children and adolescents value in lateralizing the seizure onset zone. Epilepsy Res. 2002;48:103–10.

7. Boesebeck F, Schulz R, May T, Ebner A. Lateralizing semiology predicts the seizure outcome after epilepsy surgery in the posterior cortex. Brain. 2002; 125:2320–31.

8. Tijssen CC, Bastiaensen LAK, Voskuil PHA. Epileptic eye deviation. Neuro-ophtalmol. 1993;13(1):39–44.

9. Tijssen CC, Kort PLM, Bastiaensen LAK, Voskuil PHA. Epileptic eye deviation and nystagmus. Clin Neurol Neurosurg. 1992;94(1):77.

10. Kaplan PW, Lesser RP. Vertical and horizontal epileptic gaze deviation and nystagmus. Neurology. 1989;39:1391–3.

11. Schulz R, Tomka-Hoffmeister M, WoermannFG HM, SchittkowskiMP EA, Bien CG. Epileptic monocular nystagmus and ictal diplopia as cortical and subcortical dysfunction. Epilepsy Behav Case Rep. 2013;1:89–91.

12. Munari C, Bonis A, Kochen S, Pestre M, Brunet P, Bancaud J, Chodkiewicz JP, Talairach J. Eye movement and occipital seizures in man. Acta Neurochirurgia. 1984;Suppl. 33:47–52.

13. Harris CM, Boyd S, Chong K, Harkness W, Neville BGR. Epileptic nystagmus in infancy. J Neurol Sci. 1997;151:111–4.

14. Lee SU, Suh H-I, Choi JY, Huh K, Kim H-J, Kim JS. Epileptic nystagmus: a case report and systematic review. Epilepsy Behav Case Rep. 2014;2:156–60.

15. Kellinghus C, Skidmore C, Loddenkemper T. Lateralizing value of epileptic nystagmus. Epilepsy Behav. 2008;13(4):700–2.

16. Robillard A, Saint-Hilaire JM, Mercier M, Bouvier G. The lateralizing and localizing value of adversion in epilepticseizures. Neurology. 1983;32:1241–2.

17. Wyllie E, Lüders H, Morris HH, Lesser RP, Dinner DS. The lateralizing significance of versive head and eye movementsduring epileptic seizures. Neurology. 1986;36:606–11.

18. McLachlan RS. The significance of head and eye turning in seizures. Neurology. 1987;37:1617–9.

19. Penfield W, Jasper H. Epilepsy and the Functional Anatomy of the Human Brain. Boston: Little, Brown and Co; 1954.

20. AjmoneMarsan C, Goldhammer L. Clinical ictal patterns and electrographic data in cases of partial seizures of frontalcentral-parietal-origin. In: Brazier MAB, editor. Epilepsy, its Phenomena in Man. New York: Academic; 1973. p. 235–58.

21. King DW, AjmoneMarsan C. Clinical features and ictal patterns in epileptic patients with EEG temporal lobe foci. Ann Neurol. 1977;2:138–47.

22. Rosenbaum DH, Siegel M, Rowan AJ. Contraversive seizures in occipital epilepsy: Case report and review of theliterature. Neurology. 1986;36:281–4.

23. Lynch JC. In: Squire LR, editor. Encyclopedia of Neuroscience. Berlin, Heidelberg: Springer; 2009.

24. Richard JK. Recasting the smooth pursuit eye movement system. J Neurophysiol. 2004;91:591–603.

25. Huk AC, Robert F. Dougherty, and David JH. Retinotopy and functional subdivision of human areas MT and MST. Soc Neurosci. 2002;22(16):7195–205.

26. Desimone R, Ungerleider LG. Multiple visual areas in the caudal superior temporal suclus of the macaque. J Comp Neurol. 1986;248:164–89.

27. Komatsu H, Wurtz RH. Relation of cortical areas MT and MST to pursuit eye movements. I. Localization and visual properties of neurons. J Neurophysiol. 1988;60:580–603.

28. Newsome WT, Wurtz RH, Dürsteler MR, Mikami A. Deficits in visual motion processing followingibotenic acid lesions of the middle temporal visual area of the macaque monkey. J Neurosci. 1985;5:825–40.

29. Dürsteler MR, Wurtz RH. Pursuit and optokinetic deficits following chemical lesions of cortical areas MT and MST. J Neurophysiol. 1988;60:940–65.

30. Dumoulin SO, Bittar RG, Kabani NJ, Baker CL, Goualher G, Pike B, Evans AC. A new anatomical landmark for reliable identification of human area V5/MT: a quantitative analysis of sulcal patterning. Cereb Cortex. 2000;10:454–63.

31. Malikovic A, Amunts K, Schleicher A, Mohlberg H, Eickhoff SB, Wilms M, Palomero-Gallagher N, Armstrong E, Zilles K. Cytoarchitectonic analysis of the human extrastriate cortex in the region of V5/MT+: a probabilistic, stereotaxic map of area hOc5. Cereb Cortex. 2007;17(3):562–74.

32. Shibata M, Kato T, Yoshida T, Saito K, Heike T, Awaya T. Paroxysmal gaze deviations as the sole manifestation of occipital lobe epilepsy. Seizure. 2013;22: 913–5.

33. Tusa RJ, Kaplan PW, Hain TC, Naidu S. Ipsiversive eye deviation and epileptic nystagmus. Neurology. 1990;40:662–5.

34. Albright TD, Desimone R, Gross GG. Columnar organization of directionally selective cells in visual area MT of the macaque. J Neurophysiol. 1984;51:16–31.

35. Movshon JA, Adelson EH, Gizzi MS, Newsome WT. The analysis of moving visual patterns. Exp Brain Res. 1986;11:117–52.

36. Salzman CD, Murasugi CM, Britten KH, Newsome WT. Microstimulation in visual area MT: effects on derection discrimination performance. J Neurosci. 1992;12:2331–55.

37. Krauzlis RJ. Recasting the smooth pursuit eye movement syetem. J Neurophysiol. 2004;92:591–603.

38. Nagel M, Sprenger A, Hohagen F, Binkofski F, Lencer R. Cortical mechanisms of retinal and extraretinal smooth pursuit eye movements to different target velocities. Neuroimage. 2008;41:483–92.

39. Hansraj R. Pursuit eye movements: a review. S Afr Optom. 2008;67(4):160–5.

40. Duffy CJ, Wurtz RH. Sensitivity of MST neurons to optic flow stimuli. I A continuum of response selectivity to large-field stimuli. J Neurophysiol. 1991;65:1329–45.

41. Ilg UJ, Thier P. Visual tracking neurons in primate area MST are activated by smooth-pursuit eye movements of an "imaginary" target. J Neurophysiol. 2003;90:1489–502.

42. Newsome WT, Wurtz RH, Komatsu H. Relation of cortical areas MT and MST to pursuit eye movements. II. Differentiation of retinal from extraretinal inputs. J Neurophysiol. 1988;60:604–20.

43. Lynch JC, Tian JR. Cortico-cortical networks and cortico-subcortical loops for the higher control of eye movements. Prog Brain Res. 2006;151:461–501.

44. Dukelow SP, DeSouza JF, Culham JC, van den Berg AV, Menon RS, Vllis T. Distinguishing subregions of the human MT+ complex using visual fields and pursuit eye movements. J Neurophysiol. 2001;86:1991–2000.

45. Zihl J, von Cramon DY, Mai N. Selective disturbance of movement vision after bilateral brain damage. Brain. 1983;106:313–40.

46. Miki K, Watanabe S, Kakigi R, Puce A. Magnetoencephalographicstuty of occipitotemporal activity elicited by viewing mouth movements. Clin Neurophysiol. 2004;115:1559–74.

47. Zilles K, Clarke S. Architecture, connectivity, and transmitter receptors of human extrastriate visual cortex. Extrastriate cortex in primates. US: Springer; 1997. p. 673–742.

48. Tootell RBH, Taylor JB. Anatomical evidence for MT and additional cortical visual areas in humans. Cereb Cortex. 1995;5:39–55.

49. Kolster H, Peeters R, Orban GA. The retinotopic organization of the human middle temporal area MT/V5 and its cortical neighbors. J Neurosci. 2010; 30(29):9801–20.

50. Smith AT, Wall MB, Williams AL, Singh KD. Sensitivity to optic flow in human cortical areas MT and MST. Eur J Neurosci. 2006;23:561–9.

51. Duffy CJ, Wurtz RH. Response of monkey MST neurons to optic flow stimuli with shifted centers of motion. J Neurosci. 1995;15(7 pt 2):5192–208.

52. Duffy CJ, Wurtz RH. Medial superior temporal area neurons respond tospeed patterns in optic flow. J Neurosci. 1997;17(8):2839–51.

53. Page WK, Duffy CJ. Heading representation in MST: sensory interactions and population encoding. J Neurophysiol. 2003;89(4):1994–2013.

54. Lencer P, Trillenberg P. Neurophysiology and neuroanatomy of smooth pursuit in humans. Brain Cogn. 2008;68:219–28.

4

What is the optimal sequence of decompression for multilevel noncontinuous spinal cord compression injuries in rabbits?

Chaohua Yang[1], Baoqing Yu[1], Fenfen Ma[2], Huiping Lu[2], Jianmin Huang[1], Qinghua You[3], Bin Yu[1], Jianlan Qiao[4] and Jianjun Feng[1*]

Abstract

Background: In recent years, multilevel spinal cord injuries (SCIs) have gained a substantial amount of attention from clinicians and researchers. Multilevel noncontinuous SCI patients cannot undergo the multiple steps of a one-stage operation because of a poor general condition or a lack of proper surgical approaches. The surgeon subsequently faces the decision of whether to initially relieve the rostral or caudal compression. In this study, we established a spinal cord compression model involving two noncontinuous segments in rabbits to evaluate the effects of differences in decompression order on the functional recovery of the spinal cord.

Methods: A Fogarty catheter was inserted into the epidural space through a hole in T6-7 and advanced 3 cm rostrally or caudally. Following successful model establishment, which was demonstrated by an evaluation of evoked potentials, balloons of different volumes (40 μl or 50 μl) were inflated in the experimental groups, whereas no balloons were inflated in the control group. The experimental groups underwent the first decompression in the rostral or caudal area at 1 week post-injury; the second decompression was performed at 2 weeks post-injury. For 6 weeks post-injury, the animals were tested to determine behavioral scores, somatosensory evoked potentials (SEPs) and radiographic imaging changes; histological and apoptosis assay results were subsequently analyzed.

Results: The behavioral test results and onset latency of the SEPs indicated that there were significant differences between priority rostral decompression (PRD) and priority caudal decompression (PCD) in the 50-μl compression group at 6 weeks post-injury; however, there were no significant differences between the two procedures in the 40-μl group at the same time point. Moreover, there were no significant peak-to-peak amplitude differences between the two procedures in the 50-μl compression group.

Conclusions: The findings of this study suggested that preferential rostral decompression was more beneficial than priority caudal decompression with respect to facilitating spinal cord functional recovery in rabbits with severe paraplegia and may provide clinicians with a reference for the clinical treatment of multiple-segment spinal cord compression injuries.

Keywords: Multilevel spine injuries, Somatosensory evoked potentials, Balloon compression, Decompression surgery

* Correspondence: fjjfjj369@sohu.com
[1]Department of Orthopaedics, Shanghai Pudong Hospital, Fudan University Pudong Medical Center, Shanghai 201399, China
Full list of author information is available at the end of the article

Background

Spinal cord injury (SCI), a devastating disaster to both patients and their families, is a focus of researchers worldwide. In particular, multilevel spine injuries have received considerable attention in recent years. According to statistics, 5.8% of all trauma patients suffer spinal fractures, and 21.7% of patients with spinal injuries exhibit SCIs; multilevel injuries occur in 10.4% of patients with fractures/dislocations and 1.3% of patients with SCIs [1, 2]. However, up to 26.2% of pediatric patients with SCIs exhibit multiple levels of damage [3]. In addition to trauma, multi-segmental spinal cord compression may be caused by disc herniation, posterior longitudinal ligament ossification and bone hyperplasia, as well as ligamentum flavum hypertrophy.

Consistent with the principle of treating of single-segment SCIs, the aim of surgery for the treatment of multilevel SCIs is to relieve compression and restore the integrity and stability of the spine as quickly as possible. Most patients with SCIs exhibit a critical area of injury that significantly impacts spinal cord function. In these cases, the key lesion site is the location of surgical treatment. In addition, a small number of patients may present with SCIs at multiple levels, resulting in neurological dysfunction in several segments. In these cases, it is typically difficult to determine the critical site of damage. Thus, the operative site is often determined based on the degree of compression and the experience of the surgeon.

Some patients are unable to undergo a one-stage operation on multiple areas of the body because of a poor general conditions or a lack of proper surgical approaches. In such cases, surgeons may be confused as to whether to perform rostral or caudal decompression first in patients with multilevel noncontinuous spinal cord compression injuries.

Therefore, we aimed to establish a novel model of spinal cord compression injury involving two noncontinuous segments in rabbits using a Fogarty balloon catheter and investigated the effects of different decompression sequences using somatosensory evoked potentials (SEPs), behavioral analyses and histochemical assessments. The results of our investigations will provide clinicians with a very useful reference for the clinical treatment of patients with SCIs.

Methods

Animals

Adult female New Zealand white rabbits (3–3.5 kg, Jiagan Biology, Shanghai, China) were used in this study ($n = 34$). All experimental procedures were approved by the Institutional Animal Care and Use Committee of Fudan University Pudong Medical Center.

Balloon compression model

The animals were anesthetized via an ear vein injection of 3% sodium pentobarbital (30 mg kg–1). The rabbits were subsequently placed and fixed in a prone position. The back of each animal was shaved, and a 5-cm midline incision was made over the T4–T9 spinous processes under sterile conditions. Both the soft tissue and the spinous processes of the T5–T7 vertebrae were removed. Two small holes (2 mm in diameter) were made in the vertebral arch of T6 and T7 using a micromotor (Fig. 1d). Separate grooves were drilled into the dorsal surfaces of the T6 and T7 vertebral lamina at the midline to guide the insertion of the catheter and hold it in position at the midline [4, 5]. Two 2-French Fogarty catheters (Edwards Lifesciences, California, USA) were subsequently inserted into the epidural space and advanced 3 cm cranially or caudally to ensure that the center of the balloon

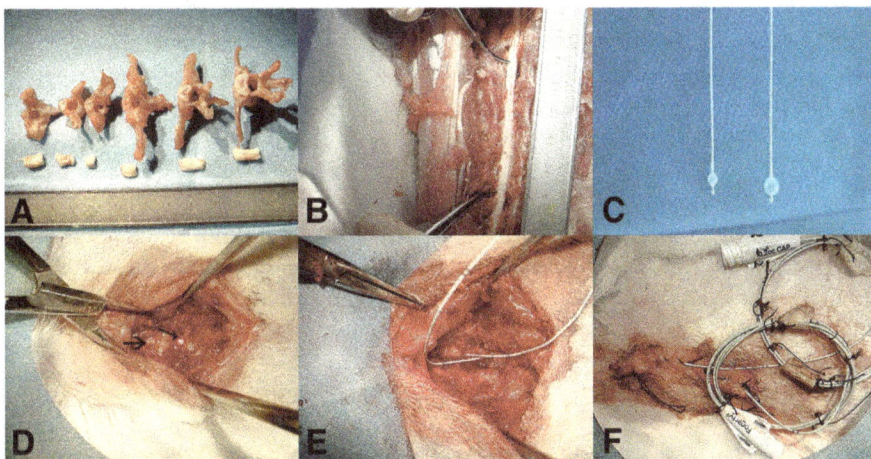

Fig. 1 Photographs showing the anatomy of the thoracic vertebrae and the surgical approach used in the model. **a** Intact rabbit thoracic vertebrae and the corresponding spinal cord segments (T1, T3, T6, T8, T10, and T12). **b** Locations of T4 and T11 in the spinal cord. **c** A 2-French Fogarty catheter was inflated with 40 μl (*left*) or 50 μl (*right*) of saline solution. **d** Two small holes were drilled in the vertebral arches of T6 and T7 (arrows indicate the sites of drilling). **e** A 2-French Fogarty catheter was inserted into the epidural space and advanced 3 cm cranially or caudally. **f** The catheter was fixed to the skin

rested at approximately the T4 or T11 level of the spinal cord (Fig. 1e). The soft tissues and skin were sutured in anatomical layers, and the end of the catheter was fixed to the skin (Fig. 1f). The SEPs of all animals were assessed before the balloon was inflated to exclude the possibility that additional damage to the spinal cord occurred during surgery. A 50% reduction in the amplitude and/or a 10% increase in the latency compared with the corresponding preoperative value was viewed as a modeling failure [6, 7].

Groups and decompression surgery

The animals that exhibited successful modeling were randomly divided into the following five groups, according to the inflation volume and the decompression sequence: a control group ($n = 6$), in which two Fogarty catheters were inserted and not inflated; a 40-µl priority rostral decompression (PRD) group ($n = 7$), which received 40 µl of saline solution and underwent PRD; a 40-µl priority caudal decompression (PCD) group ($n = 7$), which received 40 µl of saline solution and underwent PCD; a 50-µl PRD group ($n = 7$), which received 50 µl of saline solution and underwent PRD; and a 50-µl PCD group ($n = 7$), which received 50 µl of saline solution and underwent PCD. Two balloons were rapidly inflated at the same time using two Hamilton syringes. Manual bladder expression was performed at least twice daily after balloon inflation until reflex bladder activity was established, and subcutaneous injections of the antibiotic enrofloxacin (10 mg/kg/d) were administered for 3 days.

The first decompression was performed by deflating and slowly removing the catheter during the first week after injury. In the control group, the balloon was first removed in the rostral location in 3 animals and was first removed in the caudal location in the other 3 animals. At 2 weeks post-injury, the second decompression was performed using the same method that was employed for the first decompression. The rabbits were sacrificed at 4 weeks after decompression.

Behavioral analyses

Behavioral assessments were performed by two individuals blinded to the treatments at baseline, on the first day after compression, and once weekly until euthanasia. All motor and sensory testing was conducted between 08:00 am and 12:00 pm.

Reuter score

The muscle tone and motor and sensory function of the hind legs and the reflex functions of the spinal cord were assessed using Reuter scores [8] (total score of 11 points) at the above predetermined time points.

Modified Rivlin's test

All animals were assessed regarding their ability to maintain their position and the maximum angle on an inclined plane, as previously described by Rivlin [9]. Briefly, each animal was positioned horizontally on a custom-made oblique plate comprising two rectangular alloy plates connected by a hinge (the test surface consisted of a rubber surface with shallow trenches), with the body axis of the rabbit perpendicular to the longitudinal axis of the oblique plate. The oblique plate was rotated around the axis starting from the horizontal position, and the maximum angle that the animals sustained for 5 seconds without sliding down the plate was recorded two times for each direction and averaged to yield a final value.

Electrophysiological evaluations

SEPs were measured for each animal to determine the functional integrity of the spinal cord. The SEPs were recorded at baseline, at 1 h post-operation, immediately after compression, and at weeks 1, 2, 3, 4, 5 and 6 after injury. The animals were anesthetized with pentobarbital sodium (30 mg/kg) via auricular vein injections. A 3-channel Dantec-KEYPOINT electromyograph was used to generate and record the SEPs. To elicit cortical SEPs, we employed a constant current stimulator with a 3-Hz square wave of 0.2 ms in duration with a pair of subdermal electrodes inserted into the median and tibial nerves of the hind limbs. The stimulation intensity was 2–3 mA, and the effectiveness of the nerve stimulation was evaluated via visual inspection of hind limb twitches. The recordings from the skull electrodes were obtained at Cz-Fz. The recording electrode was located 2.5 mm posterior and 2.8 mm lateral to the bregma. Reference electrodes were placed along the midline of the forehead, and a subdermal needle electrode was placed at the back of the neck to serve as a ground electrode. Stimulation was initiated when the interference waveform was a smooth straight line. We averaged 600–800 SEP trials to obtain a smoother wave to improve the signal-to-noise ratio (SNR). A sensitivity of 2 µV/div and a time base of 10 ms/div were used to display the SEP responses. The SEP response was identified, and the onset latency and peak-to-peak amplitude of the response were subsequently obtained (Figs. 3, 4).

Radiographic imaging

For imaging, the animals were anesthetized as previously described. X-ray images were used to determine the balloon location (Fig. 5a–c) after modeling. The balloon catheter was filled with iohexol diluted with saline (1:1), which served as a dye for imaging the balloon size and location. Transverse computed tomography (CT) images (Fig. 5d–e) were also used to calculate the magnitude of balloon inflation and the rate of spinal cord compression within the vertebral canal. The rate of spinal canal occlusion was defined as the proportion of the anterior-posterior diameter of the vertebral canal occupied by the balloon. Magnetic resonance imaging (MRI) was performed in two animals per group at 2 weeks after SCI (after the second decompression) using a 1.5 T imaging system (Philips Medical Systems, Netherland B.V, DA Best, the Netherlands). Images of the spinal region were acquired in the sagittal plane. T2-weighted images (4000/33 [TR/TE]; section thickness: 2.5 mm, section gap: 0.2 mm, resolution ratio: 0.27 mm × 0.27 mm × 2.0 mm) were obtained to evaluate damage severity.

Tissue preparation and histological evaluations

Six weeks after injury, the rabbits were anesthetized using pentobarbital (100 mg/kg) and then intracardially perfused with PBS, followed by 4% paraformaldehyde in PBS. Two 1-cm sections of the spinal cord from the lesion epicenter at T4 and T11 were dissected and post-fixed with a 4% formaldehyde solution in liquid phosphate buffer overnight. The samples were subsequently dehydrated in graded ethanol solutions (75–100%) and embedded in paraffin. Sections with a thickness of 4 μm were collected in a series of five with a distance of 200 μm between individual sections. Transverse sections were subsequently stained with hematoxylin-eosin (H&E) and Luxol fast blue (LFB) and examined using light microscopy. The lesion area, including both the cavity size and the degree of white matter sparing, as well as the number of ventral horn motor neurons (VHMNs), was measured with Image-Pro Plus 6.0 (IPP) software (Media Cybernetics, Rockville, MD, USA). Five sections from each tissue specimen were counted, and mean values for the T4 and T11 segments in each animal were obtained.

Measurement of apoptosis in the spinal cord

To detect apoptotic cells, we performed staining using a terminal deoxynucleotidyl transferase-mediated dUTP-biotin nick end-labeling assay (TUNEL) apoptosis detection kit (Roche, Mannheim, Germany), according to the manufacturer's instructions. The sections were counter-stained with 4,6-diamino-2-phenyl indole (DAPI). Apoptosis-positive cells that appeared green under a fluorescence microscope (Fig. 8) were counted in five fields of view per section at 200× magnification. The five fields exhibiting the strongest positive expression were located in the dorsal, central canal, and ventral gray matter of the spinal cord lesions.

Statistical analysis

Statistical analyses were performed using SPSS 19.0 software (IBM, New York, NY, USA). Data were expressed as the mean ± standard deviation (SD). The Reuter score results were analyzed using the Kruskal-Wallis test, and the Rivlin's test and SEP results were analyzed via two-way analysis of variance (ANOVA) followed by Bonferroni or Tukey post-hoc test. Other data were analyzed using one-way ANOVA and the least significant difference test. $P < 0.05$ was considered statistically significant.

Results

Overall recovery of the animals after spinal cord compression

In the 50-μl compression group, 1 of 14 injured rabbits died after a mean survival time of 5 days post-injury because of the severity of its SCI, whereas all the control group and 40-μl compression group animals survived. In the 50-μl compression group, 5 of 14 rabbits exhibited hematuria during the first several days after injury. None of the control group rabbits presented with bladder dysfunction after surgery. Manual bladder expression was necessary in the 40- and 50-μl compression groups. In the 40-μl compression group, manual bladder compression was discontinued in most of the animals by the 2-week post-injury time point, whereas in the 50-μl compression group, 80% of the animals exhibited no bladder voiding at 4 weeks after injury. Several animals in the 50-μl group required manual bladder emptying throughout the entire 6-week period.

Behavioral outcomes

Reuter scores were measured in each rabbit until the end of survival (Fig. 2a). In the control group, the muscle tone, reflexes, and motor and sensory functions of the hind legs were normal after catheterization. In the 40-μl compression group, incomplete paralysis appeared in most of the animals after compression. These animals exhibited gradually spontaneous improvement by the 1-week post-injury time point compared with their initial post-injury presentations (**$p < 0.01$). Various levels of motor and sensory functional improvement were identified in most of the animals that had first undergone rostral or caudal decompression. Approximately 80% of the animals in this group exhibited a near-normal gait during the fifth week after compression surgery and subsequently reached a plateau at which no further improvement was identified; this plateau phenomenon persisted until sixth week. In contrast, the rabbits subjected to compression injury induced by 50 μl of saline solution presented with complete bilateral paraplegia from day 1 to week 1 after injury and exhibited only limited recovery. The animals in the 50-μl PRD group experienced a more rapid neurological functional recovery than the animals in the 50-μl PCD group. There were significant differences in Reuter scores between the 50-μl PRD and 50-μl PCD groups at the fourth week after

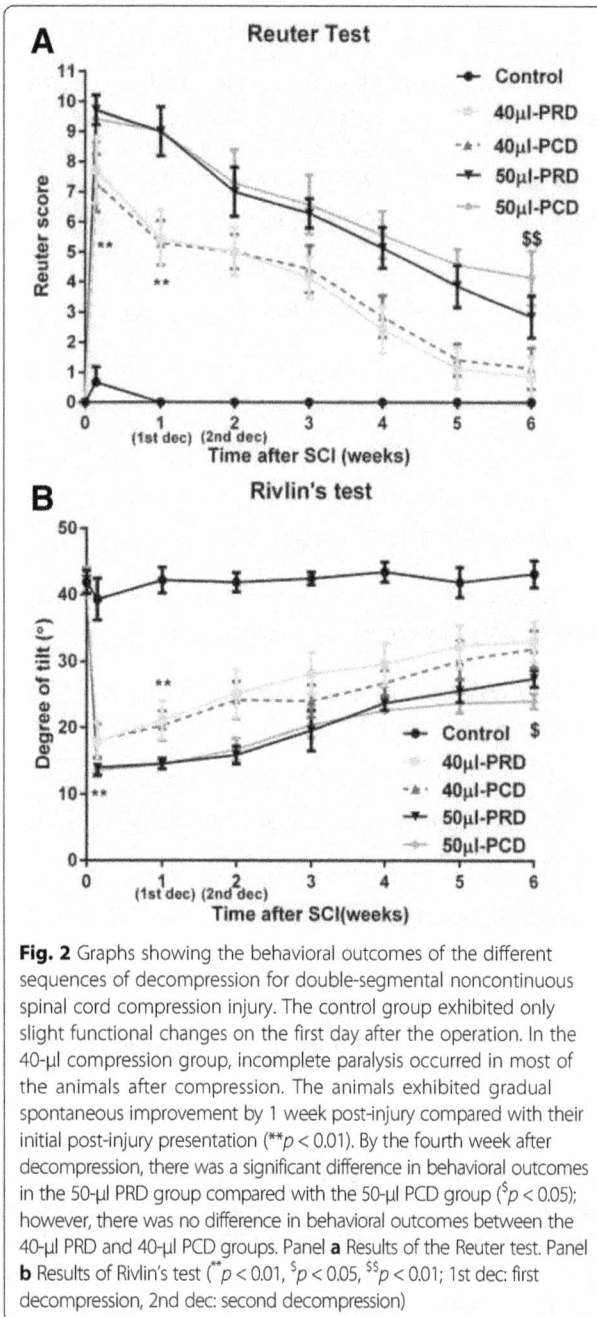

Fig. 2 Graphs showing the behavioral outcomes of the different sequences of decompression for double-segmental noncontinuous spinal cord compression injury. The control group exhibited only slight functional changes on the first day after the operation. In the 40-µl compression group, incomplete paralysis occurred in most of the animals after compression. The animals exhibited gradual spontaneous improvement by 1 week post-injury compared with their initial post-injury presentation (**$p < 0.01$). By the fourth week after decompression, there was a significant difference in behavioral outcomes in the 50-µl PRD group compared with the 50-µl PCD group ($^{\$}p < 0.05$); however, there was no difference in behavioral outcomes between the 40-µl PRD and 40-µl PCD groups. Panel **a** Results of the Reuter test. Panel **b** Results of Rivlin's test (**$p < 0.01$, $^{\$}p < 0.05$, $^{\$\$}p < 0.01$; 1st dec: first decompression, 2nd dec: second decompression)

decompression ($^{\$\$}p < 0.01$); however, there were no significant differences in Reuter scores between the 40-µl PRD and 40-µl PCD groups at the same time point.

The results of the modified Rivlin's test for all groups are presented in Fig. 2b. Initially, all animals maintained balance at a tilt ranging from 40° to 45°. The first day after injury, the control group exhibited a minimal change in its tilt score (Rivlin score = 39.3° ± 3.1°). However, the 40- and 50-µl groups exhibited significant decreases in their Rivlin scores. The animals in the 40-µl group subsequently exhibited progressive recovery by

1 week post-injury ($^{**}p < 0.01$). At the end of the observation period, the functional recovery of the 50-µl PRD group was better than that of the 50-µl PCD group ($p = 0.0344$).

Electrophysiological evaluations

SEPs were used to estimate the effects of different sequences of decompression on the ability of the spinal cord to conduct electrical impulses. Figures 3 and 4 show the changes in the SEPs for a representative animal at baseline and before and after decompression. The baseline SEP was characterized by latency after the stimulus and the peak-to-peak amplitude in all animals. The SEP amplitude was slightly decreased after catheter insertion in some rabbits ($p > 0.05$). In the control group, the SEP waveform returned to the baseline level at 1 week after the operation and remained at that level until the end of the experiment. In the 40-µl group, the mean onset latency and amplitude of the hindlimb SEPs on the first day after balloon inflation were 27.35 ± 1.23 ms and 2.52 ± 0.47 µV, respectively. However, by the 7th day after balloon inflation, the mean onset latency and amplitude of the hindlimb SEPs were 24.72 ± 1.09 ms and 3.21 ± 0.42 µV, respectively, results indicative of significant automatic recovery of neural function ($^{****}p < 0.0001$) (Fig. 4). During decompression, a small number of animals exhibited a slight reduction in the amplitude. Significant electrophysiological improvement was noted during week 4 and was sustained through week 6 (Fig. 4). The SEP responses were similar between the 40-µl PRD and 40-µl PCD groups (Fig. 4), indicating that different sequences of decompression did not influence the SEP recordings in the 40-µl groups. In the 50-µl groups, the hindlimb SEPs increased in latency such that the average SEP was 28.91 ± 1.26 ms on day 1 compared with 32.29 ± 1.81 ms at 1 week after compression. The amplitude was not significantly altered at this time. After the second decompression, the SEP latency of the animals in the 50-µl group exhibited a clear "rebound phenomenon". The change was more significant in the PCD group than in the PRD. After decompression, electrophysiological recovery proceeded more slowly in the PCD group than in the PRD group. The SEP latencies were 26.43 ± 0.89 ms and 24.33 ± 0.46 ms ($p < 0.01$) and the amplitudes were 1.68 ± 0.11 µV and 1.30 ± 0.04 µV ($p = 1.768$) in the PCD and PRD groups, respectively, at 6 weeks after injury.

Imaging results

As indicated in Fig. 5, the catheter tips were placed on the postero-lateral side of the cord in the T4 and T11 regions in the model rabbits. The rates of spinal canal occlusion under 40 µl of balloon inflation at T4 and T11 were 44.31 ± 1.79% and 44.74 ± 2.08% ($p > 0.05$), respectively,

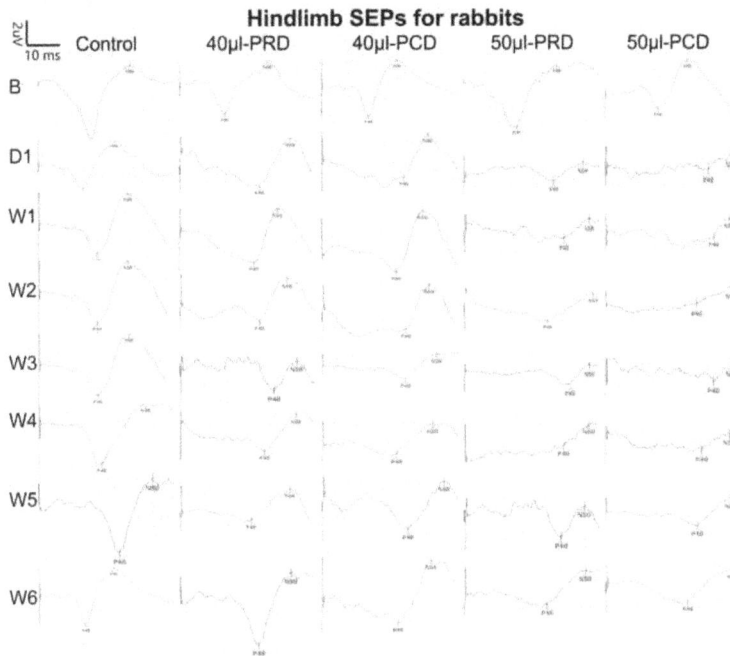

Fig. 3 Mean SEP waveforms recorded during hindlimb stimulation in the five groups over 6 weeks from the Cz-Fz. The baseline SEP waveforms recorded prior to compression injury are presented in the first row. Each column shows representative SEP waveforms that were recorded in the control, 40-μl PRD, 40-μl PCD, 50-μl PRD, and 50-μl PCD groups (from *left* to *right*). B: Baseline. D: Day. W: Week

whereas the rates under 50 μl of balloon inflation were $72.75 \pm 2.76\%$ and $72.36 \pm 3.02\%$ ($p > 0.05$), respectively (Fig. 5d-e). No lesions were evident in the MRI images of the control group. Representative T2-weighted sagittal MR images of the 40- and 50-μl groups showed that the spinal cord was surrounded by hyper-intense cerebrospinal fluid (CSF), and two hyper-intensity signals in the T4 and T11 regions were identified at 2 weeks post-SCI (Fig. 5f). In addition, the center of the lesions exhibited a completely hyper-intense signal that likely represented acute swelling of the spinal cord, which may have been the result of venous congestion, edema, and hemorrhage at the injured segments. There was no difference in damage severity between the PRD and PCD groups, as determined by visual inspection.

Histomorphological findings

To determine whether the observed differences in functional recovery were correlated with lesion extension and to investigate the potential pathophysiological mechanisms underlying these phenomena, we performed histological analysis of the injured spinal cord. Macroscopic observation noted small indentations in the spines of the animals in the 50-μl compression group during the 6-week post-injury period. Microscopically, no lesions were identified in the control group rabbits during this period. In the 40-μl compression group, in

general, the structures of the gray matter and white matter were clearly exhibited at the center of the lesions, and no necrosis was identified (Fig. 6). Furthermore, the number of VHMNs was decreased ($p < 0.05$), and vacuolar degeneration was identified around axons; there was a significant decrease in the area and density of the blue staining of the myelin sheath in the 40-μl compression group compared with the control group (Figs. 6, 7). No differences in injury severity were noted in spines treated with different decompression sequences in the 40-μl group (Fig. 7). However, more severe lesions were noted in the transverse sections of the spines in the 50-μl group than in those in the 40-μl group. At the center of the lesion, the normal structures of both the gray and the white matter were lost. Specifically, almost the entire structure of the gray matter was lost, as was part of the structure of the peripheral white matter (Fig. 6). Furthermore, instead of cavities, connective and vascular scarred tissue was present (Fig. 6). LFB staining indicated that the staining area of the myelin sheath was significantly decreased and had been replaced by continuous connective tissues. Moreover, the lesion area was infiltrated by polymorphonuclear cells and other nonneuronal cells, such as macrophages (Fig. 6). Notably, there were significant differences in the numbers of VHMNs, the sizes of the cavitations and the degree of white matter sparing in the center of the rostral lesions

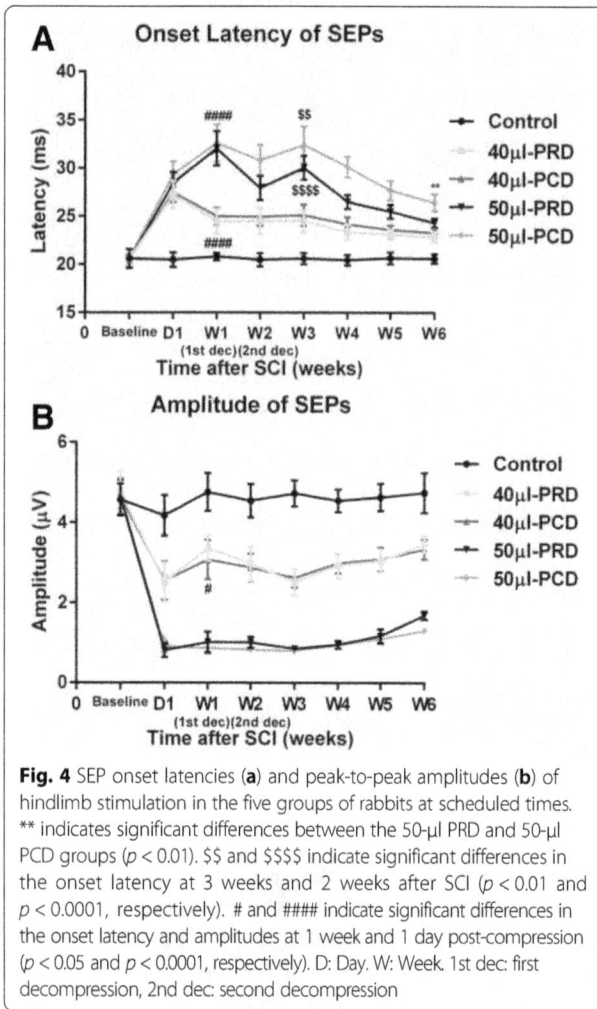

Fig. 4 SEP onset latencies (**a**) and peak-to-peak amplitudes (**b**) of hindlimb stimulation in the five groups of rabbits at scheduled times. ** indicates significant differences between the 50-μl PRD and 50-μl PCD groups ($p < 0.01$). \$\$ and \$\$\$\$ indicate significant differences in the onset latency at 3 weeks and 2 weeks after SCI ($p < 0.01$ and $p < 0.0001$, respectively). # and #### indicate significant differences in the onset latency and amplitudes at 1 week and 1 day post-compression ($p < 0.05$ and $p < 0.0001$, respectively). D: Day. W: Week. 1st dec: first decompression, 2nd dec: second decompression

between the 50-μl PRD and 50-μl PCD groups; however, there were no significant differences in these parameters in the centers of the caudal lesions (Fig. 7).

TUNEL assay to detect apoptosis

Cellular apoptosis in the spinal lesions was detected via TUNEL staining. The control group did not exhibit apoptosis-positive cells (Fig. 8a). Specific green fluorescence was identified in the nuclei of apoptotic nerve cells, and fluorescence microscopy showed that apoptotic cells were scattered throughout the SCI area. Apoptosis-positive cells were also identified at the edge of the central canal (Fig. 8). The TUNEL assay results showed that in the compression group, the number of TUNEL-positive cells was significantly increased compared with that in the spinal cord control group and that the number of TUNEL-positive cells in the 50-μl PRD group was lower than that in the 50-μl PCD group ($p < 0.0001$, Fig. 9).

Discussion

This study was the first investigation to explore the optimal sequence of decompression for multilevel non-continuous spinal cord compression injuries. Therefore, using an appropriate animal model was essential for the performance of a successful experiment. To date, sustained compression models for a single cord segment have been established via balloon compression [10, 11] and insertion of water-absorbing materials [12–14] or other hard materials [15]. In the present study, we established a double-segment spinal cord compression injury model using a balloon catheter, as this model offers several distinct advantages over other models. The balloon catheters cause minimal trauma [16] and can be reliably controlled and maintained for variable durations

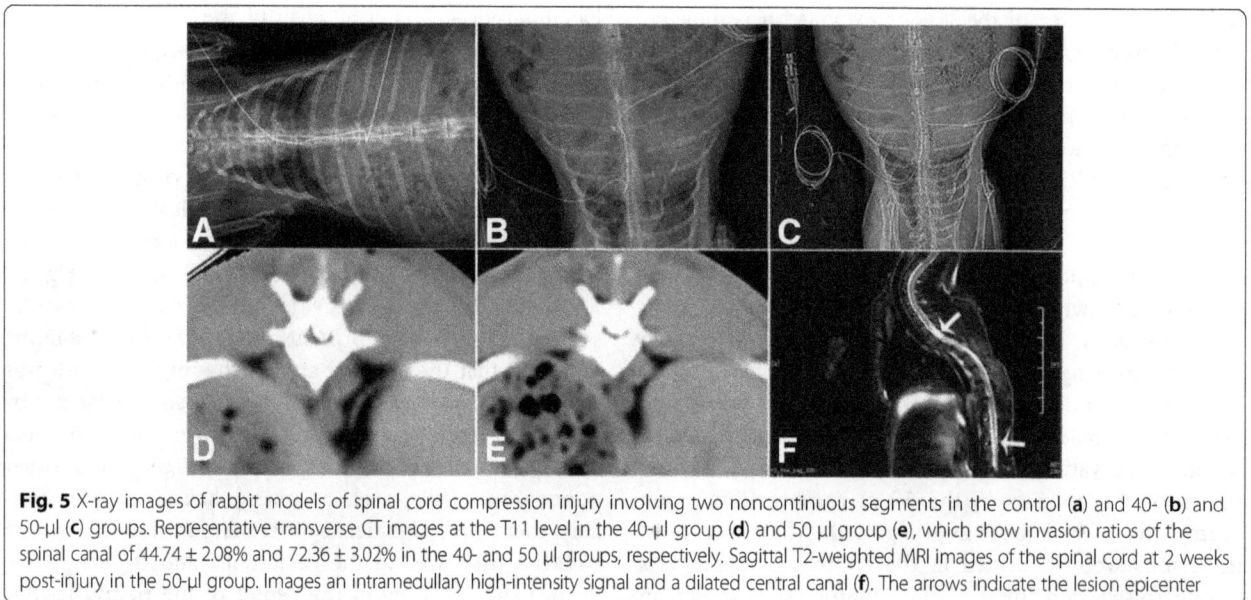

Fig. 5 X-ray images of rabbit models of spinal cord compression injury involving two noncontinuous segments in the control (**a**) and 40- (**b**) and 50-μl (**c**) groups. Representative transverse CT images at the T11 level in the 40-μl group (**d**) and 50 μl group (**e**), which show invasion ratios of the spinal canal of 44.74 ± 2.08% and 72.36 ± 3.02% in the 40- and 50 μl groups, respectively. Sagittal T2-weighted MRI images of the spinal cord at 2 weeks post-injury in the 50-μl group. Images an intramedullary high-intensity signal and a dilated central canal (**f**). The arrows indicate the lesion epicenter

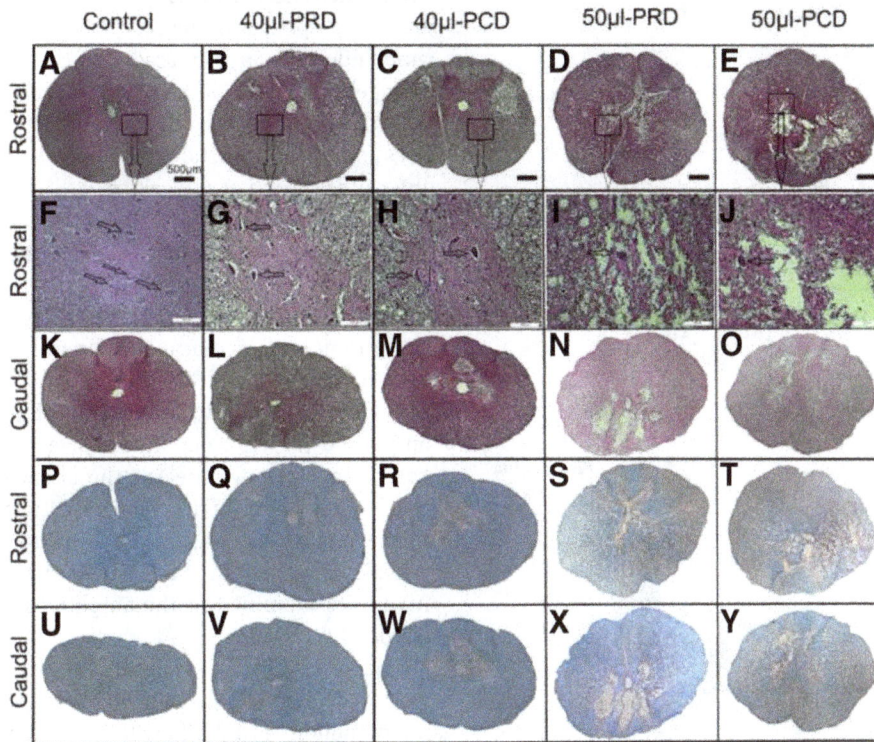

Fig. 6 Histological features of each group, as demonstrated by HE (**a-e**) and LFB (**p-y**) staining. Stained cross-sections of representative samples located rostral (**a-j, p-t**) and caudal (**k-o, u-y**) to the injury epicenter are presented. The short arrow indicates the VHMNs (magnification **a-e** and **k-y** 50×; **f-j**: 200×)

[17], which makes the use of such a model advantageous compared with other injury modalities.

The SEP results for all the rabbits that underwent catheter insertion without inflation indicated that a decreased amplitude occurred in only a small number of animals and did not reach "red flag" standards [7] and that the latency was maintained at baseline levels. These findings suggest that the model caused almost no additional spinal cord insults. During the observation period, we found that the values of the control group were not significantly different from that of the preoperative electrophysiology and behavioral results. The combination of our imaging and pathology results confirmed the safety of vertebral stabilization and placement of the balloon catheter in the spinal cord.

It is well established that balloon catheter inflation volume significantly influences injury severity [11, 18]. In the present study, the balloons were inflated to two different volumes (40 μl or 50 μl), resulting in spinal canal occupation rates of less than 50% and greater than 70%, respectively. Compression injury induced using a 50-μl inflated balloon led to extremely severe locomotor impairment (complete bilateral paraplegia), and the animals subjected to this treatment exhibited slight functional deterioration prior to the first decompression. Consistent with previous findings related to single-segment injury, we noted that use of a 40-μl balloon induced a moderate lesion; however, gradual spontaneous improvements in motor function were noted prior to the first decompression, as indicated by our observation of a shortened latency and an increased amplitude in these rabbits [4, 11, 15, 19] (Figs. 3, 4). Undoubtedly, our finding of spontaneous locomotor recovery indicates that our judgment the effects of SCI treatment is substantially limited [11].

The Reuter scoring system and modified Rivlin's test were used to quantitatively evaluate functional outcomes and behavioral analysis results in this study because of their ease of use, inter-rater reliability and sensitivity for gross motor deficits, particularly hindlimb deficits. Moreover, these scoring systems may detect relatively smaller functional changes resulting from spinal cord insults than the BBB and Tarlov scoring systems. The reliability of these tests has been verified by several studies [8, 9, 20]. Our results showed that PRD is more beneficial than PCD with respect to facilitating the recovery of neurological function in rabbits with severe paraplegia (Fig. 2). However, there were no differences in neurological recovery between the PRD and PCD rabbits subjected to 40-μl balloon inflation (Fig. 2). Our finding that moderate lesions exhibited spontaneous neurological recovery may also indicate that our judgment to the effects of decompression is limited.

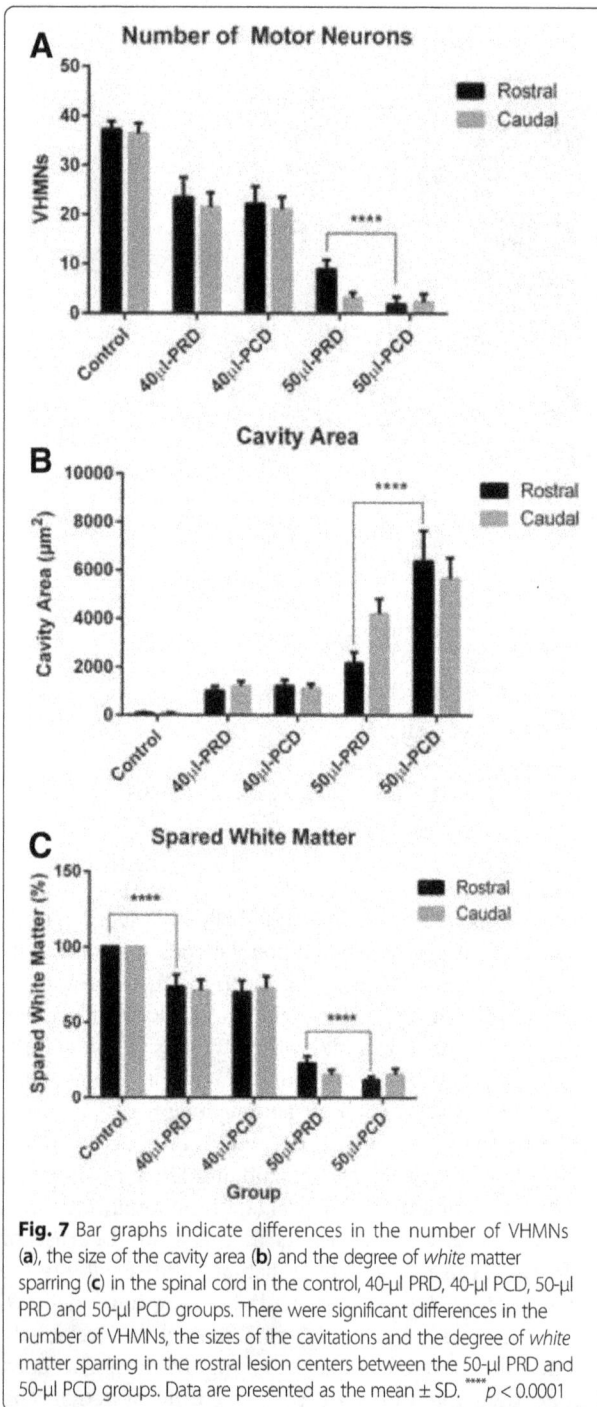

Fig. 7 Bar graphs indicate differences in the number of VHMNs (**a**), the size of the cavity area (**b**) and the degree of *white* matter sparring (**c**) in the spinal cord in the control, 40-μl PRD, 40-μl PCD, 50-μl PRD and 50-μl PCD groups. There were significant differences in the number of VHMNs, the sizes of the cavitations and the degree of *white* matter sparring in the rostral lesion centers between the 50-μl PRD and 50-μl PCD groups. Data are presented as the mean ± SD. $^{****}p < 0.0001$

SEPs, which are commonly used for intra-operative monitoring of the spinal cord [6, 21], have been introduced for the diagnosis, prognostication and quantification of the physiological integrity of the spinal cord [22, 23]. A substantial number of studies have confirmed that SEPs may serve as a biomarker of neurological status [24, 25] and indicators of ultrastructural damage [14] and that they are highly sensitive and specific

for the detection of neurological deficits [26, 27]. After SCI, the SEP responses of injured pathways exhibit a decreased amplitude and an increased latency. The degree of each change is indicative of the severity of the insult [28].

In the present study, the latency of preferential decompression in the rostral group was shorter than that in the caudal group at 6 weeks post-SCI in the rabbits with severe paraplegia (Figs. 3, 4). This result indicates that nerve conduction is faster following the release of rostral spinal cord compression, which may be a result of the sparing of more myelinated fibers (Figs. 6, 7c). However, the absence of significant differences in the amplitude between the 50-μl PRD and 50-μl PCD groups (Fig. 4) may have been due to the fact that the sensitivity of the amplitude for chronic compressive injury of the spinal cord was low; nevertheless, the latency appears to be a reliable indicator of irreversible ultrastructural damage to the spinal cord [14]. In contrast, the earliest and most reliable changes in SEPs after acute intra-operative injury are identified in the amplitude rather than in the latency [29, 30].

One unexpected yet significant finding of our study was that the SEP latency exhibited a clear "rebound phenomenon" in rabbits with severe paraplegia after the second compression. This phenomenon was more apparent in the PCD group than in the PRD group. One potential explanation for this finding is that the degree of ischemia-reperfusion injury and the inflammatory reaction after decompression [12] were more severe (the pathologic results at 6 weeks post-SCI reflect this severity to some extent) in rabbits that underwent PCD than in rabbits that underwent PRD. Interestingly, this phenomenon was not accompanied by significant behavioral functional changes (Fig. 2). This finding is partly indicative of the exquisite sensitivity of SEPs for dorsal column functionality [27].

In the current study, we also showed that X-ray and CT imaging are reliable methods for monitoring balloon location and volume during spinal surgery (Fig. 5). CT provided rapid, high-quality images of the spinal canal during surgery (Fig. 5d, e). MRI is a non-invasive technique and is the most important diagnostic method for examining spinal cord diseases. In this study, MR images showed many artifacts when balloon catheters containing metal wires were inserted into the epidural space. Catheter removal resulted in a better image of the SCI (Fig. 5f). The above phenomenon is one weakness of the catheter method and must be addressed in future research.

The histopathological and apoptosis test results suggested that the differences in functional recovery between the different groups corresponded to the extent of the spinal cord damage suffered by each group. Curiously, histopathological analysis showed almost complete

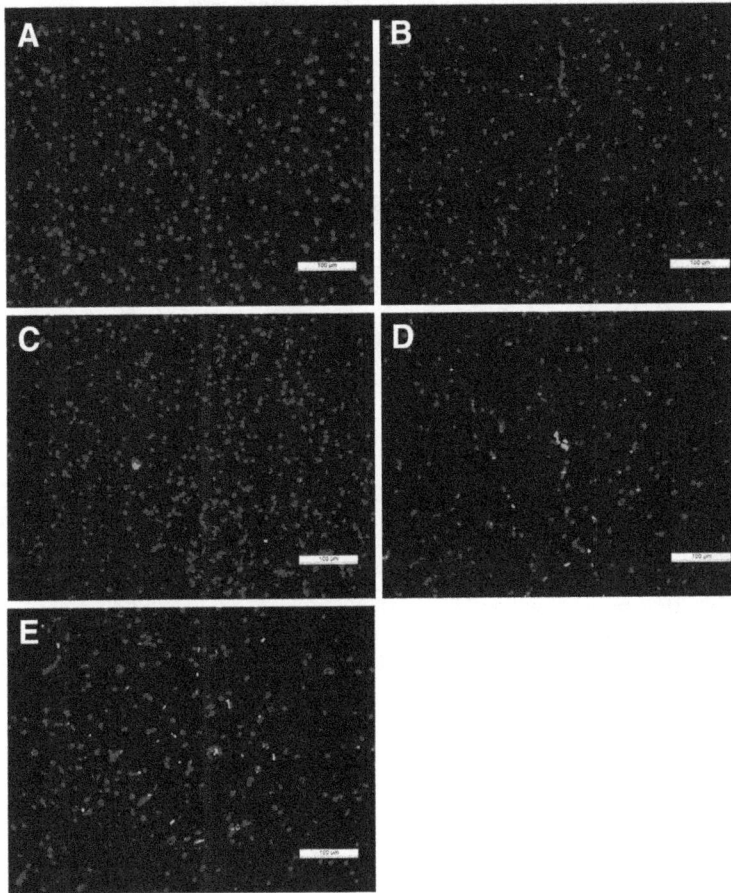

Fig. 8 TUNEL immunofluorescence staining for apoptosis in the rostral spinal cord tissue of the control (**a**), 40-μl PRD (**b**), 40-μl PCD (**c**), 50-μl PRD (**d**) and 50-μl PCD (**e**) groups. The nuclei were stained with DAPI (*blue*). The control group did not exhibit apoptosis-positive cells (*green*). The numbers of apoptotic cells were significantly increased in the 50-μl compression group compared with the 40-μl compression group. Scale bar = 100 μm

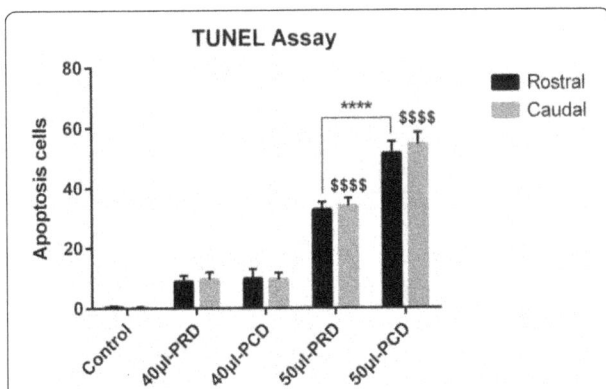

Fig. 9 Graphs illustrating the TUNEL assay results at 6 weeks post-injury in the control, 40-μl PRD, 40-μl PCD, 50-μl PRD and 50-μl PCD groups. The numbers of apoptosis-positive cells were significantly decreased in the rabbits subjected to the 50-μl compression injury when they initially underwent rostral compression release compared with the rabbits that underwent PCD. ****$p < 0.0001$, $^{$$$$}p < 0.0001$

loss of the gray matter and partial sparing of the white matter at the center of the lesion in rabbits with severe paraplegia. The area of the spared white matter corresponded to 10% of the area in intact animals. This finding is consistent with the findings of Basso et al., who found that sparing even 5–10% of the fibers at the lesion center is sufficient to help drive the segmental circuits involved in the production of basic locomotion after SCI [31]. Milder tissue lesions were identified in the cranial lesion areas of the 50-μl PRD group than in those of the 50-μl PCD group, which may be one reason why PRD was more beneficial than PCD with respect to facilitating the recovery of spinal cord function in rabbits with severe paraplegia.

Our study demonstrated for the first time that the epidural balloon-compression technique is a highly reproducible, accurate model of noncontinuous double segment injury in rabbits. Moreover, the results of the behavioral, electrophysiological, imaging, and histological analyses showed that PRD was more beneficial than PCD with respect to facilitating spinal cord function recovery in rabbits with severe paraplegia. The pathophysiological mechanism underlying this phenomenon may be that releasing rostral compression first may reduce the damage to the rostral spinal cord, allowing rostral function to recover as quickly as possible. Rostral spinal cord recovery may play a pivotal role in the overall regulation of the central and peripheral nervous systems, which may improve resistance to ischemia-reperfusion injury and attenuate the inflammatory reaction induced by the second decompression, ultimately resulting in the retention of more spinal cord function. The specific mechanism underlying this phenomenon remains to be studied further. In any case, these study results will undoubtedly provide clinicians with a very useful reference for the treatment of multilevel noncontinuous SCIs.

However, we noted some new issues that must be resolved in the future. First, the model involves drilling to insert the catheter, which requires the adjacent paraspinal muscles and spinous processes to be removed and may thus increase the chance of infection or unnecessarily damage blood vessels. This damage may be minimized using percutaneous methods and by inserting the catheter through the lumbosacral junction under fluoroscopic guidance [11]. In future studies, we will investigate the establishment of a double-segmental SCI model using a specially designed double-chamber double balloon catheter. Furthermore, blood biochemical parameters were not evaluated to assess whole-spinal cord function in the present study. Nitric oxide synthase [32, 33] (NOS) and inflammatory cytokines (TNF-α and IL-1β) [12] expressed locally during SCI have been used as indices for assessing therapeutic efficacy in previous studies but are apparently not applicable for such assessments in double-segmental SCIs.

Conclusion

In conclusion, the findings of this study suggested that preferential rostral decompression was more beneficial than priority caudal decompression with respect facilitating to spinal cord functional recovery in rabbits with severe paraplegia and may provide clinicians with a very useful reference for the clinical treatment of multiple-segment spinal cord compression injury.

Abbreviations

CT: Computed tomography; DAPI: 4,6-diamino-2-phenyl indole; LFB: Luxol fast blue; MRI: Magnetic resonance imaging; PCD: Priority caudal decompression; PRD: Priority rostral decompression; SCI: Spinal cord injury; SEPs: Somatosensory evoked potentials; TUNEL: Terminal deoxynucleotidyl transferase-mediated dUTP-biotin nick end-labeling assay; VHMNs: Ventral horn motor neurons

Acknowledgments
We thank Jianlan Qiao and Qinghua You for providing technical support.

Funding
This work was funded by the Health Service Organizations of Shanghai (20124300) and Key Disciplines Group Construction Project of Pudong Health Bureau of Shanghai (PWZxq2014-03).

Authors' contributions
JJF and BQY were responsible for the study design. CHY was responsible for performing the experiments, analyzing the data, and drafting the manuscript. FFM and HPL were responsible for revising the manuscript and writing the response letter. JLQ and QHY were responsible for collecting the imaging and pathology data, and CHY was responsible for conducting the literature review. BQY, JMH, and BY were responsible for critically revising the draft of the manuscript and for granting final approval of the version of the manuscript to be published. JJF was responsible for interpreting the data and for reviewing and revising the draft of the manuscript. All authors have read and approved the final manuscript.

Author information
The first author is currently employed in the Department of Orthopaedics, Shanghai Pudong Hospital, Fudan University Pudong Medical Center, 2800 Gongwei Road, Pudong New District, Shanghai 201399, China.

Competing interests
None of the authors have any potential conflicts of interest to disclose.

Author details
[1]Department of Orthopaedics, Shanghai Pudong Hospital, Fudan University Pudong Medical Center, Shanghai 201399, China. [2]Department of Pharmacy, Shanghai Pudong Hospital, Fudan University, Shanghai 201399, China. [3]Department of Pathology, Shanghai Pudong Hospital, Fudan University Pudong Medical Center, Shanghai 201399, China. [4]Department of Radiology, Shanghai Pudong Hospital, Fudan University Pudong Medical Center, Shanghai 201399, China.

References
1. Oliver M, Inaba K, Tang A, Branco BC, Barmparas G, Schnüriger B, et al. The changing epidemiology of spinal trauma: a 13-year review from a Level I Trauma Centre. Injury. 2012;43:1296–300. doi:10.1016/j.injury.2012.04.021.
2. Hasler RM, Exadaktylos AK, Bouamra O, Benneker LM, Clancy M, Sieber R, et al. Epidemiology and predictors of spinal injury in adult major trauma patients: European cohort study. Eur Spine J. 2011;20:2174–80. doi:10.1007/s00586-011-1866-7.
3. Mortazavi MM, Dogan S, Civelek E, Tubbs RS, Theodore N, Rekate HL, et al. Pediatric multilevel spine injuries: an institutional experience. Childs Nerv Syst. 2011;27:1095–100. doi:10.1007/s00381-010-1348-y.
4. Pedram MS, Dehghan MM, Soleimani M, Sharifi D, Marjanmehr SH, Nasiri Z. Transplantation of a combination of autologous neural differentiated and undifferentiated mesenchymal stem cells into injured spinal cord of rats. Spinal Cord. 2010;48:457–63. doi:10.1038/sc.2009.153.
5. Vanický I, Urdzíková L, Saganová K, Cízková D, Gálik J. A simple and reproducible model of spinal cord injury induced by epidural balloon inflation in the rat. J Neurotrauma. 2001;18:1399–407. doi:10.1089/08977150152725687.
6. Gonzalez AA, Jeyanandarajan D, Hansen C, Zada G, Hsieh PC. Intraoperative neurophysiological monitoring during spine surgery: a review. Neurosurg Focus. 2009;27, E6.
7. Rabai F, Sessions R, Seubert CN. Neurophysiological monitoring and spinal cord integrity. Best Practice Res Clin Anaesthesiol. 2016;30:53–68. doi:10.1016/j.bpa.2015.11.006.
8. Reuter DG, Tacker WA, Badylak SF, Voorhees WD, Konrad PE. Correlation of motor-evoked potential response to ischemic spinal cord damage. J Thorac Cardiovasc Surg. 1992;104:262–72.
9. Rivlin AS, Tator CH. Effect of duration of acute spinal-cord compression in a new acute cord injury model in rat. Surg Neurol. 1978;10:39–43.
10. Lonjon N, Kouyoumdjian P, Prieto M, Bauchet L, Haton H, Gaviria M, et al. Early functional outcomes and histological analysis after spinal cord

compression injury in rats: laboratory investigation. J Neurosurg Spine. 2010;12:106–13. doi:10.3171/2009.7.SPINE0989.

11. Chung WH, Lee JH, Chung DJ, Yang WJ, Lee AJ, Choi CB, et al. Improved rat spinal cord injury model using spinal cord compression by percutaneous method. J Vet Sci. 2013;14:329–35. doi:10.4142/jvs.2013.14.3.329.

12. Yang T, Wu L, Wang H, Fang J, Yao N, Xu Y. Inflammation level after decompression surgery for a rat model of chronic severe spinal cord compression and effects on ischemia-reperfusion injury. Neurol Med Chir (Tokyo). 2015;55:578–86. doi:10.2176/nmc.oa.2015-0022.

13. Kurokawa R, Murata H, Ogino M, Ueki K, Kim P. Altered blood flow distribution in the rat spinal cord under chronic compression. Spine (Phila Pa 1976). 2011;36:1006–9. doi:10.1097/BRS.0b013e3181eaf33d.

14. Hu Y, Wen CY, Li TH, Cheung MM, Wu EX, Luk KD. Somatosensory-evoked potentials as an indicator for the extent of ultrastructural damage of the spinal cord after chronic compressive injuries in a rat model. Clin Neurophysiol. 2011;122:1440–7. doi:10.1016/j.clinph.2010.12.051.

15. Kouyoumdjian P, Lonjon N, Prieto M, Haton H, Privat A, Asencio G, et al. A remotely controlled model of spinal cord compression injury in mice: toward real-time analysis laboratory. J Neurosurg Spine. 2009;11:461–70. doi:10.3171/2009.4.SPINE0979.

16. Benzel EC, Lancon JA, Bairnsfather S, Kesterson L. Effect of dosage and timing of administration of naloxone on outcome in the rat ventral compression model of spinal cord injury. Neurosurgery. 1990;27:597–601. doi:10.1227/00006123-199010000-00016.

17. Cao P, Zheng Y, Zheng T, Sun C, Lu J, Rickett T, et al. A model of acute compressive spinal cord injury with a minimally invasive balloon in goats. J Neurol Sci. 2014;337:97–103. doi:10.1016/j.jns.2013.11.024.

18. Lim JH, Jung CS, Byeon YE, Kim WH, Yoon JH, Kang KS, et al. Establishment of a canine spinal cord injury model induced by epidural balloon compression. J Vet Sci. 2007;8:89–94. doi:10.4142/jvs.2007.8.1.89.

19. Guizar-Sahagun G, Grijalva I, Hernandez-Godinez B, Franco-Bourland RE, Cruz-Antonio L, Martinez-Cruz A, Ibanez-Contreras A, Madrazo I. New approach for graded compression spinal cord injuries in Rhesus macaque: method feasibility and preliminary observations. J Med Primatol. 2011;40(6):401–13.

20. Dong Y, Miao L, Hei L, Lin L, Ding H. Neuroprotective effects and impact on caspase-12 expression of tauroursodeoxycholic acid after acute spinal cord injury in rats. Int J Clin Exp Pathol. 2015;8:15871–8.

21. Tamkus AA, Scott AF, Khan FR. Neurophysiological monitoring during spinal cord stimulator placement surgery. Neuromodulation. 2015;18:460–4. doi:10.1111/ner.12273.

22. Robinson LR, Micklesen PJ, Tirschwell DL, Lew HL. Predictive value of somatosensory evoked potentials for awakening from coma. Crit Care Med. 2003;31:960–7. doi:10.1097/01.CCM.0000053643.21751.3B.

23. Bazley FA, Maybhate A, Tan CS, Thakor NV, Kerr C, All AH. Enhancement of bilateral cortical somatosensory evoked potentials to intact forelimb stimulation following thoracic contusion spinal cord injury in rats. IEEE Trans Neural Syst Rehabil Eng. 2014;22:953–64. doi:10.1109/TNSRE.2014.2319313.

24. Holdefer RN, MacDonald DB, Skinner SA. Somatosensory and motor evoked potentials as biomarkers for post-operative neurological status. Clin Neurophysiol. 2015;126:857–65. doi:10.1016/j.clinph.2014.11.009.

25. Morris SH, El-Hawary R, Howard JJ, Rasmusson DD. Validity of somatosensory evoked potentials as early indicators of neural compromise in rat model of spinal cord compression. Clin Neurophysiol. 2013;124:1031–6. doi:10.1016/j.clinph.2012.10.023.

26. Nuwer MR, Dawson EG, Carlson LG, Kanim LE, Sherman JE. Somatosensory evoked potential spinal cord monitoring reduces neurologic deficits after scoliosis surgery: results of a large multicenter survey. Electroencephalogr Clin Neurophysiol. 1995;96:6–11. doi:10.1016/0013-4694(94)00235-D.

27. Thirumala P, Zhou J, Krishnan R, Manem N, Umredkar S, Hamilton DK, et al. Diagnostic accuracy of evoked potentials for functional impairment after contusive spinal cord injury in adult rats. J Clin Neurosci. 2016;25:122–6. doi:10.1016/j.jocn.2015.10.010.

28. Agrawal G, Kerr C, Thakor NV, All AH. Characterization of graded multicenter animal spinal cord injury study contusion spinal cord injury using somatosensory-evoked potentials. Spine (Phila Pa 1976). 2010;35:1122–7. doi:10.1097/BRS.0b013e3181be5fa7.

29. Cheung WY, Arvinte D, Wong YW, Luk KD, Cheung KM. Neurological recovery after surgical decompression in patients with cervical spondylotic myelopathy - a prospective study. Int Orthop. 2008;32:273–8. doi:10.1007/s00264-006-0315-4.

30. Hu Y, Ding Y, Ruan D, Wong YW, Cheung KM, Luk KD. Prognostic value of somatosensory-evoked potentials in the surgical management of cervical spondylotic myelopathy. Spine (Phila Pa 1976). 2008;33:E305–10. doi:10.1097/BRS.0b013e31816f6c8e.

31. Basso DM, Beattie MS, Bresnahan JC, Anderson DK, Faden AI, Gruner JA, et al. MASCIS evaluation of open field locomotor scores: effects of experience and teamwork on reliability. Multicenter Animal Spinal Cord Injury Study. J Neurotrauma. 1996;13:343–59. doi:10.1089/neu.1996.13.343.

32. Huang SH, Wu SH, Lee SS, Chang KP, Chai CY, Yeh JL, et al. Fat grafting in Burn scar alleviates neuropathic pain via anti-inflammation effect in scar and spinal cord. PLoS ONE. 2015;10:e0137563–e137563. doi:10.1371/journal.pone.0137563.

33. Su YF, Lin CL, Lee KS, Tsai TH, Wu SC, Hwang SL, et al. A modified compression model of spinal cord injury in rats: functional assessment and the expression of nitric oxide synthases. Spinal Cord. 2015;53:432–5. doi:10.1038/sc.2014.245.

5

An unusual delusion of duplication in a patient affected by Dementia with Lewy bodies

Paolo Solla[1*†] iD, Gioia Mura[2†], Antonino Cannas[1], Gianluca Floris[1], Davide Fonti[1], Gianni Orofino[1], Mauro Giovanni Carta[3†] and Francesco Marrosu[1,2†]

Abstract

Background: Dementia with Lewy bodies (DLB) is the second most frequent diagnosis of progressive degenerative dementia in older people. Delusions are common features in DLB and, among them, Capgras syndrome represents the most frequent disturbance, characterized by the recurrent and transient belief that a familiar person, often a close family member or caregiver, has been replaced by an identical-looking imposter. However, other delusional conditions near to misidentification syndromes can occur in DLB patients and may represent a major psychiatric disorder, although rarely studied systematically.

Case presentation: We reported on a female patient affected by DLB who presented with an unusual delusion of duplication. Referring to the female professional caregiver engaged by her relatives for her care, the patient constantly described the presence of two different female persons, with a disorder framed in the context of a delusion of duplication.
A brain 99Tc-hexamethylpropyleneamineoxime SPECT was performed showing moderate hypoperfusion in both occipital lobes, and associated with marked decreased perfusion in parieto-fronto-temporal lobes bilaterally.

Conclusions: An occipital hypoperfusion was identified, although in association with a marked global decrease of perfusion in the remaining lobes. The role of posterior lobes is certainly important in all misidentification syndromes where a natural dissociation between recognition and identification is present. Moreover, the concomitant presence of severe attentional and executive deficits evocative for a frontal syndrome and the marked global decrease of perfusion in the remaining lobes at the SPECT scan also suggest a possible dysfunction in an abnormal connectivity between anterior and posterior areas.

Keywords: Dementia with Lewy bodies, Delusion of duplication, Misidentification syndromes, Capgras syndrome

Background

Dementia with Lewy bodies (DLB) is a progressive degenerative dementia, with core features characterized by fluctuating cognitive symptoms with pronounced variations in attention and alertness, recurrent visual hallucinations and associated features of parkinsonism [1], which is recognized as the second most common form of severe cognitive impairment in older people [2].

Delusions are common features in DLB, and patients affected by this condition are firmly hold on their false beliefs also in the presence of strong contradictory evidence. Among delusional disturbances in DLB, Capgras syndrome represents the most frequent disorder affecting approximately 17% of DLB patients and is characterized by the recurrent and transient belief that a familiar person, often a close family member or caregiver, has been replaced by an identical-looking imposter [3]. Capgras syndrome belongs to delusional misidentification syndromes (see Additional file 1: Table S1), among which two major groups were proposed, based on content-specific misidentifications [4, 5]: the Capgras type (also including

* Correspondence: paosol29@yahoo.it
†Equal contributors
[1]Department of Neurology, Movement Disorders Center, Institute of Neurology, University of Cagliari, SS 554 Bivio per Sestu, Monserrato 09042, Cagliari, Italy
Full list of author information is available at the end of the article

the Fregoli delusion, a delusional belief that one or more familiar persons, usually persecutors following the patient, are masquerading as several other people) and the Clonal Pluralization type. In the last, patients firmly belief that multiple exact copies of places, objects, self or others exist, such as in the misidentification of reflection, in the reduplicative paramnesia, and in the clonal pluralization of the self [6–8]. However, other delusional conditions near to misidentification syndromes can occur in several patients with DLB and may represent a major psychiatric disorders, although rarely studied systematically. Here we reported on a female patient affected by DLB who presented with an unusual delusion of duplication.

Case presentation

A 77-year-old woman had a history of DLB since 2013 when she was 75. She has a primary school education and was a retired saleswoman. Previous clinical history was unremarkable, she did not assume any medication, and there was no family history of psychiatric or movement disorders. Her initial motor symptoms, started approximately six months before the first examination, were bilateral bradykinesia, followed by rigidity and mild postural instability with associated marked hypomimia and mild hypophonia. Her relatives signaled also a history of likely rapid eye movement sleep behavior (RBD) disorder. Mood and affect were normal, with the exception of mild symptoms of apathy described mainly as a lack of motivation. She was initially treated with levodopa/carbidopa 400/100 mg daily with good initial improvement of parkinsonian symptoms. In agreement with the patient, no medications were introduced to treat RBD symptoms, which were considered not significant by the same patient.

However, three months later, she noticed a moderate increase of her motor symptoms and selegiline 10 mg daily was added. After another month, we were contacted by her relatives because she has started to present a significant cognitive impairment with fluctuating episodes of confusion and visual hallucinations, and, although less marked, with delusional jealousy and persecutory ideas, sometimes with behavioral problems (aggressiveness). Brain MRI was normal and without significant atrophy. Her dementia work-up did not reveal any reversible causes, while results of laboratory tests were normal. Although clinical feature were not suggestive for prion disease or epilepsy, an EEG was done and was normal.

A neuropsychological evaluation was done (Table 1) which showed a moderate-severe cognitive impairment mainly characterized by severe attention and executive deficits and frontal syndrome, with associated severe deficit of visual-spatial functions. Rey Copy and the Clock drawing tests are reported in Fig. 1. Moderate/severe impairment in long-term verbal and visual-spatial

memory recall was registered with deficit of fluency for semantic categories (mainly due to attentional fluctuations). A brain 99Tc-hexamethylpropyleneamineoxime single-photon emission computed tomography (SPECT) was performed showing moderate hypoperfusion in both occipital lobes, and associated with marked decreased perfusion in parieto-fronto-temporal lobes bilaterally (Fig. 2). At this time, she was diagnosed as DLB.

Thus, delusional jealousy and persecutory ideas were treated with the simultaneous suspension of selegiline and the introduction of quetiapine 12,5 mg/daily. In the following two weeks, both disappearance of these delusions and the normalization of behavioral problems were observed, although a moderate impairment of bradykinesia and rigidity was noted.

However, after four months, her family members reported the appearance of an unusual delusion, characterized by the fact that the patient, referring to the female professional caregiver engaged by her relatives for her care, constantly described the presence of two different female persons, sometimes with different physical characteristics, sometimes similar, with a disorder framed in the context of a delusion of duplication. It was reported, in fact, that the patient always talked about the "two ladies", despite the complaints of family members who indicated the obvious presence of a single person, without substantial criticism of the delusional disorder by the patient. Also in the absence of the professional caregiver, the aberrant conviction of the existence of two different ladies was constantly present, while the caregiver was never recognized as a unique person by the patient. In this respect, during the conversation the patient said: "Today I have arrived to the hospital with my son, without the two ladies who usually take care of me.", "They are nice people, even if they do not speak much. I do not remember their names, but both speak with a foreign accent". When we asked if they were both with blond hair, her response was: "I do not remember exactly the color of their hair, but it seems to be of a different color".

Thus, levodopa was decreased to 200 mg/daily, with no disappearance of the delusion of duplication, but with a clear worsening of parkinsonism. At a follow-up visit, two months later, with the same professional caregiver present during the interview, the patient was referring to her as if it actually were two people. The delusional disorder of duplication was not present in relation to other people or other patient's relatives. No visual or auditory hallucinations were referred.

Discussion

Here, we have described a particular delusion of duplication quite different both to the classical Capgras syndrome described in DLB and to the typical clonal pluralization syndromes. In fact, the delusion was not characterized by

Table 1 Neuropsychological findings of the subject at evaluation

Test	Raw score	Adjusted score and/or (Cut-off)	Equivalent score and/or classification
MMSE	18/30	17.7 (>24)	Impaired
ADL	3/6		Impaired
IADL	3/6		Impaired
Frontal assessment battery	10/18	11.5 (>13.4)	0
Stroop Test			
Time Interference	93.5	80.25 (<36.91)	0
Error interference	15	13 (<4.23)	0
Attentional matrices	25	30.75 (>31)	0
Trail making test	NP		Impaired
Digit span forward	4	4,65 (>4.26)	2 - Normal
Digit span backward	3	3.77 (>2.66)	2- Normal
Rey Auditory Verbal Learning Test			
Learning	27/75	37 (>28.53)	3 - Normal
Recall	0/15		0
Recognition (False recognition)	15/15 (6)		Impaired
Test of Corsi			
Direct	2	2.68 (>3.46)	0 - Impaired
Forward	3	3.42 (>3.08)	2 - Normal
Phonological verbal fluency	31	40 (>16)	4 - Normal
Semantic verbal fluency	10	20 (>25)	0 - Impaired
Modified Card Sorting Test (MCST)	NP		Impaired
Rey figure (Copy)	0	(>23.74)	0 - Impaired
Immediate recall	1	8.6 (>6.44)	1 -At lower limit
Delay recall	0	(>6.33)	0 - Impaired-
Simple Figure Copy	3	4.3 (>7.18)	0 - Impaired
Clock Test	0	>3	Impaired

Legend. Raw score, score test; Adjusted score: obtained by subtracting or adding the contribution of patient's age and education; Equivalent score: adjusted scores converted to a five-point interval scale, ranging from 0 to 4 equivalent scores. Score 0 was equal or lower than the outer tolerance limit (5%), NP, not performable

the patients's belief that her professional caregiver was been replaced by an identical imposter, but, on the contrary, by the duplication of the same person. Furthermore, in Capgras syndrome, the imposter commonly has features that are very similar to those of the original

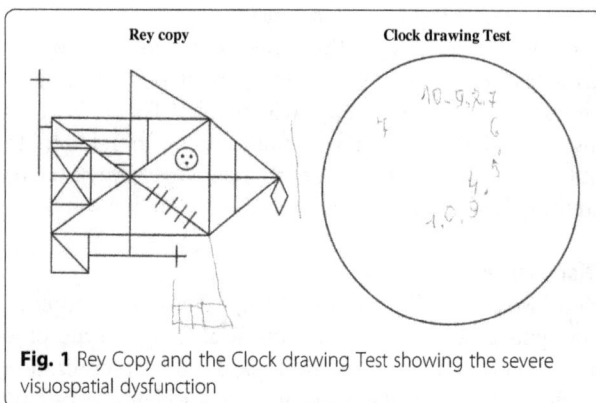

Fig. 1 Rey Copy and the Clock drawing Test showing the severe visuospatial dysfunction

person, although subtle physical differences are used to differentiate the original person from the imposter. In our case, according the description made by the patient herself, the core of the delusional idea was not characterized by the perception of an imposter, but was simply described as a phenomenon of reduplication. This delusion was not simply an unusual psychotic symptom driven uniquely by medication, because an important reduction of levodopa/carbidopa dosage did not change its clinical presentation, while a total suspension of dopaminergic treatment was impossible for the worsening of parkinsonian symptoms.

Another striking difference with Capgras syndrome is represented by the person involved in the appearance of this delusion of duplication. In fact, while in Capgras syndrome, patients report that one or more well-known persons (usually family members) have been replaced by substitutes [4], it is interesting to note that this delusion of duplication was referred only to the professional

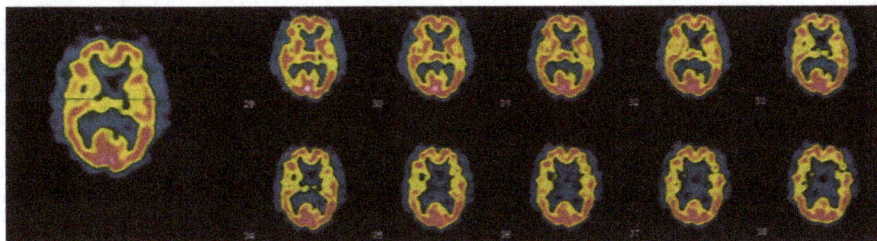

Fig. 2 Brain ^{99}mTc-hexamethylpropyleneamineoxime single-photon emission computed tomography (SPECT) imaging shows moderate hypoperfusion in both occipital lobes, and associated with marked decreased perfusion in parieto-fronto-temporal lobes bilaterally. SPECT images were generated in the transaxial plane, with direction of the slices from feet to head

caregiver and not to family members. In this context, it should be considered as the caregiver is at the same time both the nearest and the more extraneous person. On the other hand, the clonal pluralization syndromes are characterized by the false belief of the existence of an identical copy (clone) of the patient's self or of other individuals; in our case, the patient believed that there was another caregiver in addition to that real, but she did not refer to her as an exact copy, rather than as she was a different individual. This particular form of reduplicative delusion could explain why the patient did not show persecutory ideas neither toward the real caregiver nor the "other" caregiver: simply, she believed to have two caregivers.

This phenomenon of reduplication appears very interesting because its similarity to a type of hallucinatory disorder raises the question on its clear operating framework between these psychiatric conditions. However, the previous presence of other delusional disturbances and the fact that this belief, with a duration longer than two months, was fixed and not amenable to change in light of conflicting evidence, in addition to the absence of any other hallucinatory problem, depose with greater evidence to a classification within the spectrum of delusions, according to the DSM 5 [9]. In any case, it should be remembered as a previous study found a strong relationship between Capgras syndrome and visual hallucinations [3].

Another issue concerns the possible neurobiological mechanisms that may contribute to the appearance of this delusion of duplication. In fact, several studies have addressed their attention to Capgras syndrome, but other misidentification syndromes have been scarcely studied. With regard to Capgras syndrome, proposed alterations include the presence of impairment in facial processing [10, 11], dysfunction of working memory [12], altered connectivity among associative areas and limbic/paralimbic structures [13], bilateral dysfunction of fronto-temporal connectivity [14, 15], and right hemispheric hypo function [16, 17].

In our patient with this peculiar delusion of duplication, an occipital hypoperfusion was identified, although

in association with a marked global decrease of perfusion in the remaining lobes. In this context, it should be kept in mind as a deficiency in occipital hypoperfusion is more frequently seen in DLB with respect to other dementia such as Alzheimer disease [18]. The role of posterior lobes is certainly important in all misidentification syndromes where a natural dissociation between recognition and identification is present and is confirmed by the findings of severe deficit of visual-spatial functions observed at the neuropsychological evaluation and typical of a posterior cerebral areas dysfunction. However, the concomitant presence of severe attentional and executive deficits evocative for a frontal syndrome and the marked global decrease of perfusion in the remaining lobes at the SPECT scan also suggest a possible dysfunction in an abnormal connectivity between anterior and posterior areas.

Moreover, the presence of a significant impairment in visual-spatial functions and in visual-spatial memory recall is in agreement with previous neuropsychological findings on delusional misidentifications reporting a low efficiency in the complex visuospatial organization tasks and in non-verbal memory [19]. In this context, there is a clear evidence for impaired visuoperceptual functions in the appearance of misidentificative psychotic symptoms in patients affected by Alzheimer's disease [20].

Conclusions

In conclusion, we have described an unusual delusion of duplication in a patient affected by LBD. Neural correlates of this peculiar delusion of duplication in LBD still remain largely unclear, and future researches are required to better identify possible neurobiological mechanisms that may contribute to the appearance of this peculiar type of delusion.

Abbreviations
DLB: Dementia with Lewy bodies; MRI: Magnetic resonance imaging; RBD: Rapid eye movement sleep behavior; SPECT: Single-photon emission computed tomography

Acknowledgements
None.

Funding
No funding was obtained for this study.

Authors' contributions
PS contributed to the conception and design of the paper, to the acquisition, to the analysis and interpretation of data, wrote the first draft of the manuscript and was involved in its final drafting. GM contributed to the design of the paper, to the acquisition, to the analysis and interpretation of data, wrote the first draft of the manuscript and was involved in its final drafting. AC revised the manuscript and was involved in its final drafting. GF contributed to the design of the paper, wrote the first draft of the manuscript and was involved in its final drafting. GO revised the manuscript and was involved in its final drafting. DF revised the manuscript and was involved in its final drafting. MGC contributed to design of the paper, revised critically the manuscript and was involved in its final drafting. FM contributed to design of the paper, revised critically the manuscript and was involved in its final drafting. All authors read and approved the final manuscript, and were involved in the decision to submit the manuscript for publication.

Competing interests
The authors declare that they have no competing interests.

Author details
[1]Department of Neurology, Movement Disorders Center, Institute of Neurology, University of Cagliari, SS 554 Bivio per Sestu, Monserrato 09042, Cagliari, Italy. [2]Department of Medical Sciences and Public Health, University of Cagliari, Cagliari, Italy. [3]Chair of Quality of Care and Applied Medical Technologies, Department of Public Health, Clinical and Molecular Medicine, University of Cagliari, Monserrato, Italy.

References
1. McKeith IG, Dickson DW, Lowe J, Emre M, O'Brien JT, Feldman H, et al. Diagnosis and management of dementia with Lewy bodies: third report of the DLB Consortium. Neurology. 2005;65(12):1863–72.
2. Vann Jones SA, O'Brien JT. The prevalence and incidence of dementia with Lewy bodies: a systematic review of population and clinical studies. Psychol Med. 2014;44:673–83.
3. Thaipisuttikul P, Lobach I, Zweig Y, Gurnani A, Galvin JE. Capgras syndrome in Dementia with Lewy Bodies. Int Psychogeriatr. 2013;25(5):843–9.
4. Murai T, Toichi M, Yamagishi H, Sengok A. What is meant by 'misidentification' in delusional misidentification syndromes. Psychopathology. 1998;31:313–7.
5. Salvatore P, Bhuvaneswar C, Tohen M, Khalsa HM, Maggini C, Baldessarini RJ. Capgras' syndrome in first-episode psychotic disorders. Psychopathology. 2014;47(4):261–9.
6. Politis M, Loane C. Reduplicative paramnesia: a review. Psychopathology. 2012;45:337–43.
7. Voros V, Tényi T, Simon M, Trixler M. "Clonal pluralization of the self": a new form of delusional misidentification syndrome. Psychopathology. 2003;36(1):46–8.
8. Ranjan S, Chandra PS, Gupta AK, Prabhu S. Clonal pluralization of self, relatives and others. Psychopathology. 2007;40:465–7.
9. The Diagnostic and Statistical Manual of Mental Disorders (5th ed.; DSM–5; American Psychiatric Association, 2013)
10. Walther S, Federspiel A, Horn H, Wirth M, Bianchi P, Strik W, Muller TJ. Performance during face processing differentiates schizophrenia patients with delusional misidentifications. Psychopathology. 2010;43:127–36.
11. Phillips ML, David AS. Facial processing in schizophrenia and delusional misidentification: cognitive neuropsychiatric approaches. Schizophr Res. 1995;17:109–14.
12. Papageorgiou C, Lykouras L, Ventouras E, Uzunoglu N, Christodoulou GN. Abnormal P300 in a case of delusional misidentification with coinciding Capgras and Fregoli symptoms. Prog Neuropsychopharmacol Biol Psychiatry. 2002;26:805–10.
13. Weinstein EA. Classification of delusional misidentification syndromes. Psychopathology. 1994;27:130–5.
14. Joseph AB, O'Leary DH, Wheeler HG. Bilateral atrophy of the frontal and temporal lobes in schizophrenic patients with Capgras syndrome: a case-control study using computed tomography. J Clin Psychiatry. 1990;51:322–5.
15. Feinberg TE, Roane DM. Delusional misidentification. Psychiatr Clin North Am. 2005;28(3):665–83. 678-9.
16. Cutting J. Delusional misidentification and the role of the right hemisphere in the appreciation of identity. Br J Psychiatry Suppl. 1991;14:70–5.
17. Weinstein EA, Burnham DL. Reduplication and the syndrome of Capgras. Psychiatry. 1991;54(1):78–88.
18. Lobotesis K, Fenwick JD, Phipps A, Ryman A, Swann A, Ballard C, McKeith IG, O'Brien JT. Occipital hypoperfusion on SPECT in dementia with Lewy bodies but not AD. Neurology. 2001;56(5):643–9.
19. Paillère-Martinot ML, Dao-Castellana MH, Masure MC, Pillon B, Martinot JL. Delusional misidentification: a clinical, neuropsychological and brain imaging case study. Psychopathology. 1994;27(3-5):200–10.
20. Reeves SJ, Clark-Papasavas C, Gould RL, Fytche D, Howard RJ. Cognitive phenotype of psychotic symptoms in Alzheimer's disease: evidence for impaired visuoperceptual function in the misidentification subtype. Int J Geriatr Psychiatry. 2015;30(12):1147–55.

6

Juglone induces apoptosis of tumor stem-like cells through ROS-p38 pathway in glioblastoma

Jinfeng Wu[1†], Haibo Zhang[2†], Yang Xu[2], Jingwen Zhang[2,4], Wei Zhu[2], Yi Zhang[2], Liang Chen[2*], Wei Hua[2*] and Ying Mao[2,3,5,6]

Abstract

Background: Juglone is a natural pigment, which has cytotoxic effect against various human tumor cells. However, its cytotoxicity to glioma cells, especially to tumor stem-like cells (TSCs) has not been demonstrated.

Methods: TSCs of glioma were enriched from U87 and two primary cells (SHG62, and SHG66) using serum-free medium supplemented with growth factors, including bFGF, EGF and B27. After treatment of juglone with gradient concentrations (0, 10, 20, and 40 μM), the viability and apoptosis of TSCs were evaluated by WST-8 assay and flow cytometry. Reactive oxygen species (ROS) was labeled by the cell-permeable fluorescent probe and detected with flow cytometry. ROS scavenger (NAC) and p38-MAPK inhibitor (SB203580) were applied to resist the cytotoxic effect. Caspase 9 cleavage and p38 phosphorylation (P-p38) were quantified by western blot. Juglone as well as temozolomide (TMZ) were administrated in intracranial xenografts and MR scan was performed every week to evaluate the anti-tumor effect in vivo.

Results: Juglone could obviously inhibit the proliferation of TSCs in glioma by decreasing cell viability ($P < 0.01$) and inducing apoptosis ($P < 0.01$), which was accompanied by increased caspase 9 cleavage in a dose-dependent manner ($P < 0.01$). In the meantime, juglone could generate ROS significantly and increase p38 phosphorylation ($P < 0.01$). In addition, pretreatment with ROS scavenger or p38-MAPK inhibitor could reverse juglone-induced cytotoxicity ($P < 0.01$). More importantly, juglone could also suppress tumor growth in vivo and improve the survival of U87-bearing mice compared with control ($P < 0.05$), although TMZ seemed to have better effect.

Conclusions: Juglone could inhibit the growth of TSCs in gliomas through the activation of ROS-p38-MAPK pathway in vitro, and the anti-glioma effect was validated in vivo, which offers a potential therapeutic agent to gliomas.

Keywords: Juglone, Glioma, Tumor stem-like cells, Apoptosis, Reactive oxygen species

Background

As one of the most deadly primary brain tumors, glioblastoma (GBM) has the characteristics of rapid growth and high invasiveness. The median survival time of GBM has been prolonged to about 14.6 months even after comprehensive treatments of surgery, chemotherapy and radiotherapy [1]. After many endeavors, temozolomide (TMZ) emerged as a feasible first-line chemotherapeutic agent through DNA alkylation in glioma cells, which was validated by phase III clinical trial [2, 3]. However, some tumors without MGMT methylation have been reported to be resistant to TMZ, and thus limiting its efficiency [4]. In the meantime, a subgroup of quiescent tumor stem-like cells (TSC) have been demonstrated to re-initiate tumor growth after TMZ treatment [5]. Bevacizumab (anti-VEGFA), which could only benefit proneural subtype of GBM [6], has also not been encouraging. Therefore, it is necessary to find some novel chemotherapeutic agents targeting GBM.

* Correspondence: clclcl95@sina.com; hs_glioma@126.com
†Equal contributors
²Department of Neurosurgery, Huashan Hospital, Fudan University, #12 Middle Wurumuqi Road, Shanghai 200040, People's Republic of China
Full list of author information is available at the end of the article

Natural products have recently received much attention as potential therapeutic agents, e.g., matrine as a cell cycle blocker [7], camptothecin as a proliferation inhibitor [8], and podophyllotoxin as an apoptosis inducer [9]. Similarly, juglone, a lipid-soluble drug, has been widely used as a chemotherapeutic agent in Chinese herbal medicine against various tumors, including leukaemia [10], melanoma [11], gastric cancer [12] and pancreatic cancer [13] through the activation of apoptotic caspase cascade and the increase of ROS (reactive oxygen species) [14, 15]. Recently, juglone has been found to inhibit cell proliferation and to reduce the invasiveness of C6 rat glioma cells in vitro [16]. However, if it could exert a cytotoxic effect in vivo remains unknown.

TSCs in glioma could not be completely eliminated even through combined treatment modality, and thus become the main reason of chemotherapy resistance and the root of tumor relapse [17]. Therefore, we explored the anti-tumor effect of juglone to glioma TSCs and its potential mechanism in this study. Furthermore, we also compared its effect with TMZ in order to provide an available alternative for patients after chemotherapeutic treatment failure.

Methods
Glioma stem-like cells culture
U87 was purchased from American Type Culture Collection (Manassas, VA). GBM primary cells (SHG62 and SHG66) were established in our laboratory previously [18]. The glioma TSCs were cultured in serum-free medium (DMEM/F12) supplemented with growth factors, including 10 ng/mL bFGF (basic Fibroblast Growth Factor), 20 ng/mL EGF (Epidermal Growth Factor), and B-27 (1:50 dilution; Life Technologies, Carlsbad). Cell cultures were maintained in a 5% CO_2 humidified incubator at 37 °C.

Cell viability assays
Juglone (St Louis, MO) was dissolved in dimethyl sulfoxide (DMSO) and diluted in DMEM/F12. The final working concentration of DMSO was 100 mM. Cell viability was measured by the WST-8 assay (Kumamoto, Japan) following optimized manufacturer's recommendation. Briefly, cells were seeded at a density of 2×10^4cells/200ul/well in 96-well plates, and then incubated overnight in serum-free medium. The cells were pretreated with and without NAC (a ROS scavenger, 2 mM), or SB203580 (an inhibitor of p38-MAP kinase, 5 μM) for 1 h. Then the cells were treated with different concentrations of juglone (0, 10, 20, and 40 μM). After 48 h incubation, 20 μl WST-8 was added to each well, and the cells were incubated for another 6 h. The optical density (OD) was detected at 450 nm with microplate spectrophotometer (BD Biosciences, San Jose, CA). The percentage of viable cells was determined by the formula:

ratio (%) = [OD (juglone) - OD (blank)/OD (control) -OD (blank)] × 100. The experiment were triplicated, and each contained six replicates.

Cell apoptosis and death assay
For cell apoptosis assay, GBM cells in serum-free medium were treated with juglone (0, 20, and 40 μM) for 48 h, 1×10^5 cells were harvested and incubated in 100 μL labeling solution (5 μL of Annexin V FITC, 5 μL of PI, 10 μL of 10 × binding buffer and 80 μL of H_2O) in darkness at room temperature for 15 min, after that, 400 μL of binding buffer was added to stop the staining reaction. For cell death assay, the cells were pretreated with or without NAC (Sigma Aldrich, 2 mM), or SB203580 (Sigma Aldrich, 5 μM) for 1 h. Then the cells were treated with juglone (0, 40 μM) for 48 h. Following incubation, cells were collected and fixed in 70% ethanol for 24 h at 4 °C. After that, the cells were resuspended in 500 μL phosphate buffer solution (PBS) containing RNaseA (10 mg/mL, 50 μL) and PI (2 mg/mL, 10 μL). The mixture was incubated in the dark at 37 °C for 30 min. For cell apoptosis and death assay, cells were then analyzed on a FACS Calibur cytometer (Becton Dickinson, San Joe CA). The data were analyzed using FlowJo software V6.0 (Tree star, Ashland OR). Early apoptotic cells are defined as annexin V^+/PI^-, whereas late apoptotic/necrotic cells are defined as annexin V^+/PI^+. The extent of cell death was determined by evaluating the sub G1 fraction. The experiments were triplicated.

Evaluation of ROS generation
ROS was labeled by the cell-permeable fluorescent probe (2',7'- Dichloro- fluorescein diacetate, DCFDA, Sigma Aldrich) and detected with flow cytometry. Briefly, cells were exposed to various concentrations of juglone (0, 20, and 40 μM) for 24 h and then loaded with DCFDA (10 μM) in serum-free medium. Following incubation at 37 °C for 30 min, cells were washed with PBS and fluorescence was measured with flow cytometry. The mean fluorescence intensity (MFI) data was analyzed by FlowJo software. The MFI experiments were repeated three times.

Western blot assay
Cells were treated with different concentrations of juglone (0, 20, and 40 μM) for 48 h. Total protein extracts were obtained from lysis buffer (150 mM NaCL, 1% NP-40, 0.5% sodium deoxycholate, 0.1% SDS, and 50 mM Tris-Cl pH 8.0, 2 ug/mL aprotinin, 2 ug/mL leupeptin, 40 mg/mL of phenylmethylsulfonyl fluoride, 2 mM DTT). The protein concentration was determined by the Bradford assay (BioRad, Hercules, CA), and samples were separated on SDS-PAGE, and then transferred onto polyvinylidene difluoride (PVDF) membranes. The

membranes were immunoblotted with primary Abs against cleaved caspase 9 (Cell Signaling Technology, 1:1000), P-p38 (Cell Signaling Technology,1:1000), and β-actin (Cell Signaling Technology,1:10000) overnight at 4 °C, followed by horseradish peroxidase (HRP) conjugated secondary Ab (BioRad,1:3000). Detection was carried out using Supersignal West Femto Chemiluminescent Substrate (Pierce, Rockford, IL). β-actin was taken as reference and the band intensities were quantified using UN-SCAN-IT gel analysis software (Silk Scientific, Orem, UT).

Cytotoxicity of juglone on glioma stem-like cells in vivo

Female BALB/c-nu mice (8–10 week) were obtained from SlacLaboratoryAnimal Company (Shanghai, China). Animal experiment was conducted according to protocols approved by the Institutional Animal Care and Use Committee at Fudan University. Animals were housed with a 12 h light/dark cycle, and acclimated to their environment as least 1 week prior to experimentation. Micewere anesthetized intraperitoneally with 10% chloral hydrate and stereotactically inoculated with 1×10^5 U87 stem-like cells in 10uL PBS *via* micro-syringe into the right forebrain (2.5 mm lateral and 1 mm anterior to bregma, at a 3 mm depth from the skull surface). 3 days after the inoculation, the mice were randomly distributed into three groups, including vehicle control group, juglone treatment group, and TMZ treatment group. The number of animals in each group was 8. Juglone or TMZ was dissolved in DMSO and diluted in PBS; the final concentration of DMSO was 20 mg/ml [19]. PBS containing the same concentration of DMSO was used as vehicle control. Juglone treatment group was injected intraperitoneally with juglone (1 mg/kg) every 3 days, while TMZ treatment group was injected intraperitoneally with TMZ (25 mg/kg) every day. The total drug injections were 5 times per animal. The mice were monitored every three days,and the tumor were evaluated weekly using enhanced MR scan (1.5 T, gadolinium,Bayer Schering Pharma AG,0.2 ml/kg).

Statistics

All data were presented as the mean ± standard deviation (SD). Data analysis was performed by one-way analysis of variance (*ANOVA*). For comparison of two groups, a student's *t*-test was used. Differences with P values < 0.05 were considered to be statistically significant.

Results

Juglone is cytotoxic to glioma stem-like cells

The stem-like cell viability of U87, SHG62 and SHG66 were evaluated by WST-8 assay after treatment with juglone for 48 h. As shown in Fig. 1b, juglone (10, 20, 40 μM) could dramatically decrease the viability of glioma stem-like cells as compared to the control ($P < 0.01$), and the cell viability fell significantly to 65.3 ± 5.06% and 40.7 ± 8.21% after treated with higher concentration of juglone. Meanwhile, stem-like cell spheres formation decreased gradually after juglone treatment in a dose-dependent manner, accompanied with cell shrinkage, reduction of cell adherence (Fig. 1c).

Juglone could induce glioma stem-like cells apoptosis

To determine if juglone could induce apoptosis, the percentage of Annexin V$^+$PI$^-$ and Annexin V$^-$PI$^+$ U87 stem-like cells after concentration gradients (0, 20, and 40 μM) were measured with flow cytometry. As shown in Fig. 2a

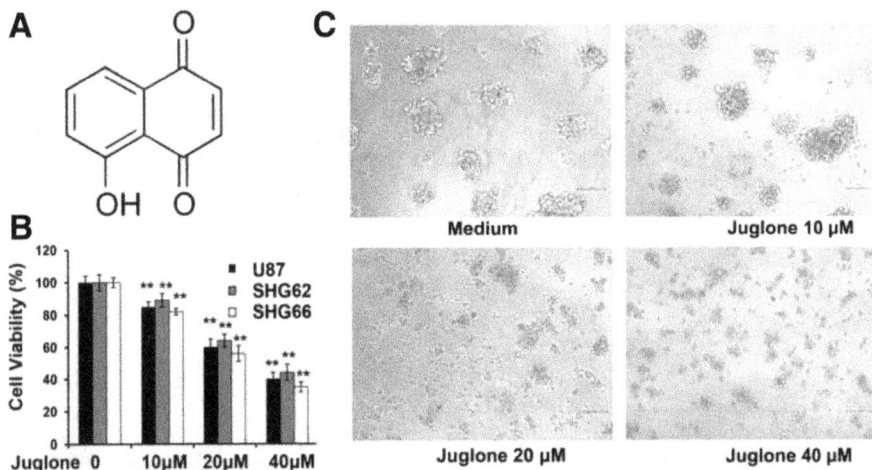

Fig. 1 Juglone could decrease cell viabilityof glioma stem- like cells in vitro. **a** Chemical structure of juglone. **b** Cell viability (U87, SHG62 and SHG66) decreased obviously after treatment with juglone at various concentrations (10, 20, and 40 μM) as compared to control (**$P < 0.01$). **c** The cell morphology (100×) of juglone-treated U87 showed that stem-like cell spheres formation decreased gradually after juglone treatment in a dose-dependent manner

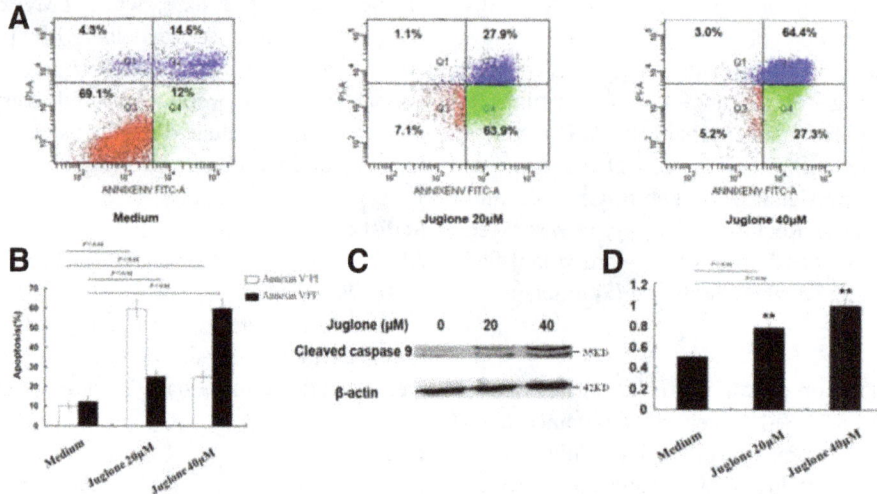

Fig. 2 Juglone could induce apoptosis of glioma stem-like cells. **a** FACS analysis indicated that juglone could significantly induce apoptosis at different concentrations. **b** Statistic analysis indicated that juglone could significantly induce both early apoptosis and late apoptosis as compared to the control. **c** Juglone increased caspase 9 cleavage. **d** Quantification of caspase 9 cleavage with western blot (**$P < 0.01$)

and b, juglone (20 μM) increased percentage of Annexin V^+PI^- and Annexin V^-PI^+ cells by $49.1 \pm 9.15\%$ and $11.1 \pm 7.15\%$ as compared to control ($P < 0.01$). However, juglone (40 μM) increased the percentage of Annexin V^+PI^- and Annexin V^-PI^+ cells by $12.1 \pm 7.35\%$ and $51.1 \pm 8.52\%$ as compared to control ($P < 0.01$). In the meantime, juglone could increase caspase 9 cleavage (Fig. 2c and d), which indicated juglone-induced apoptosis.

Juglone could generate ROS and activate p38-MAPK pathway

Juglone-induced ROS generation was obvious in a dose-dependent manneras compared to vehicle control ($P < 0.01$) (Fig. 3a and b). As demonstrated by western blot (Fig. 3c and d), juglone (20, 40 μM) treatment significantly increased p38 phosphorylation ($P < 0.01$),which indicated p38-MAPK pathway activation in TSCs.

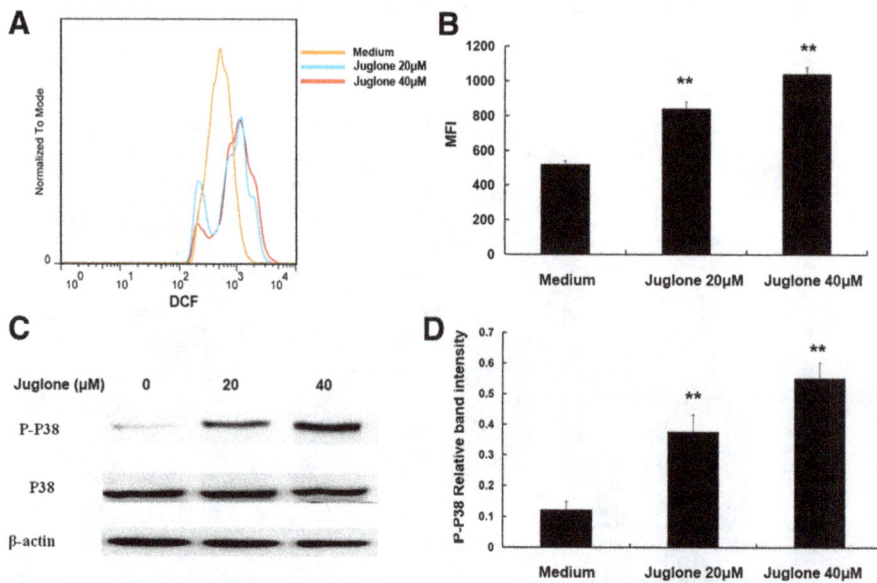

Fig. 3 Juglone could generate ROS and activate p38 phosphorylation. **a** Flow cytometry showed that juglone-induced ROS generation was increased in a dose-dependent manner. **b** Statistical data of ROS MFI in different groups (**$P < 0.01$). **c** Juglone treatment significantly increased p38 phosphorylation in a dose-dependent manner. **d** Statistical data of P-p38 protein at different concentrations using western blot (**$P < 0.01$)

NAC and SB203580 pretreatment could reverse juglone-induced growth inhibition of glioma stem-like cells

As demonstrated by WST-8 assay (Fig. 4a), juglone (40 μM) treatment could decreased cell viability by $65 \pm 2.53\%$ ($P < 0.01$), whereas NAC and SB203580 could reversed the cytotoxic effect of juglone by $75 \pm 3.18\%$ ($P < 0.01$) and $58 \pm 3.92\%$($P < 0.01$). Cell death data (Fig. 4b and c) showed that treatment with juglone (40 μM) increased cell death by $17 \pm 3.87\%$ ($P < 0.01$), while NAC and SB203580 pretreatment could reverse juglone-mediated increases of cell death by $12.4 \pm 2.33\%$ ($P < 0.01$) and $7.1 \pm 2.91\%$ ($P < 0.01$). All those results indicated that ROS-p38-MAPK pathway was involved in the juglone-induced cytotoxicity.

Juglone could reduce glioma growth in vivo and improve the survival of glioma-bearing mice

Brain tumor models were successfully established, and the anti-glioma effect of juglone in vivo was investigated.

Both juglone and TMZ could markedly retard glioma growth in vivo confirmed by the MR scan results (Fig. 5a). In the meantime, juglone and TMZ could both significantly increase the survival time of glioma-bearing mice as compared to control ($P = 0.025$, $P = 0.017$, respectively. Figure 5b) and juglone could increase the survival time by about 23.6%. Obviously, TMZ had a better cytotoxic effect than juglone in vivo. All these results demonstrated that juglone could be an effective anti-glioma agent.

Discussion

Since TSCs are responsible for resistance to chemotherapy [5], novel therapeutic strategies targeting specifically to TSCs are urgently needed. Spectrum Collection Library (MicroSource, Gaylordsville, CT) was designed to screen small compounds for anti-tumor chemotherapeutic agents, and obtusaquinone (one natural product) was identified to have pro-apoptotic effect on TSCs in vitro and to suppress tumor in vivo [20]. However, the suppression ratio was not as high as expected, and many new promising agents needed confirmation by clinical

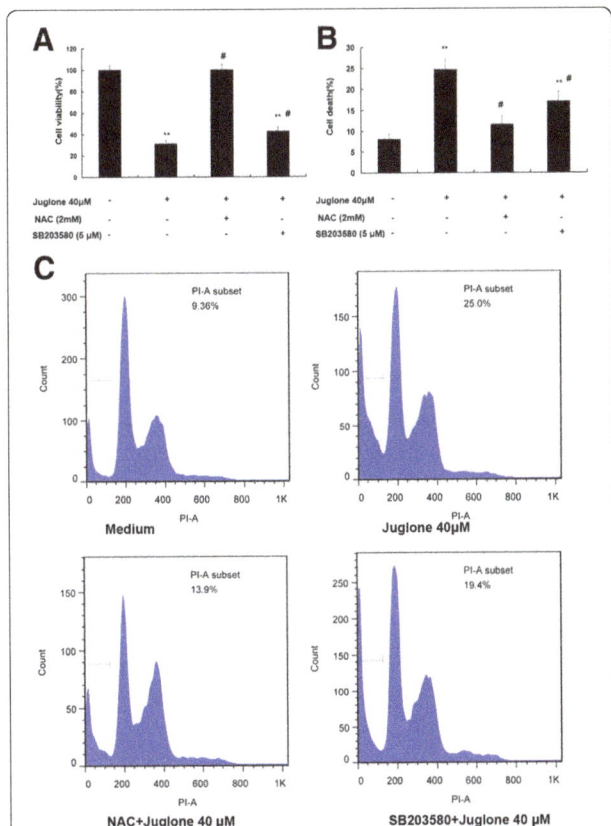

Fig. 4 Pretreatment with NAC and SB203580 could reverse juglone-induced inhibition of glioma stem-like cells. **a** Statistic analysis indicated that NAC or SB203580 could resist juglone-induced cell viability decrease (**$P < 0.01$). **b** Statistic analysis indicated that NAC or SB203580 could resist juglone-induced cell death (**$P < 0.01$). **c** Flow cytometry showed that NAC or SB203580 pretreatment could reverse the decrease of cell viability and the increase of cell death induced by juglone (**$P < 0.01$)

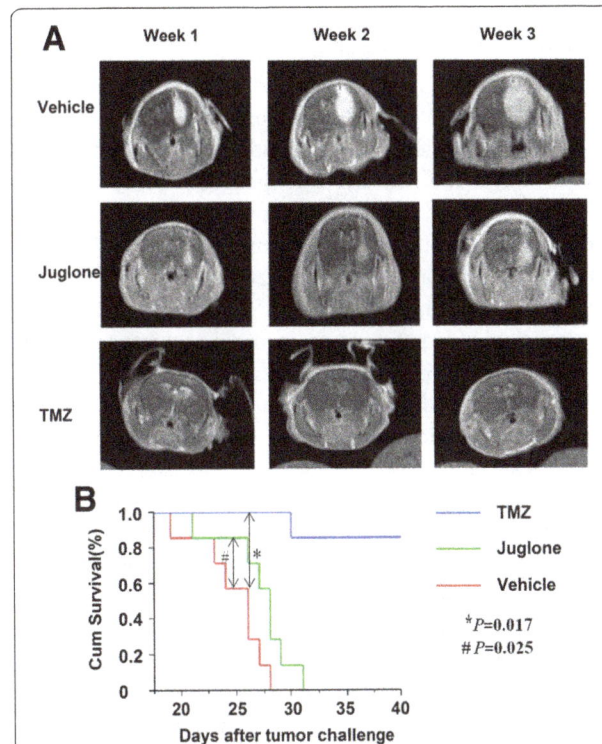

Fig. 5 Juglone could retard glioma growth in vivo and prolong the survival time of glioma-bearing mice. **a** MR images showed that juglone group (1 mg/kg), as TMZ group (25 mg/kg) ($P = 0.017$),could also retarded glioma growth in vivo comparing with control group ($P = 0.025$). **b** Juglone treatment could improve, though less significant than TMZ, the survival status of glioma-bearing miceas compared with control ($P < 0.05$)

studies. Here, we reported a natural pigment-juglone, a lipid-soluble drug, which could easily pass the blood brain barrier and exert anti-tumor effect against GBM cells, especially against TSCs in vitro and in vivo.

In current study, juglone treatment could inhibit TSCs growth by inducing apoptosis. We also observed that juglone treatment could increase caspase 9 cleavage which was consistent with previous study [14]. Juglone treatment could induce apoptosis of glioma cells at both early and late stage. These results indicated that juglone could exert different biological function under different concentrations.

Many possible mechanisms have been reported to be involved in the juglone-induced anti-tumor effect, among which ROS-based pathways were investiagted the most [10, 12]. Tumor cells presented higher level of ROS than normal cells [21]. In addition, high ROS concentration could induce cell apoptosis and necrosis in relation with the severity and the duration of exposure [22]. Therefore, many ROS-inducing agents are currently used in clinical trials for different tumors [21, 23]. These agents could not only act as direct inhibitors of cancers, but also sensitize tumor cells to chemotherapies [24]. In this study, we evaluated the growth inhibition and apoptosis induction by juglone in human GBM TSCs in vitro and in vivo, and we also confirmed that ROS was involved in juglone-induced apoptosis. These findings were further supported by the pretreatment with NAC, which could block the cytotoxicity of juglone as a ROS scavenger. Previous studies indicated that ROS could induce the activation of the p38-MAPK pathway, which is involved with apoptosis [25, 26]. In this study, we also found that juglone could activate the p38-MAPK pathway *via* ROS generation, and pretreatment with SB203580 could reverse the ROS-induced effect. Besides p38-MAPK pathway, many other pathways could be activated by ROS, such as ROS-AMPK-mTOR pathway and ROS-ERK/AKT-p53 pathway [27, 28], which need to be validated in gliomas. Juglone could also exert cytotoxic effect as a Pin-1 (Peptidyl-prolyl cis/trans isomerase 1) inhibitor through caspase cascade in nasopharyngeal carcinoma [29], which need further research. Therefore, juglone might inhibit TSCs through multiple mechanisms.

There were also some limitations in this study. Juglone could exert better anti-glioma effect than TMZ in vitro (data not shown). However, the cytotoxic effect of juglone was poorer than that of TMZ in vivo, which is partially due to the various anti-tumor mechanisms. In the meantime, the dosage of juglone was low (1 mg/kg) in animal experiment due to the consideration of the side effects. So, we can modify specific chemical groups to reduce its side effects while maintaining its cytotoxicity. The elaboration of anti-tumor mechanism by juglone and better understanding of TSCs would also contribute to the future treatment of gliomas. At least, juglone could offer us

another alternative for GBM patients with TMZ resistance or failure, which needs further clinical investigation.

Conclusions

Juglone could inhibit proliferation and induce apoptosis of glioma stem-like cells in vitro and in vivo, which was mediated through the activation of ROS-p38- MAPK pathway. So, juglone might serve as a potential chemotherapeutic agent for gliomas.

Abbreviations
GBM: Glioblastoma; MFI: Mean fluorescence intensity.; ROS: Reactive oxygen species; TMZ: Temozolomide; TSCs: Tumor stem-like cells

Acknowledgments
None.

Funding
In this study, the test of cell viability, apoptosis and death were supported by the Program of International Science & Technology Cooperation of China (Grand No. 2014DFA31470), the evaluation of reactive oxygen species (ROS) and the in vivo research were supported by the National Natural Science Foundation of China (Grand No. 81611130223 and 81572483) and the submission process was supported by China Postdoctoral Science Foundation (Grand No.2015 M5815).

Authors' contributions
JW performed the cell culture studies and the statistical analysis. HZ participated in the test of cell viability, apoptosis as well as death and drafted the manuscript. YX and JZ performed the evaluation of reactive oxygen species (ROS). WZ, YZ and YM participated in the design of the study. LC and WH conceived of the study, participated in its design and coordination, and helped to draft the manuscript. All the authors had read and approved the final manuscript.

Competing interests
The authors declare that they have no competing interests.

Author details
[1]Department of Dermatology, Huashan Hospital, Fudan University, #12 Middle Wurumuqi Road, Shanghai 200040, People's Republic of China. [2]Department of Neurosurgery, Huashan Hospital, Fudan University, #12 Middle Wurumuqi Road, Shanghai 200040, People's Republic of China. [3]Institutes of Biomedical Sciences, Fudan University, #131 Dong'an Road, Shanghai 200040, People's Republic of China. [4]Department of Ultrasound, Hebei General Hospital, #348 West Heping Road, Shijiazhuang, Hebei Province 050000, People's Republic of China. [5]State Key Laboratory of Medical Neurobiology, School of Basic Medical Sciences and Institutes of Brain Science, Fudan University, Shanghai 200040, People's Republic of China. [6]The Collaborative Innovation Center for Brain Science, Fudan University, Shanghai 200040, People's Republic of China.

References
1. Wen PY, Kesari S. Malignant gliomas in adults. N Engl J Med. 2008;359(5): 492–507.
2. Stupp R, Mason WP, van den Bent MJ, Weller M, Fisher B, Taphoorn MJ, Belanger K, Brandes AA, Marosi C, Bogdahn U. Radiotherapy plus concomitant and adjuvant temozolomide for glioblastoma. N Engl J Med. 2005;352:987–96.
3. Friedman HS, Kerby T, Calvert H. Temozolomide and treatment of malignant glioma. Clin Cancer Res. 2000;6:2585–97.
4. Dullea A, Marignol L. MGMT testing allows for personalised therapy in the temozolomide era. Tumour Biol. 2016;37:87–96.

5. Chen J, Li Y, Yu TS, McKay RM, Burns DK, Kernie SG, Parada LF. A restricted cell population propagates glioblastoma growth after chemotherapy. Nature. 2012;488:522–6.

6. Sandmann T, Bourgon R, Garcia J, Li C, Cloughesy T, Chinot OL, Wick W, Nishikawa R, Mason W, Henriksson R. Patients With Proneural Glioblastoma May Derive Overall Survival Benefit From the Addition of Bevacizumab to First-Line Radiotherapy and Temozolomide: Retrospective Analysis of the AVAglio Trial. J Clin Oncol. 2015;33:2735–44.

7. Zheng K, Li C, Shan X, Liu H, Fan W, Wang Z. A study on isolation of chemical constituents from Sophora flavescens Ait. and their anti-glioma effects. Afr J Tradit Complement Altern Med. 2014;11:156–60.

8. Zhou Y, Zhao HY, Jiang D, Wang LY, Xiang C, Wen SP, Fan ZC, Zhang YM, Guo N, Teng YO. Low toxic and high soluble camptothecin derivative 2–47 effectively induces apoptosis of tumor cells in vitro. Biochem Biophys Res Commun. 2016;472:477–81.

9. Mei X, Jiang YG, Lu JJ, Wu KZ, Cao B, Chen H. Anti-MDR tumor mechanism of CIP-36, a podophyllotoxin derivative. Yao Xue Xue Bao. 2011;46:1193–8.

10. Xu HL, Yu XF, Qu SC, Qu XR, Jiang YF, Sui da Y. Juglone, from Juglans mandshruica Maxim, inhibits growth and induces apoptosis in human leukemia cell HL-60 through a reactive oxygen species-dependent mechanism. Food Chem Toxicol. 2012;50:590–6.

11. Aithal BK, Kumar MR, Rao BN, Udupa N, Rao BS. Juglone, a naphthoquinone from walnut, exerts cytotoxic and genotoxic effects against cultured melanoma tumor cells. Cell Biol Int. 2009;33:1039–49.

12. Ji YB, Qu ZY, Zou X. Juglone-induced apoptosis in human gastric cancer SGC-7901 cells via the mitochondrial pathway. Exp Toxicol Pathol. 2011;63:69–78.

13. Avci E, Arikoglu H, Erkoc Kaya D. Investigation of juglone effects on metastasis and angiogenesis in pancreatic cancer cells. Gene. 2016;588:74–8.

14. Zhang W, Liu A, Li Y, Zhao X, Lv S, Zhu W, Jin Y. Anticancer activity and mechanism of juglone on human cervical carcinoma HeLa cells. Can J Physiol Pharmacol. 2012;90:1553–8.

15. Jha BK, Jung HJ, Seo I, Suh SI, Suh MH, Baek WK. Juglone induces cell death of Acanthamoeba through increased production of reactive oxygen species. Exp Parasitol. 2015;159:100–6.

16. Meskelevicius D, Sidlauskas K, Bagdonaviciute R, Liobikas J, Majiene D. Juglone exerts cytotoxic, anti-proliferative and anti-invasive effects on Glioblastoma multiforme in a cell culture model. Anticancer Agents Med Chem. 2016;16(9):1190–7.

17. Qiang L, Yang Y, Ma YJ, Chen FH, Zhang LB, Liu W, Qi Q, Lu N, Tao L, Wang XT. Isolation and characterization of cancer stem like cells in human glioblastoma cell lines. Cancer Lett. 2009;279:13–21.

18. Hua W, Yao Y, Chu Y, Zhong P, Sheng X, Xiao B, Wu J, Yang B, Mao Y, Zhou L. The CD133+ tumor stem-like cell-associated antigen may elicit highly intense immune responses against human malignant glioma. J Neurooncol. 2011;105:149–57.

19. Perazzoli G, Prados J, Ortiz R, Caba O, Cabeza L, Berdasco M, Gonzalez B, Melguizo C. Temozolomide Resistance in Glioblastoma Cell Lines: Implication of MGMT, MMR, P-Glycoprotein and CD133 Expression. PLoS One. 2015;10:e0140131.

20. Badr CE, Van Hoppe S, Dumbuya H, Tjon-Kon-Fat LA, Tannous BA. Targeting cancer cells with the natural compound obtusaquinone. J Natl Cancer Inst. 2013;105:643–53.

21. Trachootham D, Alexandre J, Huang P. Targeting cancer cells by ROS-mediated mechanisms: a radical therapeutic approach? Nat Rev Drug Discov. 2009;8:579–91.

22. Thiyagarajan V, Sivalingam KS, Viswanadha VP, Weng CF. 16-hydroxy-cleroda-3,13-dien-16,15-olide induced glioma cell autophagy via ROS generation and activation of p38 MAPK and ERK-1/2. Environ Toxicol Phar. 2016;45:202–11.

23. Pang Y, Qin G, Wu L, Wang X, Chen T. Artesunate induces ROS-dependent apoptosis via a Bax-mediated intrinsic pathway in Huh-7 and Hep3B cells. Exp Cell Res. 2016;347(2):251–60.

24. Karthikeyan S, Hoti SL, Nazeer Y, Hegde HV. Glaucarubinone sensitizes KB cells to paclitaxel by inhibiting ABC transporters via ROS-dependent and p53-mediated activation of apoptotic signaling pathways. Oncotarget. 2016;7(27):42353.

25. Liu WH, Chang LS. Reactive oxygen species and p38 mitogen-activated protein kinase induce apoptotic death of U937 cells in response to Naja nigricollis toxin-gamma. J Cell Mol Med. 2009;13:1695–705.

26. Lee MW, Park SC, Yang YG, Yim SO, Chae HS, Bach JH, Lee HJ, Kim KY, Lee WB, Kim SS. The involvement of reactive oxygen species (ROS) and p38 mitogen-activated protein (MAP) kinase in TRAIL/Apo2L-induced apoptosis. FEBS Lett. 2002;512:313–8.

27. Tang H, Li J, Liu X, Wang G, Luo M, Deng H. Down-regulation of HSP60 Suppresses the Proliferation of Glioblastoma Cells via the ROS/ AMPK/ mTOR Pathway. Sci Rep. 2016;6:28388.

28. Aroui S, Dardevet L, Ben Ajmia W, de Boisvilliers M, Perrin F, Laajimi A, Boumendjel A, Kenani A, Muller JM, De Waard M. A Novel Platinum-Maurocalcine Conjugate Induces Apoptosis of Human Glioblastoma Cells by Acting through the ROS-ERK/AKT-p53 Pathway. Mol Pharm. 2015;12:4336–48.

29. Xu M, Cheung CC, Chow C, Lun SW, Cheung ST, Lo KW. Overexpression of PIN1 Enhances Cancer Growth and Aggressiveness with Cyclin D1 Induction in EBV-Associated Nasopharyngeal Carcinoma. PLoS One. 2016;11:e0156833.

7

Mild encephalitis/encephalopathy with reversible splenial lesion (MERS) in adults

Junliang Yuan[1†], Shuna Yang[1†], Shuangkun Wang[2], Wei Qin[1], Lei Yang[1] and Wenli Hu[1*]

Abstract

Background: Mild encephalitis/encephalopathy with reversible splenial lesion (MERS) is a rare clinico-radiological entity characterized by the magnetic resonance imaging (MRI) finding of a reversible lesion in the corpus callosum, sometimes involved the symmetrical white matters. Many cases of child-onset MERS with various causes have been reported. However, adult-onset MERS is relatively rare. The clinical characteristics and pathophysiologiccal mechanisms of adult-onset MERS are not well understood. We reviewed the literature on adult-onset MERS in order to describe the characteristics of MERS in adults and to provide experiences for clinician.

Methods: We reported a case of adult-onset MERS with acute urinary retension and performed literature search from PubMed and web of science databases to identify other adult-onset MERS reports from Januarary 2004 to March 2016. Preferred Reporting Items for Systematic Reviews and Meta-Analyses (PRISMA) guideline was followed on selection process. And then we summarized the clinico-radiological features of adult-onset MERS.

Results: Twenty-nine adult-onset MERS cases were reviewed from available literature including the case we have. 86. 2% of the cases (25/29) were reported in Asia, especially in Japan. Ages varied between 18 and 59 years old with a 12: 17 female-to-male ratio. The major cause was infection by virus or bacteria. Fever and headache were the most common clinical manifestation, and acute urinary retention was observed in 6 patients. All patients recovered completely within a month.

Conclusion: Adult-onset MERS is an entity with a broad clinico-radiological spectrum because of the various diseases and conditions. There are similar characteristics between MERS in adults and children, also some differences.

Keywords: Mild encephalitis/encephalopathy with reversible splenial lesion, Adult-onset MERS, Encephalitis, Encephalopathy, Corpus callosum, Reversible plenial lesion

Background

Tada et al. first identified the concept of mild encephalitis/encephalopathy with reversible splenial lesion (MERS) as a rare clinico-radiological syndrome in 2004 [1, 2]. In general, patients with MERS presented with mild central nervous system symptoms such as consciousness disturbance, seizures and headache and recovered completely within a month [1, 3]. MERS is divided into two types according to the lesion location. MERS type I, the typical form, most involves a singular lesion in the midline of the splenium of the corpus callosum (SCC), while MERS type II most commonly presents lesions in the symmetrical cerebral white matter or the anterior aspect of the corpus callosum with similar signal manifestations [4, 5]. The typical magnetic resonance imaging (MRI) features are transient high-signal-intensity on T2-weighted images (T2WI), fluid-attenuated inversion recovery images (FLAIR), and diffusion-weighted images (DWI), decreased apparent diffusion coefficient (ADC) value of the lesion on ADC maps, and hyper-isointense signals on T1-weighted imaging (T1WI) sequences without contrast enhancement [1, 4, 6]. Previous studies have identified that MERS can be triggered by infection including influenza virus [7], rotavirus [8], mumps virus [9], Mycoplasma

* Correspondence: huwenli@sina.com
†Equal contributors
[1]Department of Neurology, Beijing Chaoyang Hospital, Capital Medical University, Chaoyang District, Beijing, China
Full list of author information is available at the end of the article

pneumoniae [10] or Legionella pneumophila [11]. In addition to infection, MERS has also been reported to be associated with the administration of antiepileptic drugs [12–14].

Many child-onset MERS cases have been reported, most in Asia, especially Japan [1, 15]. However, adult-onset MERS is relatively rare. Here we reported a case of adult-onset MERS with acute urinary retention. It has been speculated that the characteristics of MERS in adults are different from that in children. So we utilized this opportunity to review the literature on adult-onset MERS in order to describe the clinico-radiological features and establish a clinical position of the disease.

Methods

Case presentation

A previously healthy 37-year-old man was admitted to our hospital due to a 9-day history of headache and vomiting. Ten days prior to admission, he suddenly developed a fever of 40 °C, diarrhea and headache. After taking oral antipyretics, he still had a fever of 38–39 °C. Three days before admission, his body temperature returned to normal. Two days before admission, he suffered acute urinary retention and was treated by temporary transurethral catheterization at another hospital. One day before admission, he came to our hospital for acute urinary retention and the catheter was kept. Neurological examination revealed nuchal rigidity positive. Chemistry panel and urine analysis showed no abnormalities except for an elevated blood white cell counts (10.99×10^9/L), C-reactive protein level (9.41 mg/L) and decreased serum sodium (131.8mml/L). Routine immunological screening and tumor markers were negative. Lumbar puncture showed an elevated cerebrospinal fluid (CSF) pressure of 190mmH$_2$O. CSF examination demonstrated an increase in white blood cells (97/ul) and protein content (124 mg/dl). The CSF etiological examination was negative. Oligoclonal bands, IgG index and myelin basic protein were within the normal ranges in CSF. Paraneoplastic antibodies were negative. Cranial MRI scans taken on the day after admission showed abnormal signals in SCC, which was hyperintense on T2WI and DWI imaging, decreased on ADC, isointense on T1WI with no contrast enhancement (Fig. 1). The plain and enhancement spinal cord MRI showed no obvious abnormalities. He received intracranial pressure reduction, antiviral, anti-inflammatory and experimental anti-tuberculosis. His urinary retention and fever resolved within 10 days. The follow-up MRI scan taken 14 days after the initial examination showed previous lesion disappeared (Fig. 2). He was discharged home without neurological complications. The final diagnosis was MERS with acute urinary retention.

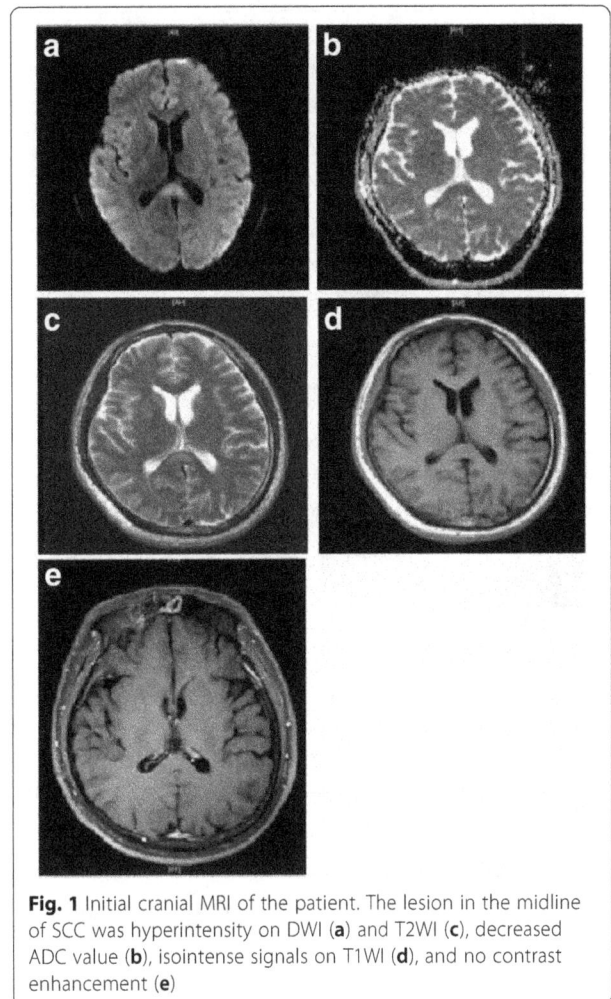

Fig. 1 Initial cranial MRI of the patient. The lesion in the midline of SCC was hyperintensity on DWI (**a**) and T2WI (**c**), decreased ADC value (**b**), isointense signals on T1WI (**d**), and no contrast enhancement (**e**)

Literature search and selection

To better understand the characteristics of adult-onset MERS, we performed a literature search to identify other reports (reviews, case reports or case series) from Januarary 2004 to March 2016, using the PubMed and web of science databases with the following terms, 'mild encephalitis/encephalopathy with reversible splenial lesion'/'MERS'/'reversible splenial lesion'. All pertinent English language articles were retrieved. A hand-search by reviewing the reference sections of the retrieved articles was also performed. The non-English language articles, child-onset MERS reports and not getting full-text articles were excluded. We followed the Preferred Reporting Items for Systematic Reviews and Meta-Analyses (PRISMA) guideline on selection process.

Data extraction

Two investigators collected data from the selected articles. The following information were extracted: last name of the first author, country where the study was

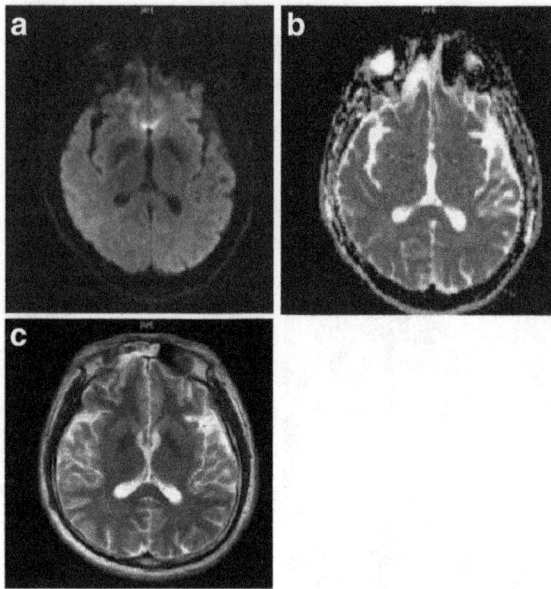

Fig. 2 Follow up cranial MRI. The follow up cranial MRI showed no lesion on any sequence (**a**: DWI, **b**: ADC, **c**: T2WI)

performed, the reported patient's age, gender, CNS symptoms, neurological examination, etiology, auxiliary examination, therapy and outcome.

Results of literature review

A total of 435 articles between Jan", auary 2004 and March 2016 were identified by preliminary electronic literature search and hand search. The selection process was presented in Fig. 3. The characteristics of the included cases were presented in Table 1 and Table 2.

Of the 29 adult-onset MERS patients, 11 were from Japan, 8 from China, 3 from Turkey, 2 from Germany, 2 from Korea, 1 from France, 1 from India and 1 from America. From a geographical point of view, 86.2% of the countries were in Asia (25/29), especially in Japan (11/29).

The age of onset varied between 18 and 59 years old, with an average of 31. Twelve patients were females (41.38%) with a 12:17 female-to-male ratio. Fifteen patients had identified causes, including 5 virus infections, 3 pneumoniae, and 1 mycoplasma infection. One patient developed MERS due to Amanita phalloides toxication, one because of tick-bites. One patient had emotional and behavioral changes presenting with auditory hallucinations within 10 days after C-section.

Fever had preceded or simultaneously presented with neurologic symptoms in 24 patients. Twelve patients complained of headache while having MERS, and disturbance of consciousness was observed in 15 cases. Seizure occurred in 4 cases, and acute urinary retention in 6 patients. 75.9% of the patients (22/29) had an isolated lesion in the splenium of the corpus callosum.

Six patients had lesions in both splenium and extracallosal. One patient had lesions in the entire corpus callosum. Lumbar punctures were performed in 23 patients, 15 of which had elevated CSF WBCs. Sixteen patients had their serum sodium reported, 6 of which had decreased levels. EEG was performed in 23 patients, 14 of which were abnormal.

The patients were treated with antiviral therapy, antibiotics, corticosteroids, IVIG, intravenous osmotic diuretic and isotonic fluid. Thirteen patients received corticosteroids therapy, 5 of which received a methylprednisolone pulse therapy. No case resulted in neurological sequelae.

Discussion

We reported a previously healthy 37-year-old man who suffered MERS associated with acute urinary retention. A lesion in the SCC resulting in acute urinary retention has rarely been reported. We considered acute disseminated encephalomyelitis (ADEM) being the main differential diagnosis. In comparison with the lesions in MERS which show no contrast enhancement and usually disappear quickly [1], the corpus callosum lesions in ADEM are usually asymmetrical, contrast-enhancing, extend to the white matter and spinal cord [16], and resolve over weeks to months. Our patient's cranial MRI showed an isolated abnormal signal in the SCC with no contrast enhancement. His spinal cord MRI showed no obvious abnormalities. The follow-up MRI scan revealed normalized findings within two weeks. So the patient was diagnosed as MERS instead of ADEM.

At first, a reversible isolated SCC lesion on MRI was diagnosed as MERS [1]. Recent studies suggested additional similar lesions in the cerebral white matter and anterior aspects of the corpus callosum in some encephalitis/encephalopathy patients should also been regarded as MERS (type 2 MERS) [4, 5]. Since the radiologic range of MERS had been expanded, patient no.7, 8, 10, 12, 15, 21 and 29 were included in the literature review.

Similar to child-onset MERS, most adult-onset MERS patients were also reported in Asia, including Japan, China and India. Interestingly, the majority cases were reported in recent five years. The phenomenon may be related to ethnics and social factors, as well as lack of diagnostic awareness and criteria before 2011. The common neurological manifestations of MERS in adult were headache and disturbance of consciousness. However, disturbance of consciousness and seizures were the most common neurological symptoms in children [15]. We suspect that it is related to children's immature central nervous system and blood brain barrier.

The pathogenesis of MERS is still unknown. There are several hypotheses, including intramyelinic edema, axonal damage, hyponatemia, and oxidative stress [1, 17, 18]. High signal intensity on DWI and decreased ADC values

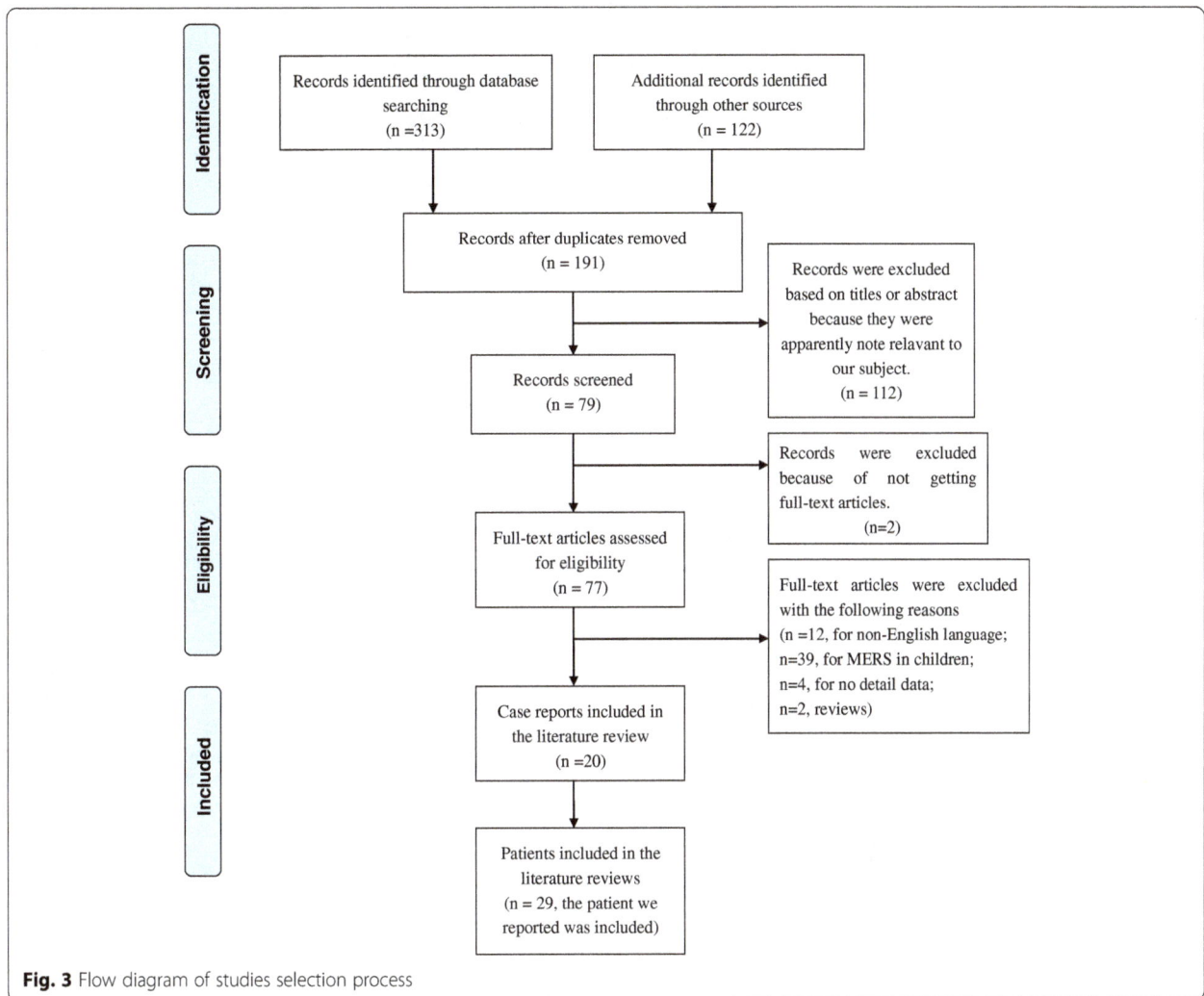

Fig. 3 Flow diagram of studies selection process

of white matter have been observed in MERS. The possible explanation for this is intrmyelinic edema resulting from separation of myelin layers [19, 20] and local infiltration of inflammatory cells [1, 3]. In this review, we found that more than half (15/23) cases had elevated white cells in the CSF. A previous small sample study reported that patients with MERS has an elevated IL-6 and IL-10 levels in CSF, however, the sample is not enough for any conclusions to be drawn [17]. ADC may return to normal within a week if the intramyelinic edema or inflammatory infiltrate resolves quickly. Takanashi et al. [21] reported that most patients with MERS had mild hyponatremia with a mean serum sodium level (131.0 ± 4.1 mmol/L) lower than that of the healthy group. Our review revealed that 6/16 MERS patients had hyponatremia upon admission. All these indicate that hyponatremia might be a possible cause of MERS. Taken all together, MERS is a rare syndrome with unclear pathogenesis. None of the existing hypotheses explains why MERS specially involves the site splenium.

In any patients presenting with symptoms of encephalitis/encephalopathy who are found to have lesions in the white matter, ADEM should be included in the differentials [1, 4, 22, 23]. ADEM is a post-infectious inflammatory disorder which can present with seizures, focal neurological signs or altered mental status days to weeks after the presumed infections [24]. MRI with contrast shows various enhancements of the lesions in ADEM depending on the stages of the acuity [24]. Other differential diagnoses include posterior reversible encephalopathy syndrome (usually hypertension-related and has subcortical white matter lesion), multiple sclerosis (characteristic relapsing-remitting course), Marchiafava-Bignami disease (often seen in alcoholism), ischemia (usually irreversible and has vascular territory distributions), diffuse axonal injury (head trauma-related), lymphoma (positive contrast enhancement), and extrapontine myelinolysis (happens with electrolyte abnormality) [25].

Even though the evidence of methylprednisolone pulse therapy and IVIG's efficacy on MERS is still lacking, they

Table 1 Information of 29 adult-onset MERS cases

Reported by, location, reference	Case no.	Sex, age (years)	symptomsis	Neurological examination	Etiology
Beijing Chaoyang Hospital, China	1	M, 37	Fever, UT	cervical rigidity (+)	NQ
Tada et al. [1] Japan	2	F, 59	Fever, vertigo, lethargy	NS	NQ
	3	F, 18	Fever, seizure, delirium	NS	NQ
	4	M, 19	Fever, cough, delirium, seizure	NS	NQ
	5	F, 25	Fever, vesicular, headache, drowsiness, nausea	NS	VZV
	6	M, 22	Fever, hallucination, delirium	NS	NQ
Jun-ichi et al. [22] Japan	7	M, 31	Headache, fever, drowsiness, disorientation, memory disturbance	drowsiness, disorientation, memory disturbance	NQ
Jeong-Seon et al. [6] Korea	8	M, 59	Dysarthria, drowsiness,fever	Normal	NQ
Nida Tascilar et al. [27] Turkey	9	F, 26	Fever, headache, phonophobia, photophobia, dizziness, UT	Neck stiffness (+), positive Kernig's sign, right truncal and gait ataxia	NQ
Makiko et al. [28] Japan	10	F, 23	Fever, headache, UT	Unsteady gait, patellar tendon reflexes, plantar reflexes, abdominal wall reflexes diminished	NQ
Henning Vollmann et al. [29] Germany	11	M, 42	Fever, vomit, headache	Mild ataxia, disturbance of gait	Tick-bites
Dimitri Renard et al. [30] France	12	M, 43	Stuporous state	GCS E4M5V2, mutism, persistent hiccup	Anti-Yo rhombenceh-halitis
Shingo Mitraki et al. [31] Japan	13	M, 29	Consciousness disturbance	Drowsy, disoriented	pneumonia
Hideki Shibuya et al. [10] Japan	14	M, 30	Fever, consciousness disturbance	Glasgrow coma scale: E4V1M6	Mycoplasma- pneumoniae
Balasubramanyam Shankar et al. [32] India	15	F, 28	Fever, vomiting, paresthesia	Drowsy, neck rigidity, up going plantar reflex	NQ
Soon Young Ko et al. [33] Korea	16	M, 30	Fever, alalia	dysarthra	Nonfulminant hepatitis A
Makoto Hibino et al. [34] Japan	17	F, 24	Fever, diarrhea, abdominal pain, weakness of right upper extremity	Right-side hemiparesis, hemianesthesia, Chaddock (+)	adenovirus
Yuji Tomizawa et al. [11] Japan	18	M, 49	Fever, gait difficulty	Wide-based gait, fine postural tremors, mildly exaggerate deep tendon reflexes	Legionella pneumophila-serogroup 2
Robert M et al. [35] America	19	M, 41	Fever, headache, delirium, consciousness disturbance, tremor, gait instability, paresthesias, UT	Slow thought, mild difficulty finding words, intention tremor of the left arm, dysmetria of lower extremities, broad-based gait	ipilimumba
Jing Jing Pan et al. [36] China	20	F, 18	Fever	(–)	NQ
	21	M, 26	Fever, acute UT	Nuchal rigidity (+)	NQ
	22	F, 23	Fever, headache, disturbance of consciousness	Kerning (+)	C-section
	23	M, 21	Fever, headache, acute UT, intestinal obstruction	Kerning (+)	NQ

Table 1 Information of 29 adult-onset MERS cases (*Continued*)

Shuo Zhang et al. [37] China	24	F, 26	Headache, fever, seizure, somnolence	Somnolence	Mycoplasm-a
	25	F, 34	Dizziness, fever, somnolence	Somnolence	Mumps virus
	26	M,25	Headache, fever, cognitive impairment, behavioral disorders, confusion	Cognitive impairment, behavioral disorders, confusion	Herpes simplex virus
Eylem Degirmenci et al. [38] Turkey	27	M, 27	Headache, apathy, nausea, vomiting	Bilateral papilledema, mildly altered mental status	NQ
Naila Alakbarvova et al. [39] Turkey	28	M, 46	Headache, vomiting, nausea, diarrea, abdominal pain, generalized tonic-clonic seizure	Confusing with time disorientation	Amanita phalloides intoxication
Matthias Gawlitza et al. [40] Germany	29	F, 28	disorientated	Disorientated, confusion	Hemolytic uremic syndrome

M male, *F* female, *UT* urinary retention, *NS* no statement, *NQ* no required, *VZV* varicella zoster virus

Table 2 Auxiliary examination and treatment of 29 adult-onset MERS cases

Case no.	Initial examination				MRI	EEG	Treatment
	WBC (10⁹/L)	CRP (g/L)	Serum sodium (mmol/L)	CSF WBC (10⁶/L)			
1	10.99	9.41	131.8 (hyponatremia)	97	SCC	NE	mannitol, low dose methylprednisolone, ACV, anti-tuberculosis
2	NS	NS	NS	500	SCC	Slow BA	ACV, antibiotics
3	NS	NS	NS	17	SCC	Slow BA and spikes	PB, PSL
4	NS	NS	NS	Normal	SCC	Slow BA	ACV, PHT, PSL
5	NS	NS	NS	NE	SCC	NE	ACV
6	NS	NS	NS	Normal	SCC	Slow BA	ACV, antibiotics, PSL
7	18.8	17.0	NS	253	Entire CC and peripheral WM	NS	antibiotics
8	normal	normal	normal	normal	SCC and frontal WM	NS	No specific therapy
9	normal	normal	normal	408	SCC	normal	Ceftriaxone, ACV, ampicillin, catheterization
10	normal	normal	normal	normal	SCC, WM	NS	Methylprednisolone pulse, PSL, catheterization
11	NS	normal	132 (hyponatremia)	33	SCC	NS	Ceftriaxone, ACV, symptomatic therapy of headache and fever
12	NS	normal	133 (hyponatremia)	6	SCC, frontoparie-tal WM, putamina, thalami	Diffuse slowing wave	Antiepileptic treatment, methylprednisolone pulse, immunoglobulin treatment
13	elevated	elevated	NS	normal	Entire CC	NS	methylprednisolone pulse, immunoglobulin treatment
14	NS	NS	NS	NS	SCC	NS	Levofloxacin
15	NS	NS	NS	60	SCC, bilateral WM	Slow activity, frontal sharp wave	Empirical corticosteroids and ACV
16	3.48	NS	138	NS	SCC	abnormal	hemodialysis
17	normal	12.21	normal	NE	SCC	NS	No specific therapy
18	elevated	22.9	130	3	SCC	NS	Antibiotics
19	normal	normal	normal	128	SCC	NS	oral PSL and methylprednisolone pulse
20	6.08	normal	137.0	90	SCC	abnormal	methylprednisolone pulse, oral PSL
21	7.10	normal	130.2	100	SCC, insula, caudate nucleus	abnormal	Oral methylprednisolone and PSL
22	11.20	normal	138.6	12	SCC	abnormal	Oral methylprednisolone and PSL
23	8.20	normal	126.5	80	SCC	abnormal	Oral PSL
24	NS	NS	NS	3	SCC	Occipital slow waves	Mannitol, diazepam, macrolides antibiotics and moxifloxacin
25	NS	NS	NS	7	SCC	Occipital slow waves	Interferon, ribavirin
26	NS	NS	NS	112	SCC	Occipital slow waves	Ganciclovir, mannitol, antibiotics
27	normal	normal	normal	150	SCC	NS	Acetazolamide, antibiotics, oseltamivir
28	17.8	NQ	normal	normal	SCC	NS	Risperidone, clozapine, venlafaxine and diazepam, antipsychotic and intoxication treatment
29	NS	NS	NS	NS	SCC	NS	eculizumab

WBC white blood cell, *CRP* C-reactive protein, *CSF* cerebrospinal fluid, *EEG* electroencephalography, *NE* no examined, *NS* no statement, *BA* basic activity, *ACV* acyclovir, *PB* Phenobarbital, *PHT* phenytoin, *PSL* prednisolone, *WM* white matters

are recommended for patients with infectious encephalopathy regardless of the pathogen or clinicl-radiological syndromes [26]. In this review, only five MERS patients were treated with methylprednisolone pulse therapy and two with IVIG treatment. However, all patients without methylprednisolone pulse therapy or IVIG recovered clinically completely, which suggests that those treatments may not be necessary.

Conclusion

In conclusion, we reported a case of an adult-onset MERS with acute urinary retention. Taken together with the previously reported cases, we suggest that MERS in adults is an entity with a broad clinico-radiological spectrum and the prognosis is good. From a geographical point of view, most adult-onset MERS patients were also reported in Asia. The common neurological manifestations were headache and disturbance of consciousness. There are similar characteristics between MERS in adults and children, also some differences.

Abbreviations
ADC: Apparent diffusion coefficient; ADEM: Acute disseminated encephalomyelitis; CSF: Cerebrospinal fluid; EEG: Electroencephalogram; MERS: Mild encephalitis/encephalopathy with reversible splenial lesion; SCC: Splenium of the corpus callosum

Acknowledgment
None.

Funding
This work is supported by National Natural Science Foundation of China (Grant No. 81271309) and Beijing Municipal Administration of Hospitals' Youth Programme (QML20150303).

Authors' contributions
JLY provided the adult-onset MERS case. WLH conceived and designed the experiments. SNY performed the literature search and drafted the manuscript. SKW performed the studies selection process. WQ and LY collected data from the selected articles. All authors have read and approved the final manuscript to be published.

Competing interests
The authors declare that they have no competing interests.

Author details
[1]Department of Neurology, Beijing Chaoyang Hospital, Capital Medical University, Chaoyang District, Beijing, China. [2]Department of Radiology, Beijing Chaoyang Hospital, Capital Medical University, Beijing, China.

References
1. Tada H, Takanashi J, Barkovich A, et al. Clinically mild encephalitis/encephalopathy with a reversible splenial lesion. Neurology. 2004;63:1854–8.
2. Garcia-Monco JC, Cortina IE, Ferreira E, et al. Reversible splenial lesion syndrome (RESLES): what's in a name? J Neuroimaging. 2011;21:e1–e14.
3. Takanashi J-i. Two newly proposed infectious encephalitis/encephalopathy syndromes. Brain Dev. 2009;31:521 8.
4. Takanashi J, Barkovich A, Shiihara T, et al. Widening spectrum of a reversible splenial lesion with transiently reduced diffusion. Am J Neuroradiol. 2006;27:836–8.
5. Notebaert A, Willems J, Coucke L, Van Coster R, Verhelst H. Expanding the spectrum of MERS type 2 lesions, a particular form of encephalitis. Pediatr Neurol. 2013;48:135–8.
6. Cho J-S, Ha S-W, Han Y-S, et al. Mild encephalopathy with reversible lesion in the splenium of the corpus callosum and bilateral frontal white matter. J Clin Neurol. 2007;3:53–6.
7. Takanashi J-i, Barkovich AJ, Yamaguchi K-i, Kohno Y. Influenza-associated encephalitis/encephalopathy with a reversible lesion in the splenium of the corpus callosum: a case report and literature review. Am J Neuroradiol. 2004;25:798–802.
8. Fuchigami T, Goto K, Hasegawa M, et al. A 4-year-old girl with clinically mild encephalopathy with a reversible splenial lesion associated with rotavirus infection. J Infect Chemother. 2013;19:149–53.
9. Takanashi J-i, Shiihara T, Hasegawa T, et al. Clinically mild encephalitis with a reversible splenial lesion (MERS) after mumps vaccination. J Neurol Sci. 2015;349:226–8.
10. Shibuya H, Osamura K, Hara K, Hisada T. Clinically mild encephalitis/encephalopathy with a reversible splenial lesion due to Mycoplasma pneumoniae infection. Intern Med. 2012;51:1647–8.
11. Tomizawa Y, Hoshino Y, Sasaki F, et al. Diagnostic utility of Splenial lesions in a case of Legionnaires' disease due to Legionella pneumophila Serogroup 2. Intern Med. 2015;54:3079–82.
12. Kim SS, Chang K-H, Kim ST, et al. Focal lesion in the splenium of the corpus callosum in epileptic patients: antiepileptic drug toxicity? Am J Neuroradiol. 1999;20:125–9.
13. Polster T, Hoppe M, Ebner A. Transient lesion in the splenium of the corpus callosum: three further cases in epileptic patients and a pathophysiological hypothesis. J Neurol Neurosurg Psychiatry. 2001;70:459–63.
14. Maeda M, Shiroyama T, Tsukahara H, Shimono T, Aoki S, Takeda K. Transient splenial lesion of the corpus callosum associated with antiepileptic drugs: evaluation by diffusion-weighted MR imaging. Eur Radiol. 2003;13:1902–6.
15. Karampatsas K, Spyridou C, Morrison IR, Tong CY, Prendergast AJ. Rotavirus-associated mild encephalopathy with a reversible splenial lesion (MERS)—case report and review of the literature. BMC Infect Dis. 2015;15:1.
16. Barkovich AJ. Pediatric neuroimaging: Lippincott Williams & Wilkins, 2005.
17. Miyata R, Tanuma N, Hayashi M, et al. Oxidative stress in patients with clinically mild encephalitis/encephalopathy with a reversible splenial lesion (MERS). Brain Dev. 2012;34:124–7.
18. Takanashi J-i, Maeda M, Hayashi M. Neonate showing reversible splenial lesion. Arch Neurol. 2005;62:1481–2.
19. Engelbrecht V, Scherer A, Rassek M, Witsack HJ, Mödder U. Diffusion-weighted MR imaging in the brain in children: findings in the normal brain and in the brain with white matter diseases 1. Radiology. 2002;222:410–8.
20. Phillips MD, McGraw P, Lowe MJ, Mathews VP, Hainline BE. Diffusion-weighted imaging of white matter abnormalities in patients with phenylketonuria. Am J Neuroradiol. 2001;22:1583–6.
21. Takanashi J-i, Tada H, Maeda M, Suzuki M, Terada H, Barkovich AJ. Encephalopathy with a reversible splenial lesion is associated with hyponatremia. Brain Dev. 2009;31:217–20.
22. Takanashi J-i, Hirasawa K-i, Tada H. Reversible restricted diffusion of entire corpus callosum. J Neurol Sci. 2006;247:101–4.
23. Hong JM, Park MS, Jun D. Transient splenial lesion of the corpus callosum in patients with infectious disease. J Korean Neurol Assoc. 2005;23:667–70.
24. Dyken PR. Viral diseases of the nervous system. Pediatr Neurol. 1994;1:499–501.
25. Friese S, Bitzer M, Freudenstein D, Voigt K, Küker W. Classification of acquired lesions of the corpus callosum with MRI. Neuroradiology. 2000;42:795–802.
26. Mizuguchi M, Yamanouchi H, Ichiyama T, Shiomi M. Acute encephalopathy associated with influenza and other viral infections. Acta Neurol Scand. 2007;115:45–56.
27. Tascilar N, Aydemir H, Emre U, Unal A, Atasoy HT, Ekem S. Unusual combination of reversible splenial lesion and meningitis-retention syndrome in aseptic meningomyelitis. Clinics. 2009;64:932–7.
28. Kitami M, Kubo S-i, Nakamura S, Shiozawa S, Isobe H, Furukawa Y. Acute urinary retention in a 23-year-old woman with mild encephalopathy with a reversible splenial lesion: a case report. J Med Case Rep. 2011;5:159.

29. Vollmann H, Hagemann G, Mentzel H-J, Witte OW, Redecker C. Isolated reversible splenial lesion in tick-borne encephalitis: a case report and literature review. Clin Neurol Neurosurg. 2011;113:430–3.

30. Renard D, Taieb G, Briere C, Bengler C, Castelnovo G. Mild encephalitis/encephalopathy with a reversible splenial, white matter, putaminal, and thalamic lesions following anti-Yo rhombencephalitis. Acta Neurol Belg. 2012;112:405-7.

31. Mitaki S, Onoda K, Ishihara M, Nabika Y, Yamaguchi S. Dysfunction of default-mode network in encephalopathy with a reversible corpus callosum lesion. J Neurol Sci. 2012;317:154–6.

32. Shankar B, Narayanan R, Muralitharan P, Ulaganathan B. Evaluation of mild encephalitis/encephalopathy with a reversible splenial lesion (MERS) by diffusion-weighted and diffusion tensor imaging. BMJ case reports. 2014; 2014:bcr2014204078.

33. Ko SY, Kim BK, Kim DW, et al. Reversible splenial lesion on the corpus callosum in nonfulminant hepatitis a presenting as encephalopathy. Clin Mol Hepatol. 2014;20:398–401.

34. Hibino M, Horiuchi S, Okubo Y, Kakutani T, Ohe M, Kondo T. Transient Hemiparesis and Hemianesthesia in an atypical case of adult-onset clinically mild encephalitis/encephalopathy with a reversible Splenial lesion associated with adenovirus infection. Intern Med. 2014;53:1183–5.

35. Conry RM, Sullivan JC, Nabors LB. Ipilimumab-induced encephalopathy with a reversible splenial lesion. Cancer Immunol Res. 2015;3:598–601.

36. Pan JJ, Zhao Y-y, Lu C, Hu YH, Yang Y. Mild encephalitis/encephalopathy with a reversible splenial lesion: five cases and a literature review. Neurol Sci. 2015;36:2043–51.

37. Zhang S, Ma Y, Feng J. Clinicoradiological spectrum of reversible splenial lesion syndrome (RESLES) in adults: a retrospective study of a rare entity. Med. 2015;94(6):e512.

38. Degirmenci E, Degirmenci T, Cetin EN, Kıroğlu Y. Mild encephalitis/encephalopathy with a reversible splenial lesion (MERS) in a patient presenting with papilledema. Acta Neurol Belg. 2015;115:153–5.

39. Alakbarova N, Eraslan C, Celebisoy N, Karasoy H, Gonul AS. Mild encephalitis/encephalopathy with a reversible splenial lesion (MERS) development after Amanita phalloides intoxication. Acta Neurol Belg. 2015:1–3.

40. Gawlitza M, Hoffmann KT, Lobsien D. Mild encephalitis/encephalopathy with reversible Splenial and Cerebellar lesions (MERS type II) in a patient with hemolytic uremic syndrome (HUS). J Neuroimaging. 2015;25:145–6.

8

Lumbar puncture as possible cause of sudden paradoxical herniation in patient with previous decompressive craniectomy

Liang Shen[1], Sheng Qiu[1], Zhongzhou Su[1], Xudong Ma[1] and Renfu Yan[1,2*]

Abstract

Background: Lumbar puncture is often used for the diagnosis and treatment of subarchnoid hemorrhage, infection of Cerebro-spinal Fluid (CSF), hydrocephalus in neurosurgery department patients. It is general that paradoxical herniation followed by lumbar puncture is quite rare in decompressive craniectomy cases; the related reports are very few. Moreover, most of the paradoxical herniation cases are chronic, which often occur weeks or even months after the lumbar puncture, to date, barely no reports on the acute onset paradoxical herniation have been found.

Case presentation: Two traumatic brain injury patients with decompressive craniectomy (DC) and hydrocephalus suffered from a sudden paradoxical herniation after lumbar puncture. The symptoms of herniation were improved by treated with Trendelenburg position and rapid intravenous infusion.

Conclusions: Lumbar puncture may have a potential risk of inducing sudden paradoxical herniation in patients with DC. CSF drainage during lumbar puncture should be in small volume for patients with DC. Once a paradoxical herniation occurs after lumbar puncture, an immediate Trendelenburg position and rapid intravenous infusion treatment may be effective.

Keywords: Case report, Lumbar puncture, Herniation, Decompressive craniectomy

Background

Decompressive craniectomy (DC) is a simple yet useful emergency surgery for patients with uncontrollable intracranial pressure (ICP) to decrease ICP, especially for patients with high risks of herniation. Paradoxical herniation is a rare but life-threatening complication after DC. Paradoxical herniation is an intracranial hypotensive herniation in the direction of opposite site of the DC with subsequent brainstem compression resulting from atmospheric pressure along with brain gravity [1]. This kind of herniation with an uncommon mesencephalon compression [2] is one of the most serious sinking skin flap syndrome (SSFS). Besides, the traditional managements reducing the intracranial pressure for herniation

may exacerbate paradoxical herniation, therefore, timely diagnosis and correct treatments are significantly important to combat this condition. Paradoxical herniation may also occur and become worse in patients with intracranial infection following lumbar puncture or hydrocephalus after ventriculoperitoneal shunting [3]. However, only few cases have been reported in public that paradoxical herniation may be occurred as a rare complication in patients with DC following lumbar puncture [4]. Here, we have reported and analyzed rare sudden paradoxical herniation after lumbar punctures for postoperative hydrocephalus in two traumatic brain injury (TBI) patients with a purpose to warn that lumbar puncture is a hazard in these circumstance, and once the herniation occurs it may be reversed by placing in Trendelenburg position and intravenous fluids supplements.

* Correspondence: yanrenfu62@163.com
[1]Department of Neurosurgery, Huzhou Central Hospital, 198 Hongqi Road, Huzhou, Zhejiang 313000, China
[2]School of Medicine, Huzhou University, 759 East Second Ring Road, Huzhou, Zhejiang 313000, China

Case presentation

Patient A

A 29-year-old man with unconsciousness after TBI was sent and treated to our hospital in two hours after the injury, the Glasgow Coma Scale (GCS) score was used to estimate coma severity based on Eye (4), Verbal (5), and Motor (6) criteria of 5 (E1V1M3). There was a difference in diameter of pupils with 3.0 mm on the right side, and 4.0 mm on the left side; and the light reflex of eyes was disappeared. Emergency brain computed tomography (CT) revealed that patient had acute subdural hematoma in the left frontotemporal, a hemorrhagic contusion in the left frontal temporal lobe, skull fracture in the posterior occipital with epidural hematoma in the posterior fossa. Then, the patient had underwent emergent hematoma exclusion in the left frontal temporal, followed by DC. Six months later, the young man got a Glasgow Outcome Scale (GOS) of 5, Activity of Daily Living Scale (ADL) of 18, but the CT had disclosed a progressive hydrocephalus compared with three months ago. Considering the disturbance of CSF hydrodynamics, we had expected to perform cranioplasty. Before the skull repair, we conducted a lumbar puncture to release cerebrospinal fluid (CSF) and to detect and rule out the possibility of intracranial infection. Two hours later after 30 ml CSF release, the man had complained of progressively worsening dizziness and headache, and then he fell into a coma, based on the symptoms, we felt suspected paradoxical herniation might occur. Thus, the patient was placed in the Trendelenburg position and given sufficient hydration immediately. A following brain CT in three days had showed skin flap sank, but no obvious midline shift had been found. By then, the patient's consciousness had been gradually restored, and the patient got a GCS of 15 two weeks later. The cranioplasty has not been performed for this patient in the next few years for some personal reasons. Five years later, repeated brain CT has revealed complete resolution of the midline shift, and the hydrocephalus improved itself without cranioplasty or ventriculoperitoneal shunt (Fig. 1), and the man has got a GOS of 5 and has a favorable recovery with ADL of 14.

Patient B

A 56-year-old man was diagnosed with severe TBI with a GCS of 3. Pupil diameter was 4.0 mm on the right side, 2.0 mm on the left side, and pupillary reactions to light were absent. Subsequently, life-saving surgeries that cleaning subdural hematoma in the right frontal temporal lobe, DC and ventricular drainage were performed. During the course of the treatment, the patient was in a coma with a GCS of 8 (E2V1M5). The CT scanning showed a hydrocephalus in the third week after the initial surgery, accordingly, lumbar puncture was performed with an initial ICP of 200 mmHg. Subsequently, 30 ml CSF was released slowly to see immediate effects on outcome improvement. However, the man had shown some abnormal symptoms one hour later: shortness of

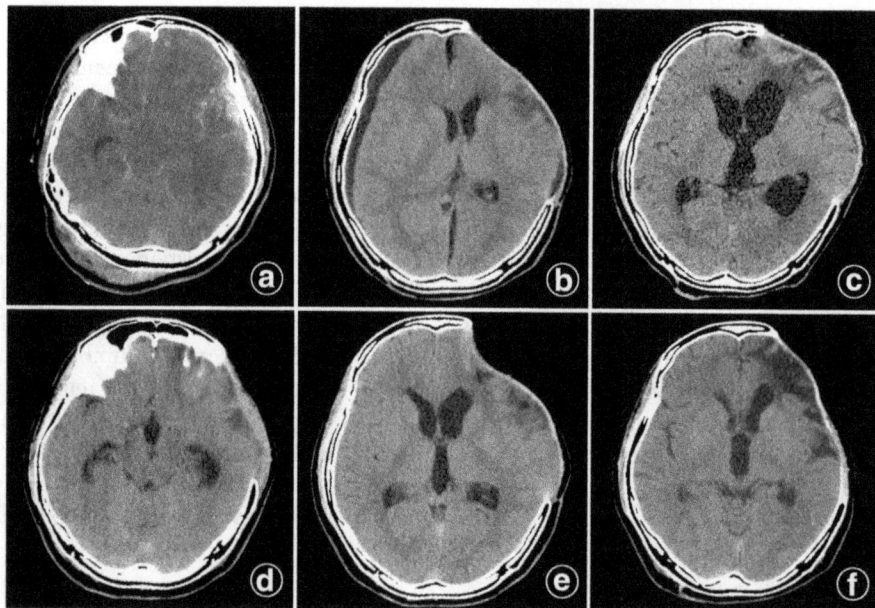

Fig.1 a A acute subdural hematoma in the left frontotemporal. **b** A repeated CT two months after the initial surgery. **c** A progressive hydrocephalus three months later. **d, e** Three days after placing the patient in a Trendelenburg position and giving sufficient hydration, the patient had a SSFS but no obvious midline shift. **f** Five years later, hydrocephalus improved itself without cranioplasty or ventriculoperitoneal shunt

breath, unequal size of both pupils diameters, SSFS. A Trendelenburg position and rapid saline infusion were conducted before an immediate CT scan, which showed the paradoxical herniation had occurred (Fig. 2). Two hours later, two pupil diameters were equal and pupil light reaction had become normal, the symptoms of hydrocephalus didn't get any improvement and the consciousness disorder gradually become deepen and worsen; after many unsuccessful treatment attempts, the man was pronounced dead few weeks later due to other complications.

Discussion

To our knowledge, most of TBI patients may have a secondary damage, which play a critical role in prognosis and has the potential to provoking death. These damage factors included subdural hematomas, intracerebral hematomas, cerebral swelling from vasospasm after subarachnoid hemorrhages, elevation of ICP. DC is generally conducted immediately in the setting of uncontrollable ICP [2]. However, TBI patients with DC may have numerous complications [5], and some of which were rare but dangerous, for example, SSFS and paradoxical herniation [4, 6–8]. The pathophysiology of paradoxical herniation has been postulated to be secondary to a large craniectomy defect exposing the intracranial contents to the external positive atmospheric pressure. This may cause also CSF disease, including post-trauma hydrocephalus. In our paper report, we have reported that two DC TBI patients with hydrocephalus, have suffered from paradoxical herniation within

a few hours following lumbar puncture. The lumbar puncture may be a hazard for DC patients with hydrocephalus or intracranial infection, and it should be performed with a caution when it is necessary.

Intracranial contents exposing following craniectomy may make patients have a presentation of skin flap depression, which was known as SSFS [9]. Several decades ago, Nakamura and colleagues [10] had reported a case that performing ventriculoperitoneal shunt for hydrocephalus and cranioplasty, yet the implanted plate had to be removed due to infection in the end. It should be noted that SSFS normally occur the neurological deterioration get exacerbated, but it may reversed by making patient lying flat or in the Trendelenburg position. The paradoxical herniation risk over time may exist in this "open box" state. The proposed mechanism of paradoxical herniation may be that atmospheric pressure and the brain gravity overwhelm over the natural buoyancy that CSF provided to the brain; the brain has become collapsed after the DC, and the brain stem has get compressed [3, 4]. Doubtlessly, lumbar CSF drainage is just an effective approach in the setting of subarachnoid hemorrhage, intracranial infection. If the drainage volume is more than 200 ml/24 h, patients undergoing DC would have a high risk of SSFS [4]. Moreover, according to some reports, paradoxical herniation is a complication which occurs until days or weeks later after the lumber puncture [11, 12]. These two cases that we reported had hydrocephalus after the DC surgery; and lumbar puncture was performed to explore whether

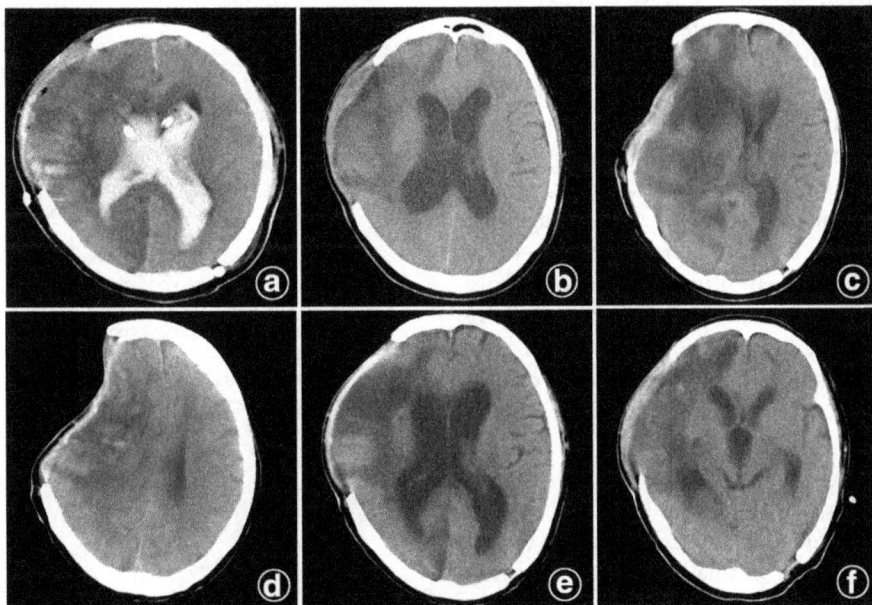

Fig. 2 a A CT after the surgery of subdural hematoma in the frontal temporal lobe cleaning, craniectomy and ventricular drainage. **b** CT showed a hydrocephalus three-week later after the surgery. **c, d** The patient had a SSFS and midline shift after the lumbar puncture. **e, f** After placing the patient in a Trendelenburg positon and giving intravenous fluid, SSFS and midline shift disappeared one day later

hydrocephalus had worsened the consciousness or if there were any intracranial infections. A lumbar puncture releasing slowly about 30 ml CSF leading to an acute onset paradoxical herniation within a few hours followed the drainage was observed. We believe that a rapid spontaneous CSF leak that a large volume of CSF poured out into the paraspinal soft tissues [13], was induced when conducting lumbar puncture. This proposed mechanism may explain these two cases of sudden paradoxical herniation, although we don't have sufficient image information to support this assumption.

SSFS is a visible symptom in the process of paradoxical herniation and happen in one month to one year after DC [9]. In addition to SSFS, if patients had motor symptoms, cognitive syndrome, impaired vigilance, headaches, delay in neurological progression and other neurological symptoms, an emergent CT would be undergone generally to rule out the occurrence of paradoxical herniation [4, 9]. Considering the risk of SSFS or paradoxical herniation after lumbar puncture and shunting, neurosurgeons should be aware that cranioplasty may be the first option for DC patients with hydrocephalus. From these two cases in our department, cranioplasty was not performed before the paradoxical herniation; fortunately, timely paradoxical herniation diagnosis and appropriate treatment with Trendelenburg position and rapid intravenous infusion reverse the symptoms. This brief report is a warning, especially for young neurologists and neurosurgeons, that lumbar puncture is a hazard in DC patients. It should be emphasized that the experience of our case report are limited. More relative studies are needed to clarify the mechanism of acute onset paradoxical herniation, and the treatments for those situation warrants further confirmation and exploration.

Lumbar puncture has a risk of provoking paradoxical herniation in patients with DC [8]. Correspondingly, CSF drainage procedures need to be cautiously used in patients post craniectomy. The hypertonic saline, mannitol, hyperventilation, modest cooling, CSF drainage that lowers ICP should not be taken for the treatment of paradoxical herniation, timely diagnosis, Trendelenburg position and rapid intravenous infusion are effective measures to combat this problem. Furthermore, observing the patient undergoing lumbar puncture in case of paradoxical herniation is of vital importance.

Conclusion

Lumbar puncture may have a potential risk of inducing sudden paradoxical herniation, and CSF drainage during lumbar puncture should be in small volume for patients with DC. Once a paradoxical herniation occurs after lumbar puncture, an immediate Trendelenburg position and rapid intravenous infusion treatment may be effective.

Abbreviations

ADL: Activity of daily living scale; CSF: Cerebrospinal fluid; CT: Computed tomography; DC: Decompression craniectomy; GCS: Glasgow coma scale; ICP: Intracranial pressures; SSFS: Sinking skin flap syndrome; TBI: Traumatic brain injury

Acknowledgements

None

Funding

None

Authors' contributions

RY examined the patients and conceptualized the report. LS designed the report, dealt with the resources and drafted the manuscript. SQ and ZS helped to draft the manuscript. XM helped to design the case report. All the authors read and approved the final manuscript.

Competing interests

All authors certify that they have no affiliations with or involvement in any organization or entity with any financial interest, or non-financial interest in the subject matter or materials discussed in this manuscript.

References

1.   Nasi D, Dobran M, Iacoangeli M, Di Somma L, Gladi M, Scerrati M. Paradoxical brain herniation after decompressive craniectomy provoked by drainage of subdural hygroma. World Neurosurg. 2016;91:673 e671–4.
2.   Akins PT, Guppy KH. Sinking skin flaps, paradoxical herniation, and external brain tamponade: a review of decompressive craniectomy management. Neurocrit Care. 2008;9:269–76.
3.   Creutzfeldt CJ, Vilela MD, Longstreth WT, Jr. Paradoxical herniation after decompressive craniectomy provoked by lumbar puncture or ventriculoperitoneal shunting. J Neurosurg. 2015;123:1170–5.
4.   Zhao J, Li G, Zhang Y, Zhu X, Hou K. Sinking skin flap syndrome and paradoxical herniation secondary to lumbar drainage. Clin Neurol Neurosurg. 2015;133:6–10.
5.   Stiver SI. Complications of decompressive craniectomy for traumatic brain injury. Neurosurg Focus. 2009;26:E7.
6.   Fields JD, Lansberg MG, Skirboll SL, Kurien PA, Wijman CA. "Paradoxical" transtentorial herniation due to CSF drainage in the presence of a hemicraniectomy. Neurology. 2006;67:1513–4.
7.   Oyelese AA, Steinberg GK, Huhn SL, Wijman CA. Paradoxical cerebral herniation secondary to lumbar puncture after decompressive craniectomy for a large space-occupying hemispheric stroke: case report. Neurosurgery. 2005;57:E594.
8.   Chen W, Guo J, Wu J, Peng G, Huang M, Cai C, Yang Y, Wang S. Paradoxical herniation after unilateral decompressive craniectomy predicts better patient survival: a retrospective analysis of 429 cases. Medicine. 2016;95:e2837.
9.   Annan M, De Toffol B, Hommet C, Mondon K. Sinking skin flap syndrome (or Syndrome of the trephined): a review. Br J Neurosurg. 2015;29:314–8.
10. Nakamura T, Takashima T, Isobe K, Yamaura A. Rapid neurological alteration associated with concave deformity of the skin flap in a craniectomized patient. Case report. Neurol Med Chir (Tokyo). 1980;20:89–93.
11. Samadani U, Huang JH, Baranov D, Zager EL, Grady MS. Intracranial hypotension after intraoperative lumbar cerebrospinal fluid drainage. Neurosurgery. 2003;52:148–51.
12. Vilela MD. Delayed paradoxical herniation after a decompressive craniectomy: case report. Surg Neurol. 2008;69:293–6.
13. Schievink WI. Spontaneous spinal cerebrospinal fluid leaks and intracranial hypotension. JAMA. 2006;295:2286–96.

Subarachnoid small vein occlusion due to inflammatory fibrosis—a possible mechanism for cerebellar infarction in cryptococcal meningoencephalitis

Yoshiteru Shimoda[1,2*], Satoru Ohtomo[1], Hiroaki Arai[1], Takashi Ohtoh[3] and Teiji Tominaga[2]

Abstract

Background: Cryptococcal meningoencephalitis (CM) causes cerebral infarction, typically, lacunar infarction in the basal ganglia. However, massive cerebral infarction leading to death is rare and its pathophysiology is unclear. We report a case of CM causing massive cerebellar infarction, which led to cerebral herniation and death.

Case presentation: A 56-year-old man who suffered from dizziness and gait disturbance for one month was admitted to our hospital and subsequently diagnosed with a cerebellar infarction. He had a past medical history of hepatitis type B virus infection and hepatic failure. Although the findings on magnetic resonance imaging (MRI) imitated an arterial infarction of the posterior inferior cerebellar artery, an accompanying irregular peripheral edema was observed. The ischemic lesion progressed, subsequently exerting a mass effect and leading to impaired consciousness. External and internal decompression surgeries were performed. *Cryptococcus neoformans* was confirmed in the surgical specimen, and the patient was diagnosed with CM. In addition, venule congestion in the parenchyma was observed with extensive fibrosis and compressed veins in the subarachnoid space. The patient died 26 days after admission. Autopsy revealed that pathological changes were localized in the cerebellum.

Conclusion: *C. neoformans* can induce extensive fibrosis of the subarachnoid space, which may compress small veins mechanically inducing venule congestion and massive cerebral infarction. In such cases, the clinical course can be severe and even rapidly fatal. An atypical pattern of infarction on MRI should alert clinicians to the possibility of *C. neoformans* infection.

Keywords: Cryptococcal infection, Vein occlusion, Magnetic resonance imaging, Autopsy

Background

Cryptococcal meningoencephalitis (CM) caused by *Cryptococcus neoformans* infection is the most common fungal infection of the central nervous system [1, 2]. Throughout its clinical course, *C. neoformans* induces small cerebral infarctions such as lacunar infarctions primarily in the basal ganglia [3–8]; however, massive brain infarction causing cerebral herniation has not been well described. We present a case of a patient with CM who presented with an atypical cerebellar infarction, which ultimately caused fatal cerebral herniation. Pathological and radiological findings revealed possible underlying pathogenesis.

Case presentation

A 56-year-old man presented to our department with headache, vomiting, and gait disturbance (for 1 month). He had a past medical history of hepatitis type B virus infection and hepatic failure. He had been medically

* Correspondence: yositeru8_8_8simoda@yahoo.co.jp
[1]Department of Neurosurgery, South Miyagi Medical Center, 38-1 Azanishi, Ogawara-machi, Shibata-gun, Miyagi 989-1253, Japan
[2]Department of Neurosurgery, Tohoku University Graduate School of Medicine, Sendai, Japan
Full list of author information is available at the end of the article

treated for hypertension and hepatitis for the previous 4 years. On admission, he had an impaired consciousness [Glasgow coma scale (GCS), 14]. Cerebellar ataxia and gait disturbance were evident. Diffusion weighted imaging (DWI) demonstrated multiple cerebellar infarctions at several intensities with perilesional edema of the left cerebellar hemisphere (Fig. 1a, b). Brain magnetic resonance imaging (MRI) did not reveal any prominent meningeal gadolinium enhancement or nodule (Fig. 1c). MR angiography revealed no abnormal findings. The main venous sinuses were confirmed to be patent by 3-dimensional reconstructions of MRI with gadolinium (Fig. 2). Chest X-ray did not reveal any abnormal lesions, and the results of serum examination for infectious diseases, including human immunodeficiency virus (HIV), were negative except for hepatitis B virus surface antigen.

Subsequently, the patient was diagnosed with subacute cerebellar infarction due to arteriosclerosis and was administered glycerol to control the intracranial pressure; however, 1 week after admission, his GCS decreased to 11. Computed tomography confirmed worsened cerebellar edema and hydrocephalus. External and internal decompression surgery were performed to control the intracranial pressure (Fig. 3a, d). A section of the swollen cerebellar hemisphere was removed and submitted as a surgical specimen. Additionally, external continuous ventricular drainage was performed to control hydrocephalus. Lumbar puncture to collect cerebral spinal fluid (CSF) was not performed until this time because of the risk of cerebral herniation. CSF from continuous ventricular drainage demonstrated mild inflammation (cell count, 36 /mm^3; protein, 16 mg/dl; glucose, 113 mg/dl). C. neoformans was detected in CSF as well as in the surgical specimen of the cerebellum.

Histopathologic examination of the surgical specimen revealed strong hyperplasia of the arachnoid mater (Fig. 4a). Fungi were mainly localized in the subarachnoid space and rarely in the parenchyma (Fig. 4c). Lymphocytes and multinucleated giant cells forming granulomata invaded the arachnoid and subarachnoid spaces

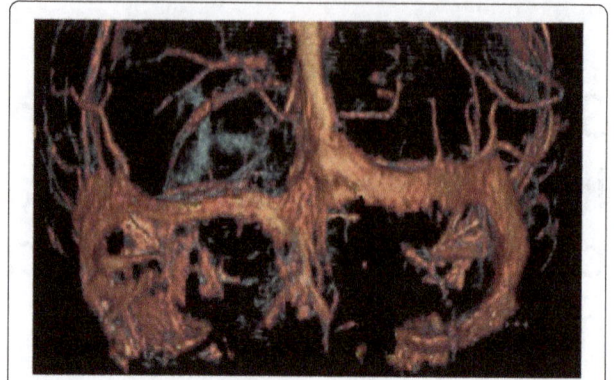

Fig. 2 Reconstruction of gadolinium enhanced magnetic resonance imaging performed on admission. Although sinus venous thrombosis was suspected to be the cause of the observed cerebellar infarction with edema, the main venous sinuses were confirmed to be patent

and pia with heavy fibrosis (Fig. 4b–f). Small arteries were occasionally observed to be occluded with internal endothelial proliferation. While there were arteries in the sample, veins were rarely observed in the subarachnoid space (Fig. 4d). In addition, venules in the parenchyma were frequently observed to be congested. The patient was diagnosed with granulomatous meningitis due to C. neoformans and was immediately treated using liposomal amphotericin B and fluconazole; however, the ischemic lesion of the cerebellum continued to bilaterally worsen along with worsening perilesional edema (Fig. 3b–f). The patient's course subsequently deteriorated. He developed renal failure and ultimately died 25 days after admission.

Autopsy confirmed that the pathological changes were confined to the central nervous system and predominantly localized at the surface of the cerebellar hemisphere. Fungal bodies were widely spread along the surface and bilaterally into the deep sulcus of the cerebellum (Fig. 4g). Few fungi were observed in the supratentorial and intraparenchymal lesions. The lesion in the arachnoid mater of the cerebellum was roughly the same as that in the surgical specimen although it was more deeply spread into the peripheral

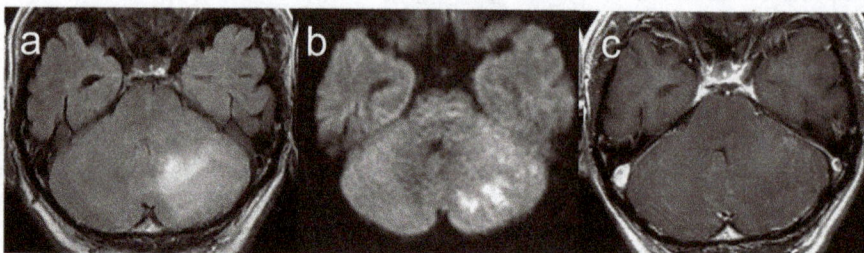

Fig. 1 Brain magnetic resonance imaging performed on admission. The findings on diffusion weighted imaging (DWI) mimicked arterial infarction of the posterior inferior cerebellar artery accompanying strong perilesional edema with almost no enhancement of the lesion. **a** Fluid-attenuated inversion recovery (FLAIR) image on admission. **b** DWI. **c** T1-weighted imaging with gadolinium enhancement

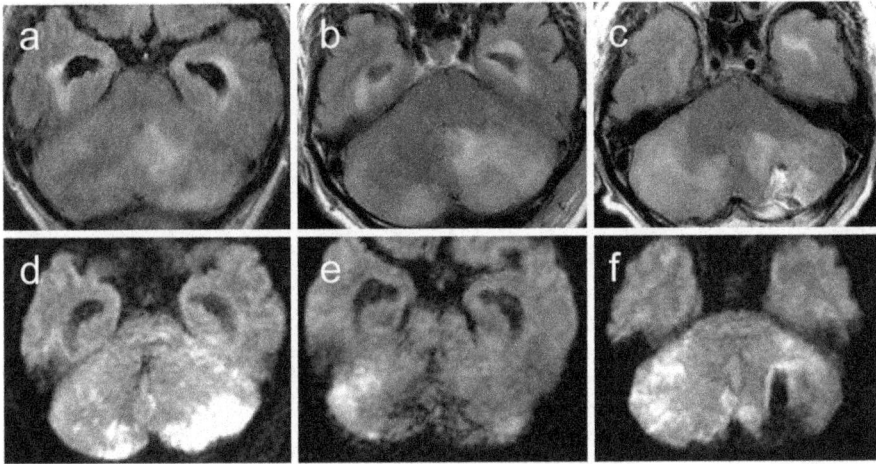

Fig. 3 Progression of cerebellar infarction in Cryptococcal meningoencephalitis. **a**, **d** FLAIR (**a**) and DWI (**d**) performed following internal and external decompression 10 days after admission. The ischemic lesion progressed to the contralateral cerebellar hemisphere with peripheral edema and ventricular dilatation unresponsive to external continuous ventricular drainage. **b**, **e**. FLAIR (**b**) and DWI (**e**) performed 17 days after admission. The ischemic and edematous lesion progressed from dorsal to ventral. **c**, **f** FLAIR (**c**) and DWI (**f**) performed 23 days after admission, 3 days before the patient died. The cerebellum had completely swollen, and tight cisterns were observed indicating brain herniation

sulcus and the granulomatous inflammation was not as severe (Fig. 4h).

Discussion

We observed two key results in this study: CM can result in massive infarction by subarachnoid small vein occlusion and an atypical infarction on MRI can be observed.

Firstly, *C. neoformans* can induce extensive subarachnoid small vein occlusion due to inflammatory fibrosis leading to poor outcomes. Generally, *C. neoformans* tends to hematogenously spread to the brain along the surface, thus inducing meningitis. When the fungi reach the perivascular space of perforating arteries, they begin to invade the perivascular space toward the deeper parts of the brain, simultaneously presenting cerebral infarction mimicking lacunar infarction; however, the mechanism of this process has not been described previously [4, 5]. In contrast, the most unprecedented finding of our case was that the fungi were present not only at the superficial subarachnoid space of the cerebellum but also diffusely spread and deeply within the sulcus (Fig. 4b–h). Peripheral subarachnoid spaces were thickened with increased internal elastic fibers (Fig. 4b–h). While small arteries showed proliferation of endothelial cells (Fig. 4d, f arrows), veins were rarely observed, which indicates that they had been compressed. Meanwhile, venules from the parenchyma were frequently observed to be congested at the entry of the fibroid subarachnoid space (Fig. 4h, arrow head). It can be speculated that the wide spread fungal involvement triggered granulomatous inflammation, which subsequently induced fibrosis. The compression of small veins in the subarachnoid space may have been due to

thickened fibroid tissue, thus blocking the venous return from the parenchyma. This may consequently lead to venous infarction with accompanying massive edema and mass effect. Although the broadly scattered fungi may underlie this pathophysiology, it was unclear how the fungi could widely invade the subarachnoid space and deeply invade the cerebellum.

Secondly, the temporal change of the infarction on MRI was unusual compared with that in the previous cases of CM. Cerebral infarctions are observed in 4–32% of patients with CM on MRI, typically lacunar at the basal ganglia [6–9]. In our case, multiple infarctions with variable phases in the left cerebellar hemisphere mimicked arterial infarctions of the posterior inferior cerebellar artery with edema on admission MRI (Fig. 1a, b). Subsequently, the ischemic lesion progressed independent of the territory of the artery (Fig. 3b–f). The lesion gradually spread from the left to the right cerebellar hemisphere and from the surface to deeper parts of the cerebellum (Fig. 3b–d). The slow progression of the initial infarction at the territory of posterior inferior cerebellar artery might may be a result of small arterial occlusion due to endothelial proliferation (Fig. 1, Fig. 4d, e), and this condition may have partly contributed to the edema. However, massive edema could not be explained by arterial occlusion alone. Together with the fact that the main venous sinuses were patent (Fig. 2) and that venules were widely congested, the massive cerebellar edema may be predominantly due to occlusion of small veins at the subarachnoid space rather than due to occlusion of large veins such as sinuses [10]. The findings on autopsy indicated that the unique

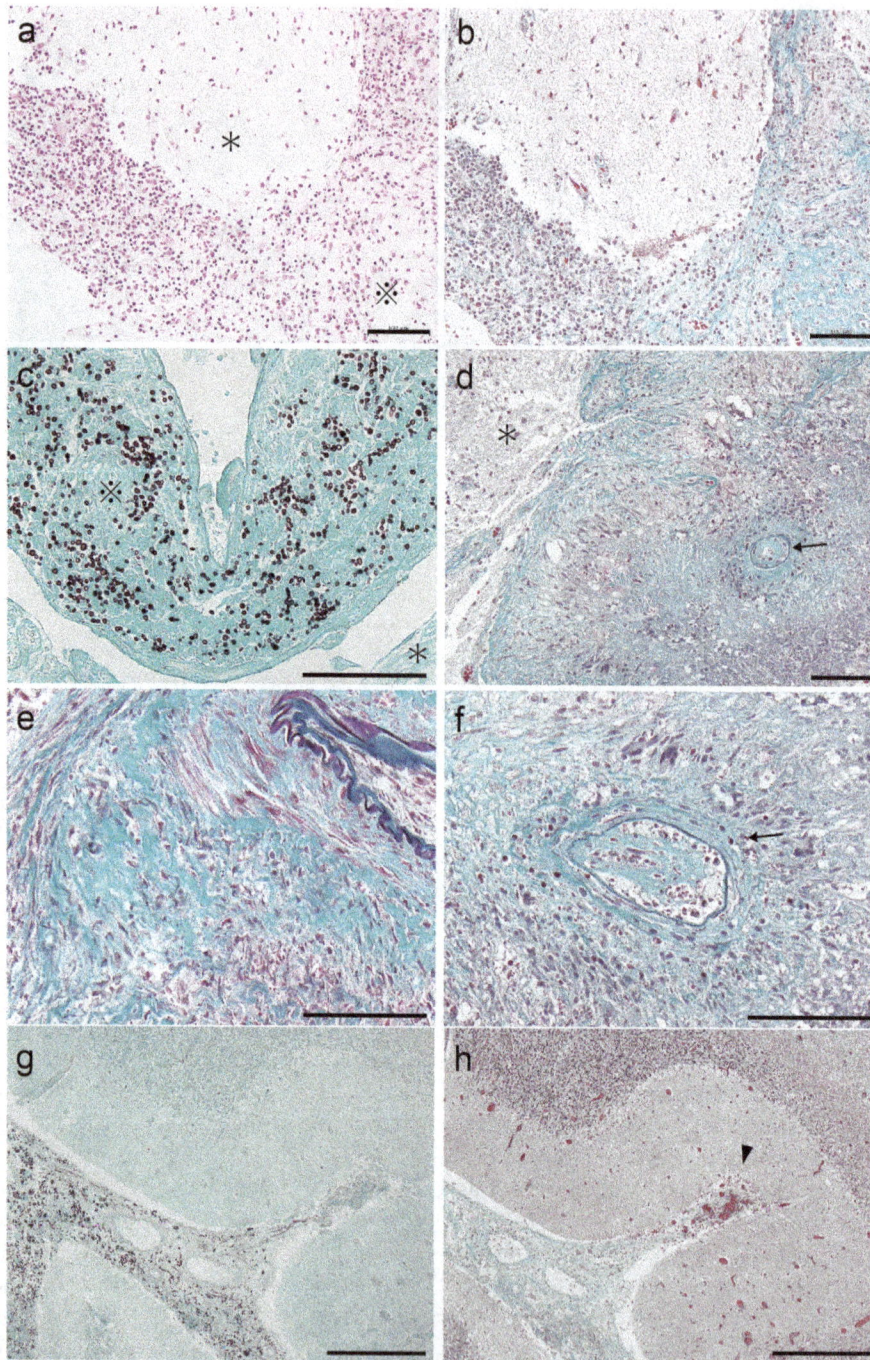

Fig. 4 Pathological findings of the cerebellum specimen. **a** Hematoxylin and Eosin staining of the left cerebellar hemisphere from the surgical specimen. The subarachnoid space was heavily thickened with inflammatory cells, which is expressed as ※. The parenchyma is expressed as *. Scale bar: 100 µm. **b** Elastica–Masson staining at the same location as in (**a**). Fibrosis was widely observed in the subarachnoid space, which appears green. Scale bar: 100 µm. **c** Grocott staining of left cerebellar hemisphere from the surgical specimen. Fungi were observed in the subarachnoid space (※) and few fungi were observed inside the parenchyma (*). Scale bar: 100 µm. **d**, **e**, **f** Elastica–Masson staining of the left cerebellar hemisphere from the surgical specimen. Strong and diffuse fibrosis was observed in the subarachnoid space (**e**). Proliferation of endothelial cells was observed inside the inner cavity of small arteries (*arrows* in **d**, **f**), which implies the slow progression of arterial occlusion. Veins were rarely observed in the subarachnoid space, which indicates that they were compressed and occluded. The parenchyma is expressed as *. Scale bar: 100 µm. **g** Grocott staining of the deep sulcus in the left cerebellar hemisphere from the autopsy specimen. The subarachnoid space was filled with fungi not only at the surface of the cerebellar hemisphere but also in the deep sulcus. Scale bar: 500 µm. **h** Elastica–Masson staining at the same location as in (**e**). Fibrosis and thickening of the subarachnoid space was observed even in the deep sulcus of the cerebellar hemisphere. Venules from the parenchyma were frequently observed to be congested at the entry to the fibrinous subarachnoid space (*arrow head*). Scale bar: 500 µm

progression of the ischemic and edematous lesion on MRI reflected the invasion of the fungi and aggressive fibrosis.

Some cases of CM are known to present with fulminant intracranial pressure elevation, which leads to brain herniation and death [11–16]. Zhu reported that cerebral herniation was observed in 30 (19.5%) of 154 non-HIV patients with CM reviewed in their study. In 30 patients who presented with cerebral herniation, 21 died within a year of the diagnosis and 11 within a week, 10 of whom died due to cerebral herniation. They also found that cerebral herniation was one of the crucial and independent factors for poor prognosis in patients with CM [11]. Thus, although cerebral herniation is known to be the most common cause of death in patients with CM, the mechanisms of herniation are not well described. Hydrocephalus due to impaired absorption or obstruction of CSF may be one of the primary reasons for cerebral herniation [12, 17]. The temporal change of the MRI and the findings from autopsy indicate that subarachnoid vein occlusion is a potential mechanism for massive brain edema and an aggressive clinical course in CM. When the fungi broadly and deeply spread into the sulcus of the cerebellum, inflammatory fibrosis widely occurs and might lead to venule congestion and, ultimately, to life threatening massive brain edema. Infarction in lesions, independent of the vascular territory, may be a sign of the progression of fibrosis of the subarachnoid space and decreased compliance of the brain. To our knowledge, this is the first case demonstrating the clinical course and pathological findings of subarachnoid vein occlusion caused by *C. neoformans*. Further reports are necessary to characterize the time course of *C. neoformans* in the central nervous system.

Conclusions

In conclusion, we suggest that CM induces subarachnoid small vein occlusion via inflammatory fibrosis, which leads to an aggressive and fatal clinical course. In this case, the temporal change in perifocal edema and ischemic lesions suggested an etiology different from that of a simple arterial infarction. Hence, CM should be considered as a cause of progressive cerebral infarction even in the absence of prior HIV.

Abbreviations
CM: Cryptococcal meningoencephalitis; DWI: Diffusion weighted image; FLAIR: Fluid-attenuated inversion recovery; GCS: Glasgow coma scale; MRI: Magnetic resonance imaging

Acknowledgments
The authors thank Enago (http://www.enago.com) for the English language review.

Funding
None of the authors have received any financial assistance for this manuscript.

Authors' contributions
YS, SO, and HA collected the data, designed, and wrote the manuscript. TT wrote and gave the final approval of the manuscript. HA and SO were involved with the clinical care of the patient. TO preformed the histological examination and interpreted the data. All authors read and approved the final manuscript.

Competing interests
The authors declare that they have no competing interests.

Author details
[1]Department of Neurosurgery, South Miyagi Medical Center, 38-1 Azanishi, Ogawara-machi, Shibata-gun, Miyagi 989-1253, Japan. [2]Department of Neurosurgery, Tohoku University Graduate School of Medicine, Sendai, Japan. [3]Department of Pathology, South Miyagi Medical Center, Shibata-gun, Miyagi, Japan.

References
1. Williamson PR, Jarvis JN, Panackal AA, Fisher MC, Molloy SF, Loyse A, et al. Cryptococcal meningitis: epidemiology, immunology, diagnosis and therapy. Nat Rev Neurol. 2017;13(1):13–24.
2. Ye S, Yang C-d. Central nervous system infections in the systemic vasculitides. Curr Opin Neurol. 2015;4(1):96–104.
3. Sarkis RA, Mays M, Isada C, Ahmed M. MRI findings in cryptococcal meningitis of the non-HIV population. Neurologist. 2015;19(2):40–5.
4. Klock C, Cerski M, Goldani LZ. Histopathological aspects of neurocryptococcosis in HIV-infected patients: autopsy report of 45 patients. Int J Surg Pathol. 2009;17(6):444–8.
5. Lee SC, Dickson DW, Casadevall A. Pathology of cryptococcal meningoencephalitis: analysis of 27 patients with pathogenetic implications. Hum Pathol. 1996;27(8):839–47.
6. Tien RD, Chu PK, Hesselink JR, Duberg A, Wiley C. Intracranial cryptococcosis in immunocompromised patients: CT and MR findings in 29 cases. AJNR Am J Neuroradiol. 1991;12(2):283–9.
7. Lan SH, Chang WN, Lu CH, Lui CC, Chang HW. Cerebral infarction in chronic meningitis: a comparison of tuberculous meningitis and cryptococcal meningitis. QJM. 2001;94(5):247–53.
8. Chen S-F, Lu C-H, Lui C-C, Huang C-R, Chuang Y-C, Tan T-Y, et al. Acute/subacute cerebral infarction (ASCI) in HIV-negative adults with cryptococcal meningoencephalitis (CM): a MRI-based follow-up study and a clinical comparison to HIV-negative CM adults without ASCI. BMC Neurol. 2011; 11(1):12.
9. Xia S, Li X, Shi Y, Liu J, Zhang M, Gu T, et al. A retrospective cohort study of lesion distribution of HIV-1 infection patients with cryptococcal meningoencephalitis on MRI: correlation with immunity and immune reconstitution. Medicine (Baltimore). 2016;95(6):e2654.
10. Senadim S, Alpaydin BS, Tekin GB, Dedei DM, Kantaroglu E, Ozturk O, et al. A rare cause of cerebral venous thrombosis: cryptococcal meningoencephalitis. Neurol Sci. 2016;37:1145–8.
11. Zhu L-P, Wu J-Q, Xu B, Ou X-T, Zhang Q-Q, Weng X-H. Cryptococcal meningitis in non-HIV-infected patients in a Chinese tertiary care hospital, 1997–2007. Med Mycol. 2010;48(4):570–9.
12. Orsini J, Blaak C, Mahmoud D, Young-Gwang J. Massive cerebral edema resulting in brain death as a complication of Cryptococcus neoformans meningitis. J Community Hosp Intern Med Perspect. 2015;5(1):26098.
13. Hamilton RL, Lane H, Browne L, Delanty N, Neill SO, Thornton J, et al. 40-year-old man with headaches and dyspnea. Brain Pathol. 2005;15(1):89–90.
14. Teo YK. Cryptococcal meningoencephalitis with fulminant intracranial hypertension: An unexpected case of brain death. Singap Med J. 2010;51: e133–6.
15. Bromilow J, Corcoran T. Cryptococcus gattii infection causing fulminant intracranial hypertension. Br J Anaesth. 2007;99:528–31.
16. Terada T. Cryptococcosis in the central nervous system in a 36-year-old Japanese man: an autopsy study. Tohoku J Exp Med. 2010;222(1):33–7.

10

Usefulness of intraoperative insular electrocorticography in modified functional hemispherectomy

Gun-Ha Kim[1,2], Joo Hee Seo[2], James E. Baumgartner[2], Fatima Ajmal[2] and Ki Hyeong Lee[2*] (iD)

Abstract

Background: The insular cortex is not routinely removed in modified functional hemispherectomy due to the risk of injury to the main arteries and to deep structures. Our study evaluates the safety and usefulness of applying intraoperative electrocorticography (ECoG) on the insular during the hemispherectomy.

Methods: We included all patients who underwent insular ECoG during a modified functional hemispherectomy from 2012 to 2015. After the surgery, the decision for further resection of the insular cortex was made based on the presence of electrographic seizures on ECoG.

Results: The study included 19 patients (age, 6.4 ± 4.7 years, mean ± standard deviation). Electrographic seizures were identified in 5 patients (26.3%). Sixteen of the 19 patients (84.2%) became seizure-free with a follow-up duration of 3.1 ± 0.6 years and no vascular complication occurred.

Conclusions: Intraoperative insular ECoG monitoring can be performed safely while providing a tailored approach for insular resection during modified hemispherectomy.

Keywords: Insular cortex, Epilepsy, Epilepsy surgery, Seizure, Child, Pediatric

Background

In the literature, the seizure outcome after hemispherectomy in children varies from 52 to 80% upon follow-up 1 year after surgery, and remains stable beyond 5 years at 58–63% [1–5]. The most common cause of surgical failure after hemispherectomy is incomplete disconnection [2]. Common areas of interest include the corpus callosum, frontal basal cortex, and insular cortex. With the use of intraoperative magnetic resonance imaging (MRI), we can complete the disconnection of the epileptic hemisphere to the remaining structures in the corpus callosum or frontal basal cortex with high reliability. Although there is a high possibility of insular involvement in intractable epilepsy suggesting hemispheric pathology, the insular cortex is not routinely removed, unless epileptogenic, due to the risk of injury to the main arteries on the

surface of the insula and deep structures such as the basal ganglia. An insular seizure is not easily distinguishable from frontal- or temporal-onset seizures based on scalp electroencephalography (EEG) or clinical semiology [6–10]. Since techniques like MRI and positron emission tomography (PET) are not sensitive enough to examine the extent of the involvement of the insular cortex in the epileptogenic zone, stereo-electroencephalography or magnetoencephalography (MEG) are often used [9, 10].

This study aimed to evaluate the safety and usefulness of applying intraoperative insular electro-corticography (ECoG) in modified functional hemispherectomy.

Methods

Patients

We included all patients who underwent intraoperative ECoG monitoring on the insular cortex during modified functional hemispherectomy, at Florida Hospital for

* Correspondence: kihyeong.lee.md@flhosp.org; kilee1024@gmail.com
[2]Comprehensive Epilepsy Center, Florida Hospital for Children and Florida Hospital, 615 E. Rollins Street, Orlando, FL 32803, USA
Full list of author information is available at the end of the article

Children, from January 2012 to September 2015, and reviewed medical records retrospectively.

Preoperative workup

Patients underwent detailed preoperative evaluation including prolonged video-EEG, 3-Tesla MRI (Siemens Healthcare, Erlangen, Germany), PET with F-18 fluoro-deoxyglucose, ictal and interictal technetium 99 m single photon emission computed tomography with subsequent subtraction ictal SPECT co-registered with MRI, and neuropsychological evaluation. If required, MEG, functional MRI, and a Wada test were performed. The surgical decision for hemispherectomy was made based on the consensus of the epilepsy board meeting.

Intraoperative procedures

Each patient underwent a modified functional hemispherectomy. After the hemispherectomy without insular resection, ECoG was recorded from frontal and temporal sides of the exposed insular cortex. We used an 8-contact strip electrodes for monitoring insular ECoG and monitored for 3–6 min on each side of insula. Total intravenous anaesthesia with Propofol and Fentanyl was used to minimize effect on cortical electrical activity during ECoG. No pharmacological activation was introduced during the recording. We removed the insular cortex if an electrographic seizure was recorded on the insular ECoG.

Pathology results and outcome

Pathological findings were reported based on the consensus of International League Against Epilepsy (ILAE) diagnostic methods commission [11]. The seizure outcome was classified based on the ILAE classifications [12].

Results

Patient profile

A total of 19 patients were included in the current study (Table 1). Five patients (26.3%) had epilepsy surgery before hemispherectomy, three (15.8%) patients had an MRI suggestive of insular involvement (Fig. 1a), and four (21.1%) patients underwent intracranial EEG monitoring to confirm hemispheric involvement, since their MRIs did not clearly show hemispheric pathology (data not shown).

Intraoperative insular electrocorticography

In the entire cohort, electrographic seizures were identified in five patients (26.3%) by post-resection intraoperative ECoG on the insular cortex (Fig. 1b), of whom one patient had previous epileptic surgery, while another had brain tumor surgery after birth. Further, of the five patients, one had Rasmussen encephalitis, one had hemimegalencephaly, and three

Table 1 Demographic data of patients with hemispherectomy

Total number of patients (N)	19
Sex, male/female (N)	8/11
Age at seizure onset, year, mean ± SD	1.2 ± 1.7
Age at surgery, year, mean ± SD	6.4 ± 4.7
Seizure duration, year, mean ± SD	5.32 ± 4.5
Number of seizures, per week, mean ± SD	28.0 ± 27.6
Epilepsy surgery prior to hemispherectomy (N)	
None	14
Lobectomy/topectomy ± corpus callosotomy	4
Corpus callosotomy only	1

N number of patients

had diffuse malformation of cortical development (MCD). The characteristics of the patient with positive insular seizure are shown in Table 2.

Consistency between MRI and ECoG

As noted in Table 3, MRI was not always predictive of the presence of an insular seizure: MR fluid-attenuated inversion recovery (FLAIR) image showed no abnormality on insular cortex in 3 of 5 patients with an insular seizure, while MRI was abnormal on insular cortex in one patient without an insular seizure.

Presence of insular seizure according to etiology

Histopathological analyses revealed MCD as the most common etiology (10/19, 52.6%, Table 4), followed by perinatal stroke (6/19, 31.6%). Of them, insular seizures were identified on ECoG in 5 patients (26.3%) and pathology showed as follows: one with hemimegalencephaly, one with Rasmussen and three with diffuse malformations of cortical development. None of six perinatal stroke patients showed electrographic seizures on the insular ECoG. However, this difference was not statistically significant ($P = 0.128$).

Outcome

In the current study, 16 of the 19 patients (84.2%) became seizure free with a median follow-up of 3.1 ± 0.6 years (mean ± standard deviation) (Table 5). Four out of 5 patients (80%) with electrographic seizures on insular ECoG became seizure-free and one patient had breakthrough seizures with the onset from basal frontal brain area. Twelve of 14 patients (80%) without insular ECoG abnormality became seizure-free. Two patients with abnormality on both imaging and ECoG and one patient with an abnormal imaging but normal ECoG became seizure-free after surgery. Two patients developed hydrocephalus, and the disconnection was incomplete in the corpus callosum or basal frontal area in

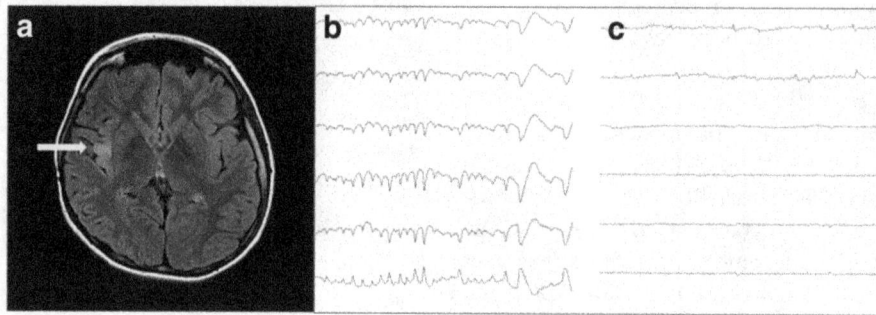

Fig. 1 Insular hyperintensity shown on fluid-attenuated inversion-recovery MRI. 3-Tesla axial fluid-attenuated inversion-recovery images at the insular level show insular hyperintensity (**a**, arrow). The patient had an electrographic seizure on frontal strip of insular ECoG (**b**), which disappeared after insular resection (**c**)

three patients. None of the patients developed peri-operative stroke.

Discussion

In the current study, although electrographic seizures were detected on the insular ECoG in five patients (5/19; 26.3%), only two of these patients demonstrated subtle high signal intensity in the insular cortex on FLAIR images. These five patients underwent removal of the insular cortex in addition to functional hemispherectomy, and 84.2% of the patients in the current cohort were seizure-free with a mean follow-up duration of 3.1 years.

We believe the use of insular ECoG should be considered in all modified hemispherectomy cases for two reasons. Firstly, there is a relatively high possibility of insular involvement in hemispherectomy candidates. The existence of bidirectional interconnections between the amygdalo-hippocampal formation and the insula was confirmed by an electrophysiological study [13]. Given that the amygdalo-hippocampal formation is the most commonly involved brain structure in intractable epilepsy, the insular cortex should be considered the critical part of the epileptic network in these children. The residual insular cortex was positively correlated with persistent postoperative seizures in failed hemispherectomy patients [14].

Secondly, insular seizures could be indistinguishable from frontal or temporal lobe onset seizures [6–10]. The insular cortex is deeply located, buried in the lateral sulcus, and covered by the operculum, making it hard to detect using scalp EEG.

Although some previous research favored insular removal in hemispherectomy [15–17], others did not support it [2, 18]. Some centers routinely remove the insular cortex during hemispherectomy to prevent the potential development of persistent seizures [19, 20]. However, the routine removal of the insular cortex is not widely accepted at this point, due to the risk of injury to arteries and deep structures surrounding the insula (the average distance from the limen insulae to the putamen is only 5.7 mm [21]).

The current study also suggests the possible correlation between the pathology and the insular seizures on ECoG, although it did not reach the clinical significance.

Table 2 Characteristics of patients who had electrographic seizures on insular cortex during post-resection electrocorticography

Patient	Seizure		Past surgery	Scalp EEG		MRI	FDGPET	SPM PET	SISCOM
	Onset age, year	Frequency (per week)		Interictal	Ictal				
1	0.2	14	None	Lt/H	Lt/T, Lt/F	Hemi-megalencephaly	Lt/H	Lt/H	Lt/H
2	1.5	21	Rt/T lobectomy	Rt/F	Rt/H	Diffuse MCD	Rt/H	Rt/H	-
3	2.0	21	None	Rt/FC	Rt/FC	Diffuse MCD	Rt/H	Rt/H	-
4	5.0	70	None	Lt/H	Lt/H	Rasmussen encephalitis	Lt/H	-	-
5	0.1	70	Brain tumor resection after birth	Lt/H	Lt/H	Diffuse MCD	Lt/H	-	-

EEG electroencephalography, *FDG PET* 18 fluoro-2-deoxyglucose positron emission tomography scan, *MRI* magnetic resonance imaging, *SPM* statistical parametric mapping, *SISCOM* Subtraction ictal SPECT co-registered to MRI, *Lt* Left, *Rt* Right, *H* hemisphere, *F* frontal, *T* temporal, *FC* fronto-central, *MCD* malformations of cortical development, – not available

Table 3 Consistency between FLAIR MRI and intraoperative insular electrocorticography (N)

	High signal intensity on insular cortex on FLAIR image	
	Present	Absent
Insular seizure Present 2		3
Absent 1		13

N number of patients, FLAIR Fluid-attenuated inversion recovery

Except one patient with Rasmussen encephalitis, all 4 patients with electrographic seizures on insular ECoG had a developmental etiology; three had MCD and one had hemimegalencephaly. None of the five perinatal stroke patients showed insular seizure. These results suggest that developmental malformation commonly occurs in a more diffuse pattern, increasing the chances of insular cortex involvement. Due to the small number of patients in each pathology group, further research is required to validate the correlation between pathology and the involvement of the insular cortex in the epileptic network.

Our data support the use of insular ECoG as a safe and sensitive method to detect insular involvement in hemispherectomy patients. None of the 19 patients developed stroke or infection.

Limitations in the current study must be noted. The average duration of postoperative follow-up was less than 5 years. A recent multicenter study suggested that complications such as hydrocephalus could occur even after 8.5 years [22] and seizure outcome may change with a longer duration of follow-up [4]. In addition, intraoperative ECoG findings are not always predictive of postoperative seizure recurrence. Only a randomized controlled study could answer whether insular ECoG truly contributes to a better surgical outcome following hemispherectomy.

Table 4 Presence of insular seizure according to pathology

Pathology	Total patients	Presence of Insular seizure on ECoG (N)	p-value
Developmental			0.128
Malformation of cortical development	10	3	
Hemimegalencephaly	1	1	
Inflammation			
Rasmussen encephalitis	2	1	
Vascular			
Perinatal stroke	6	0	

N number of patients, ECoG electrocorticography
Fisher's exact test, statistical significance with p < 0.05

Table 5 Seizure outcome and surgical complication (total patients = 19)

Seizure-free	
Total	16/19 (84.2%)
Patients with insular seizure on ECoG	4/5 (80%)[a]
Complication	
Stroke	0
Infection	0
Hydrocephalus	2
Incomplete resection[b]	3

Data are number (%) or number unless otherwise stated. Mean follow-up duration of 3.1 (±0.6) years; [a] One patient had breakthrough seizures from basal frontal area of brain. [b] Incomplete resection on corpus callosum or basal frontal area, ECoG electrocorticography

Conclusions

Intraoperative insular ECoG monitoring could be performed safely without adding risk while providing a tailored approach to insular removal. Patients with developmental malformation may benefit from this approach.

Abbreviations
ECoG: Electrocorticography; EEG: Electroencephalography; FLAIR: Fluid-attenuated inversion recovery; ILAE: International League Against Epilepsy; MCD: Malformations of cortical development; MRI: Magnetic resonance imaging; PET: Positron emission tomography

Acknowledgements
None.

Funding
This research received no specific grant from any funding agency in the public, commercial, or not-for-profit sectors.

Authors' contributions
GHK acquired the data, conducted all of the data analyses and wrote the article. JHS and FA helped providing data, interpreted the data, and checked the final version of the article. KHL and JEB conceptualized the study design, analyzed and interpreted the data and revised the article. All of the authors read and approved the final version of the manuscript.

Author details
[1]Department of Pediatrics, College of Medicine, Korea University, Seoul, South Korea. [2]Comprehensive Epilepsy Center, Florida Hospital for Children and Florida Hospital, 615 E. Rollins Street, Orlando, FL 32803, USA.

References
1. Hamad AP, Caboclo LO, Centeno R, Costa LV, Ladeia-Frota C, Carrete Junior H, Gomez NG, Marinho M, Yacubian EMT, Sakamoto AC. Hemispheric surgery for refractory epilepsy in children and adolescents: outcome regarding seizures, motor skills and adaptive function. Seizure. 2013;22(9):752–6.
2. González-Martínez JA, Gupta A, Kotagal P, Lachhwani D, Wyllie E, Lüders HO, Bingaman WE. Hemispherectomy for catastrophic epilepsy in infants. Epilepsia. 2005;46(9):1518–25.

3. Lettori D, Battaglia D, Sacco A, Veredice C, Chieffo D, Massimi L, Tartaglione T, Chiricozzi F, Staccioli S, Mittica A. Early hemispherectomy in catastrophic epilepsy: a neuro-cognitive and epileptic long-term follow-up. Seizure. 2008;17(1):49–63.

4. Moosa AN, Gupta A, Jehi L, Marashly A, Cosmo G, Lachhwani D, Wyllie E, Kotagal P, Bingaman W. Longitudinal seizure outcome and prognostic predictors after hemispherectomy in 170 children. Neurology. 2013;80(3):253–60.

5. Jonas R, Nguyen S, Hu B, Asarnow R, LoPresti C, Curtiss S, De Bode S, Yudovin S, Shields W, Vinters H. Cerebral hemispherectomy hospital course, seizure, developmental, language, and motor outcomes. Neurology. 2004; 62(10):1712–21.

6. Ryvlin P, Minotti L, Demarquay G, Hirsch E, Arzimanoglou A, Hoffman D, Guénot M, Picard F, Rheims S, Kahane P. Nocturnal hypermotor seizures, suggesting frontal lobe epilepsy, can originate in the insula. Epilepsia. 2006;47(4):755–65.

7. Dobesberger J, Ortler M, Unterberger I, Walser G, Falkenstetter T, Bodner T, Benke T, Bale R, Fiegele T, Donnemiller E. Successful surgical treatment of insular epilepsy with nocturnal hypermotor seizures. Epilepsia. 2008;49(1):159–62.

8. Levitt MR, Ojemann JG, Kuratani J. Insular epilepsy masquerading as multifocal cortical epilepsy as proven by depth electrode: case report. J Neurosurg Pediatr. 2010;5(4):365–7.

9. Heers M, Rampp S, Stefan H, Urbach H, Elger CE, von Lehe M, Wellmer J. MEG-based identification of the epileptogenic zone in occult peri-insular epilepsy. Seizure. 2012;21(2):128–33.

10. Dylgjeri S, Taussig D, Chipaux M, Lebas A, Fohlen M, Bulteau C, Ternier J, Ferrand-Sorbets S, Delalande O, Isnard J. Insular and insulo-opercular epilepsy in childhood: an SEEG study. Seizure. 2014;23(4):300–8.

11. Blümcke I, Thom M, Aronica E, Armstrong DD, Vinters HV, Palmini A, Jacques TS, Avanzini G, Barkovich AJ, Battaglia G. The clinicopathologic spectrum of focal cortical dysplasias: a consensus classification proposed by an ad hoc task force of the ILAE diagnostic methods Commission1. Epilepsia. 2011;52(1):158–74.

12. Wieser H, Blume W, Fish D, Goldensohn E, Hufnagel A, King D, Sperling M, Lüders H, Pedley TA. Proposal for a new classification of outcome with respect to epileptic seizures following epilepsy surgery. Epilepsia. 2001;42(2):282–6.

13. Zonjy B, Alkhachroum A, Kahriman E, Lacuey N, Miller J, Luders H. Functional connectivity between Insula, hippocampus, and Amygdala investigated using Cortico-cortical evoked potentials (CCEPs)(S50. 005). Neurology. 2014;82(Suppl 10):S50–005.

14. Cats EA, Kho KH, Van Nieuwenhuizen O, Van Veelen CW, Gosselaar PH, Van Rijen PC. Seizure freedom after functional hemispherectomy and a possible role for the insular cortex: the Dutch experience. J Neurosurg Pediatr. 2007;107(4):275–80.

15. Cook SW, Nguyen ST, Hu B, Yudovin S, Shields WD, Vinters HV, BMVd W, Harrison RE, Mathern GW. Cerebral hemispherectomy in pediatric patients with epilepsy: comparison of three techniques by pathological substrate in 115 patients. J Neurosurg Pediatr. 2004;100(2):125–41.

16. Kaido T, Otsuki T, Kakita A, Sugai K, Saito Y, Sakakibara T, Takahashi A, Kaneko Y, Saito Y, Takahashi H. Novel pathological abnormalities of deep brain structures including dysplastic neurons in anterior striatum associated with focal cortical dysplasia in epilepsy: clinical article. J Neurosurg Pediatr. 2012;10(3):217–25.

17. Nguyen DK, Nguyen DB, Malak R, Leroux JM, Carmant L, Saint-Hilaire JM, Giard N, Cossette P, Bouthillier A. Revisiting the role of the insula in refractory partial epilepsy. Epilepsia. 2009;50(3):510–20.

18. Villemure J, Mascott C, Andermann F, Rasmussen T. Is removal of the insular cortex in hemispherectomy necessary. Epilepsia. 1989;30(Suppl):728.

19. Schramm J, Kuczaty S, Sassen R, Elger C, von Lehe M. Pediatric functional hemispherectomy: outcome in 92 patients. Acta Neurochir. 2012;154(11):2017–28.

20. Villemure J-G, Mascott CR. Peri-insular hemispherotomy: surgical principles and anatomy. Neurosurgery. 1995;37(5):975–81.

21. Tanriover N, Rhoton AL Jr, Kawashima M, Ulm AJ, Yasuda A. Microsurgical anatomy of the insula and the sylvian fissure. J Neurosurg. 2004;100(5):891–922.

22. Lew SM, Matthews AE, Hartman AL, Haranhalli N. Posthemispherectomy hydrocephalus: results of a comprehensive, multiinstitutional review. Epilepsia. 2013;54(2):383–9.

11

MOG antibody seropositivity in a patient with encephalitis: beyond the classical syndrome

Sara Mariotto[1,2*] (iD), Salvatore Monaco[1], Patrick Peschl[2], Ilaria Coledan [3], Romualdo Mazzi[3], Romana Höftberger[4], Markus Reindl[2] and Sergio Ferrari[1]

Abstract

Background: The presence of circulating anti-myelin oligodendrocyte glycoprotein antibodies (MOG-Abs) has been described in sera of patients with different inflammatory conditions of the central nervous system. In adults the core clinical feature is usually characterised by acute myelitis and/or optic neuritis. We here report an atypical case with serum and cerebrospinal fluid MOG-Abs and a clinical picture suggestive for acute encephalitis.

Case presentation: A 31-year-old Indian man presented with altered mental status, slight fever, and ataxia. Brain magnetic resonance imaging noted a widespread involvement of the white matter associated with slight cortical and subcortical damage in absence of contrast enhancement. An extensive infectious screening resulted negative while autoimmune analysis revealed the presence of MOG-Abs, detected with live cell-based assay. After treatment with intravenous immunoglobulins a marked and prompt clinical and radiological improvement was observed.

Conclusions: To date, several areas of uncertainty still remain regarding clinical features and prognosis of subjects with MOG-Abs. The description of atypical cases is crucial, since recognition of this condition leads to prompt treatment and better prognosis, as in the case here reported.

Keywords: Autoimmune diseases, Encephalitis, Anti-myelin oligodendrocyte glycoprotein antibodies (MOG-abs)

Background

Anti-myelin oligodendrocyte glycoprotein antibodies (MOG-Abs) have been reported in different inflammatory demyelinating diseases as acute disseminated encephalomyelitis (ADEM), neuromyelitis optica spectrum disorders (NMOSD), idiopathic optic neuritis, idiopathic myelitis, and atypical multiple sclerosis [1–13]. However, the whole spectrum of clinical phenotypes associated with MOG-Abs-related disorders has still to be clearly defined. Here, we present a patient with MOG-Abs and a clinical picture resembling infectious encephalitis as a possible new clinical phenotype associated with these antibodies.

* Correspondence: sara.mariotto@gmail.com
[1]Department of Neuroscience, Biomedicine and Movement Sciences, Section of Neurology, University of Verona, Verona, Italy
[2]Clinical Department of Neurology, Medical University of Innsbruck, Innsbruck, Austria
Full list of author information is available at the end of the article

Case presentation

A previously healthy 31-year-old Indian man presented to the emergency room with confusion and altered consciousness. Five days prior to onset of neurological symptoms he developed slight fever (<38 °C), sore throat and headache. His past medical history was unremarkable except for a recent stay in India for 2 months. Neurological examination disclosed a wide-based and unsteady gait and reduced level of consciousness. Diffuse papules and enanthema were also observed and spontaneously disappeared few days later. A slight increase of erythrocyte and leukocyte cell counts (13.000 cells/μL), erythrocyte sedimentation rate (30 mm/h) and C-reactive protein (48 mg/l) was noted on basic laboratory test. The patient was initially treated with acyclovir and ceftriaxone for a presumptive diagnosis of infectious encephalitis. A cerebrospinal fluid (CSF) analysis showed total protein level of 53 mg/dl, 179 cells/µL (90% mononuclear) in absence of oligoclonal IgG bands. On brain magnetic resonance imaging (MRI), fluid attenuated inversion recovery (FLAIR) and T2 diffuse hyperintensities involving thalamus, basal ganglia, internal capsule, mesial temporal lobes and brainstem associated with small hyperintensities in the subcortical, periventricular and cortical regions were noted in absence of contrast enhancement (Fig. 1a-d). Diffusion weighted images showed a mild restrictive pattern of the sopratentorial lesions affecting the left and right thalamus, the posterior limb of the internal capsule of both sides, the splenium and the posterior profile of the left trigonum. These lesions also presented medium-high apparent diffusion coefficient values and central core of low apparent diffusion coefficient, suggesting an inflammatory process. Whole spinal cord MRI was normal. A comprehensive workup for viral encephalitis and atypical infections including polymerase chain reaction for *Human immunodeficiency virus, Enterovirus, Herpes simplex 1–2-6, Epstein-Barr, Cytomegalovirus, Varicella Zoster, Toxoplasma, Mycobacterium tuberculosis, Treponema pallidum, Bartonella henselae, Human Parechovirus, West Nile, Dengue, Chikungunya,* and *Japanese encephalitis* resulted negative and also cultures for bacteria and fungi. An extensive autoimmune screening including anti-nuclear antibodies, complement levels,

thyroid function and antibodies, autoantibodies to synaptic receptors and neuronal cell surface proteins was also negative. The criteria for collagen diseases, vasculitis, Behçet and Hashimoto encephalopathy were not satisfied. No neuropil staining was observed on tissue-based screening with immunohistochemistry on rat sections. Testing for MOG-Abs with a live cell-based assay with recombinant full-length MOG expressed in HEK293 cells [14], identified MOG-Abs both in the serum (titer of 1:5120) and in the CSF (titer 1:8). Staining of rat brain tissue with serum and CSF samples resulted in a specific myelin staining already described for MOG-Abs as shown in Fig. 2 [15]. The patient was treated with intravenous immunoglobulin (IVIg) 0.5 g/kg/day for 5 days with an almost complete clinical recovery in a few days. On control MRI examination after 2 weeks a dramatic improvement of pre-existing lesion was observed (Fig. 1e-h). Only the persistence of slight unsteady gait was noted at the last clinical evaluation 2 weeks after the onset.

Discussion and conclusions

We here report an atypical presentation of MOG-Abs associated disorder with a prompt response to IVIg which satisfied the criteria of "possible encephalitis of presumed infectious origin" which also was the main presumptive clinical diagnosis [16]. Since the patient

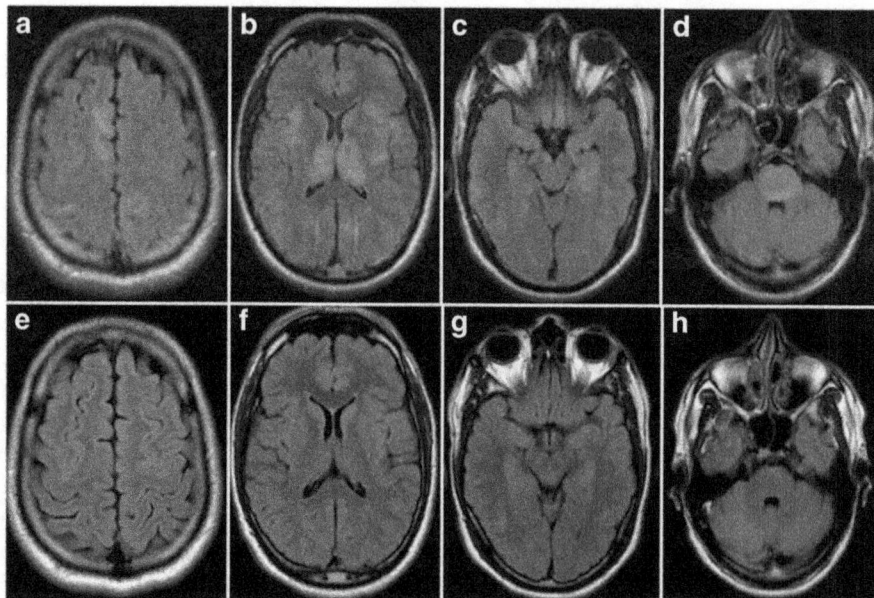

Fig. 1 FLAIR sequence from the brain MRI at onset (**a-d**) and after treatment (**e-h**). Cortical and subcortical damage (**a-b**) with severe bilateral involvement of thalamus and internal capsule (**b**), mesial temporal lobes (**c**) and pons (**d**) in absence of contrast enhancement, is seen on brain MRI performed ad onset. After treatment with IVIg a significant improvement was noted with an almost complete resolution of the cortical, thalamic and basal ganglia involvement (**e-f**) and a reduction of temporal (**g**) and brainstem lesions (**h**)

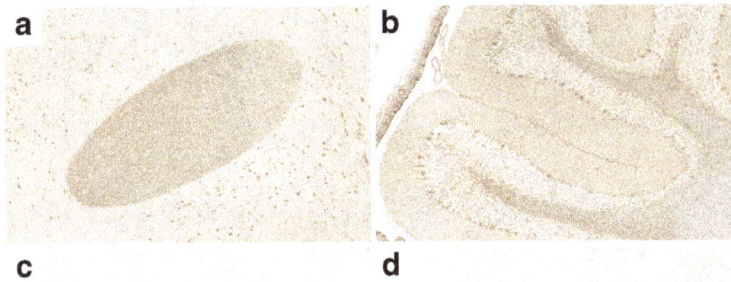

Fig. 2 Immunohistochemical analysis. Serum (dilution 1:100, MOG-IgG and IgG1 titer 1:5120, also reactive with rat and mouse MOG) and CSF (dilution 1:2, MOG-ab titer 1:8) samples were screened by immunohistochemistry on a tissue-based assay (in-house; avidin-biotin-peroxidase technique; rat brain) as described previously by Sepulveda et al. 2016 [15]. The CSF (diluted 1:2) showed a specific myelin staining in the anterior commissure (**a**) and cerebellar white matter (**b**), whereas a control sample was negative (**c**, **d**). Magnification: A, C: ×100; B, D: ×60

presented with subacute onset of altered mental status, new focal central nervous system findings and CSF pleocytosis in absence of alternative causes, he also met the revised diagnostic criteria for possible autoimmune encephalitis recently proposed [17]. However, the absence of neuropil staining on immunohistochemistry ruled out the presence of other well defined auto-antibodies or overlapping syndromes. In the case here reported, some features, as the multiple sopratentorial lesions of the white matter, basal ganglia, thalamus and brainstem, resemble those observed in ADEM. However, pleocytosis was higher than that usually observed in patients with ADEM and MRI was not totally compatible due to the type of gray and periventricular involvement and the absence of spinal cord lesions. Since criteria for ADEM have been clearly established only for pediatric cases [18] and the diagnosis in adults, also with MOG-Abs, remain challenging [17], we classified the case as "encephalitis" rather than ADEM.

Only five cases of encephalitis with MOG-Abs have been reported so far and are summarized in Table 1 [19, 20].

In these reports an autoimmune aetiology was the main presumptive diagnosis while in the case here described clinical and radiological data were suggestive of an infectious process. Moreover, all the previously reported cases presented seizures at onset or during the course of the disease and 3 out of 5 patients had optic neuritis, a feature clearly associated with MOG-Abs. The radiological features here described are also unique and in part different from the ADEM-like [19] or unilateral cortical lesions [20] previously reported. In these cases the onset was characterised by an exclusive cortical damage and in only one patient the involvement of corpus callosum, cingulate gyrus, frontal lobes, midbrain, thalamus, and nucleus basalis was noted during the follow-up [19]. In our patient we observed at onset an extensive involvement of the thalamus, basal ganglia, internal capsule, mesial temporal lobes and brainstem associated with subcortical, periventricular and cortical damage. Finally, the prompt response to IVIg is also a peculiar finding, since the other cases had a complete recovery after steroids treatment that led to the definition of "steroid- responsive encephalitis "[20]. The role of infectious agent in triggering MOG-Abs production is still a matter of debate. However, the flu-like symptoms here reported are not unexpected since attacks are preceded by infections at least once in about 40% of MOG-Abs positive cases [1]. The infection could also be responsible for the blood-brain barrier breakdown that allows the entry of autoantibodies in the central nervous system. This report confirms that MOG-Abs might denote a disease entity in its own right and that the spectrum of MOG-Abs associated diseases is wider than NMOSD and ADEM. Since a prompt and adequate treatment can lead to a favorable outcome, clinicians should be aware of this condition, also in clinical pictures suggestive for infectious encephalitis.

Table 1 Clinical, radiological and CSF data of the index case (case 1) compared with previously cases reported by Fujimori et al. (case 2) and Ogawa et al. (cases 3–6) with MOG-Abs and a presumptive diagnosis of encephalitis [19, 20]

Case	1	2	3	4	5	6
Onset	fever, headache, confusion, altered consciousness, unsteady gait	dizziness	eye pain and visual loss	seizure	involuntary movemet	headache and abnormal behavior
Seizures	no	yes	yes	yes	yes	yes
Optic neuritis	no	yes	yes	yes	no	no
Myelitis	no	no	no	no	no	no
CSF	increased cells and proteins	increased cells, negative at a second control	increased cells	increased cells	increased cells and proteins	increased cells and proteins
First Brain MRI	subcortical, periventricular, cortical, white matter, thalamus, basal ganglia, internal capsule, pons	frontal cortex	frontoparietal cortex	frontoparietal cortex	parietal cortex	emisphere cortex
Second Brain MRI	reduction of preexisting lesios	corpus callosum, cingulate gyri, frontal lobes	negative	optic nerve, emispheric cortex	negative	negative
Third Brain MRI		third ventricle, cerebral aqueduct, thalamus, nucleus basalis		negative		
Fourth Brain MRI		reduction of preexisting lesios				
Clinical symptoms	wide-based unsteady gate, reduced level of consciousness, diffuse skin swelling and pustules with enanthema	headache, paraparesis/ paraplegia, memory decline, lethargy	delirium, paranoia, hallucination, anorexia	eye pain, visual loss, dysuria	headache, disorientation	agitation, violent behavior, delirium, emotional incontinence, aphasia, hemiparesis
Treatment	acyclovir, antibiotics, immunoglobulins	methylprednisolone and acyclovir, oral prednisolone	methylprednisolone, prednisolone, antiepilepsy drugs	methylprednisolone, prednisolone, antiepilepsy drugs	acyclovir, antibiotics, antimycotic, dexamethasone, prednisolone, antiepilepsy drugs	methylprednisolone, prednisolone, antiepilepsy drugs
Relapses	no	yes	yes	no	no	yes
Outcome	almost full recovery	full recovery	full recovery	full recovery	full recovery	full recovery

Abbreviations
ADEM: Acute disseminated encephalomyelitis; CSF: Cerebrospinal fluid; FLAIR: Fluid attenuated inversion recovery; IVIg: Immunoglobulin; MOG-Abs: Anti-myelin oligodendrocyte glycoprotein antibodies; MRI: Magnetic resonance imaging; NMOSD: Neuromyelitis optica spectrum disorders

Acknowledgements
The authors thank Daniela Alberti, Alessia Farinazzo (Department of Neuroscience, Biomedicine and Movement, Section of Neurology, University of Verona, Italy), and Kathrin Schanda (Clinical Department of Neurology, Medical University of Innsbruck, Innsbruck, Austria) for their technical assistance.

Funding
Sara Mariotto is currently supported by a research fellowship of the European Academy of Neurology. Patrick Peschl and Markus Reindl are supported by a research Grant from the Fonds zur Förderung der wissenschaftlichen Forschung, Austria (FWF graduate program W1206 SPIN). This study was supported by a research grant from the Austrian Federal Ministry of Science and Economy (grant BIG WIG MS, Markus Reindl).

Authors' contributions
SMa: study design, analysis and interpretation of patient data, drafting the manuscript. SMo: revising the manuscript for content, study supervision. PP: analysis and interpretation of cell-based assay. IC: analysis and interpretation of patient data regarding the infectious origin. RM: analysis and interpretation of patient data regarding the infectious origin. RH: analysis and interpretation of histological data. MR: analysis and interpretation of data, study design, revising the manuscript for content, study supervision. SF: analysis and interpretation of data, study design, revising the manuscript for content, study supervision. All authors read and approved the final manuscript.

Competing interests
M. Reindl is an academic editor for PLoS One, The University Hospital, and Medical University of Innsbruck (Austria, Markus Reindl); receives payments for antibody assays (NMDAR, AQP4, and other autoantibodies) and for MOG and AQP4 antibody validation experiments organized by Euroimmun (Luebeck, Germany). The other authors report no competing interests.

Author details
[1]Department of Neuroscience, Biomedicine and Movement Sciences, Section of Neurology, University of Verona, Verona, Italy. [2]Clinical Department of Neurology, Medical University of Innsbruck, Innsbruck, Austria. [3]Department of Diagnostics and Public Health, Section of Infectious Diseases, University of Verona, Verona, Italy. [4]Institute of Neurology, Medical University of Vienna, Vienna, Austria.

References
1. Jarius S, Ruprecht K, Kleiter I, Borisow N, Asgari N, Pitarokoili K, Pache F, Stich O, Beume LA, Hümmert MW, Ringelstein M, Trebst C, Winkelmann A, Schwarz A, Buttmann M, Zimmermann H, Kuchling J, Franciotta D, Capobianco M, Siebert E, Lukas C, Korporal-Kuhnke M, Haas J, Fechner K, Brandt AU, Schanda K, Aktas O, Paul F, Reindl M, Wildemann B. in cooperation with the Neuromyelitis Optica Study Group (NEMOS) MOG-IgG in NMO and related disorders: a multicenter study of 50 patients. Part 2: Epidemiology, clinical presentation, radiological and laboratory features, treatment responses, and long-term outcome. J Neuroinflammation. 2016;13:280.
2. Brilot F, Dale RC, Selter RC, Grummel V, Kalluri SR, Aslam M, Busch V, Zhou D, Cepok S, Hemmer B. Antibodies to native myelin oligodendrocyte glycoprotein in children with inflammatory demyelinating central nervous system disease. Ann Neurol. 2009;66:833–42.
3. Pröbstel AK, Dornmair K, Bittner R, Sperl P, Jenne D, Magalhaes S, Villalobos A, Breithaupt C, Weissert R, Jacob U, Krumbholz M, Kuempfel T, Blaschek A, Stark W, Gärtner J, Pohl D, Rostasy K, Weber F, Forne I, Khademi M, Olsson T, Brilot F, Tantsis E, Dale RC, Wekerle H, Hohlfeld R, Banwell B, Bar-Or A, Meinl E. Derfuss Antibodies to MOG are transient in childhood acute disseminated encephalomyelitis. Neurology. 2011;77:580–8.
4. Sato DK, Callegaro D, Lana-Peixoto MA, Waters PJ, de Haidar Jorge FM, Takahashi T, Nakashima I, Apostolos-Pereira SL, Talim N, Simm RF, Lino AM, Misu T, Leite MI, Aoki M, Fujihara K. Distinction between MOG antibody-positive and AQP4 antibody-positive NMO spectrum disorders. Neurology. 2014;82:474–81.
5. Spadaro M, Gerdes LA, Mayer MC, Ertl-Wagner B, Laurent S, Krumbholz M, Breithaupt C, Högen T, Straube A, Giese A, Hohlfeld R, Lassmann H, Meinl E, Kümpfel T. Histopathology and clinical course of MOG-antibody-associated encephalomyelitis. Ann Clin Transl Neurol. 2015;2:295–301.
6. Pröbstel AK, Rudolf G, Dornmair K, Collongues N, Chanson JB, Sanderson NS, Lindberg RL, Kappos L, de Seze J, Derfuss T. Anti-MOG antibodies are present in a subgroup of patients with a neuromyelitis optica phenotype. J Neuroinflammation. 2015;12:46.
7. Waters P, Woodhall M, O'Connor KC, Reindl M, Lang B, Sato DK, Jurynczyk M, Tackley G, Rocha J, Takahashi T, Misu T, Nakashima I, Palace J, Fujihara K, Leite MI, Vincent A. MOG cell-based assay detects non-MS patients with inflammatory neurologic disease. Neurol Neuroimmunol Neuroinflamm. 2015;2:e89.
8. Baumann M, Hennes EM, Schanda K, Karenfort M, Kornek B, Seidl R, Diepold K, Lauffer H, Marquardt I, Strautmanis J, Syrbe S, Vieker S, Höftberger R, Reindl M, Rostásy K. Children with multiphasic disseminated encephalomyelitis and antibodies to the myelin oligodendrocyte glycoprotein (MOG): Extending the spectrum of MOG antibody positive diseases. Mult Scler. 2016;22:1821–9.
9. Van Pelt ED, Wong YY, Ketelslegers IA, Hamann D, Hintzen RQ. Neuromyelitis optica spectrum disorders: comparison of clinical and magnetic resonance imaging characteristics of AQP4-IgG versus MOG-IgG seropositive cases in the Netherlands. Eur J Neurol. 2016;23:580–7.
10. Siritho S, Sato DK, Kaneko K, Fujihara K, Prayoonwiwat N. The clinical spectrum associated with myelin oligodendrocyte glycoprotein antibodies (anti-MOG-Ab) in Thai patients. Mult Scler. 2016;22:964–8.
11. Spadaro M, Gerdes LA, Krumbholz M, Ertl-Wagner B, Thaler FS, Schuh E, Metz I, Blaschek A, Dick A, Brück W, Hohlfeld R, Meinl E, Kümpfel T. Autoantibodies to MOG in a distinct subgroup of adult multiple sclerosis. Neurol Neuroimmunol Neuroinflamm. 2016;3:e257.
12. Lechner C, Baumann M, Hennes EM, Schanda K, Marquard K, Karenfort M, Leiz S, Pohl D, Venkateswaran S, Pritsch M, Koch J, Schimmel M, Häusler M, Klein A, Blaschek A, Thiels C, Lücke T, Gruber-Sedlmayr U, Kornek B, Hahn A, Leypoldt F, Sandrieser T, Gallwitz H, Stoffels J, Korenke C, Reindl M, Rostásy K. Antibodies to MOG and AQP4 in children with neuromyelitis optica and limited forms of the disease. J Neurol Neurosurg Psychiatry. 2016;87:897–905.
13. Hacohen Y, Mankad K, Chong WK, Barkhof F, Vincent A, Lim M, Wassmer E, Ciccarelli O, Hemingway C. Diagnostic algorithm for relapsing acquired demyelinating syndromes in children. Neurology. 2017; doi:10.1212/WNL.0000000000004117.
14. Di Pauli F, Mader S, Rostasy K, Schanda K, Bajer-Kornek B, Ehling R, Deisenhammer F, Reindl M, Berger T. Temporal dynamics of anti-MOG antibodies in CNS demyelinating diseases. Clin Immunol. 2011;138:247–54.
15. Sepúlveda M, Armangue T, Martinez-Hernandez E, Arrambide G, Sola-Valls N, Sabater L, Téllez N, Midaglia L, Arino H, Peschl P, Reindl M, Rovira A, Montalban X, Blanco Y, Dalmau J, Graus F, Saiz A. Clinical spectrum associated with MOG autoimmunity in adults: significance of sharing rodent MOG epitopes. J Neurol. 2016;263:1349–60.
16. Venkatesan A, Tunkel AR, Bloch KC, Lauring AS, Sejvar J, Bitnun A, Stahl JP, Mailles A, Drebot M, Rupprecht CE, Yoder J, Cope JR, Wilson MR, Whitley RJ, Sullivan J, Granerod J, Jones C, Eastwood K, Ward KN, Durrheim DN, Solbrig MV, Guo-Dong L, Glaser CA, International Encephalitis Consortium. Case definitions, diagnostic algorithms, and priorities in encephalitis: consensus statement of the international encephalitis consortium. Clin Infect Dis. 2013; 57:1114–28.
17. Graus F, Titulaer MJ, Balu R, Benseler S, Bien CG, Cellucci T, Cortese I, Dale RC, Gelfand JM, Geschwind M, Glaser CA, Honnorat J, Höftberger R, Iizuka T, Irani SR, Lancaster E, Leypoldt F, Prüss H, Rae-Grant A, Reindl M, Rosenfeld MR, Rostásy K, Saiz A, Venkatesan A, Vincent A, Wandinger KP, Waters P, Dalmau J. A clinical approach to diagnosis of autoimmune encephalitis. Lancet Neurol. 2016;15:391–404.

12

Nitrous oxide induced subacute combined degeneration with longitudinally extensive myelopathy with inverted V-sign on spinal MRI

Jun Liang Yuan[1], Shuang Kun Wang[2], Tao Jiang[2*] and Wen Li Hu[1*]

Abstract

Background: Nitrous oxide (N2O), a long-standing anesthetic, is also neurotoxic by interfering with the bioavailability of vitamin B12 if abused. A few case studies have reported the neurological and psychiatric complications of N2O.

Case presentation: Here, we reported a patient of N2O induced subacute combined degeneration (SCD) with longitudinally extensive myelopathy with inverted V-sign exhibiting progressive limb paresthesia and unsteady gait.

Conclusions: This case raises the awareness of an important mechanism of neural toxicity of N2O, and clinical physicians should be well recognized this in the field of substance-related disorders.

Keywords: Nitrous oxide, Subacute combined degeneration

Background

Nitrous oxide (N2O) is a long-standing anesthetic, which also has neurotoxicity by interfering in the bioavailability of vitamin B12 if abused. A few case studies have reported the neurological and psychiatrical complications, even death, related to N2O abuse [1]. Among these complications, N2O-induced myelopathy has been regarded as the most common manifestation [1]. To the best of our knowledge, there are only 18 cases describing N2O-induced subacute combined degeneration (SCD); however, to date, only very rare cases with longitudinally extensive myelopathy with inverted V-sign or "rabbit ears" sign on spinal posterior column. We herein described a 20-year-old female who developed SCD with inverted V-sign on spinal column related to the abuse of N2O.

Case presentation

A 20-year-old woman presented with progressive paresthesia in her legs and hands, and unsteady gait for

15 days. She had inhaled N2O about 100–200 whipped cream chargers many times daily, for recreational purposes for at least one year. Neuropsychological test showed mild impairment of the cognition, and the Mini mental state examination (MMSE) score was 23. The deficit domains of the MMSE included orientation (minus 3 scores), attention and calculation (minus 4 scores). Neurological examination revealed distal slight weakness, decreased vibration and proprioception, bilateral hyporeflexia, sensory ataxia, positive Babinski sign and Romberg sign.

Laboratory tests revealed decreased level of folic acid (4.40 ng/ml, reference range > 5.4 ng/ml), but the others were normal, including red blood cell, hemoglobin, mean corpuscular volume, serum vitamin B12 (800 pg/ml, reference range 211–911 pg/ml) and homocysteine (8μmmol/L, reference range 0-15 μmol/L). The antibodies of human immunodeficiency virus and neurosyphilis were negative. The results of cerebrospinal fluid test (CSF) were normal for leucocyte count (5/μL, reference range 0–8/L), glucose (3.1 mmol/μL, reference range 2.5–4.5 mmol/L), and protein concentration (33 mg/dl, reference range 15–45 mg/dl). The

* Correspondence: jiangtao@bjcyh.com; huwenli@sina.com
[2]Department of Radiology, Beijing Chaoyang Hospital, Capital Medical University, Beijing 100020, China
[1]Department of Neurology, Beijing Chaoyang Hospital, Capital Medical University, Beijing 100020, China

Nitrous oxide induced subacute combined degeneration with longitudinally extensive myelopathy...

81

inflammatory, immune and infectious biomarkers of both CSF and serum were also unremarkable.

The cranial MRI yielded normal findings. The spinal cord MRI showed abnormal longitudinally extensive T2 weighted hyperintensities involving the posterior columns from C1 through T12, with inverted V or "rabbit ears" sign on cervical spinal MRI, but without contrast enhancement (Figs. 1 and 2). Electromyography showed multiple peripheral neurogenic damage, also with decreased nerve conduction velocity and abnormal somatosensory evoked potential. However, visual evoked potential showed normal response.

Three months later, with a high dose of supplementation of intramuscular vitamin B12 injections (1 mg per day) and the cessation of N2O exposure, the symptoms of sensation and gait resolved markedly, and the cognitive function fully recovered (MMSE 30). The abnormal hyperintensities of spinal MRI also dissolved with three months' follow up (Figs. 3 and 4). The diagnosis of N2O induced SCD was supported by clinical history, clinical manifestations, MRI findings, the distinct relationship between N2O exposure, also with the favorable prognosis by the vitamin B12 supplementation.

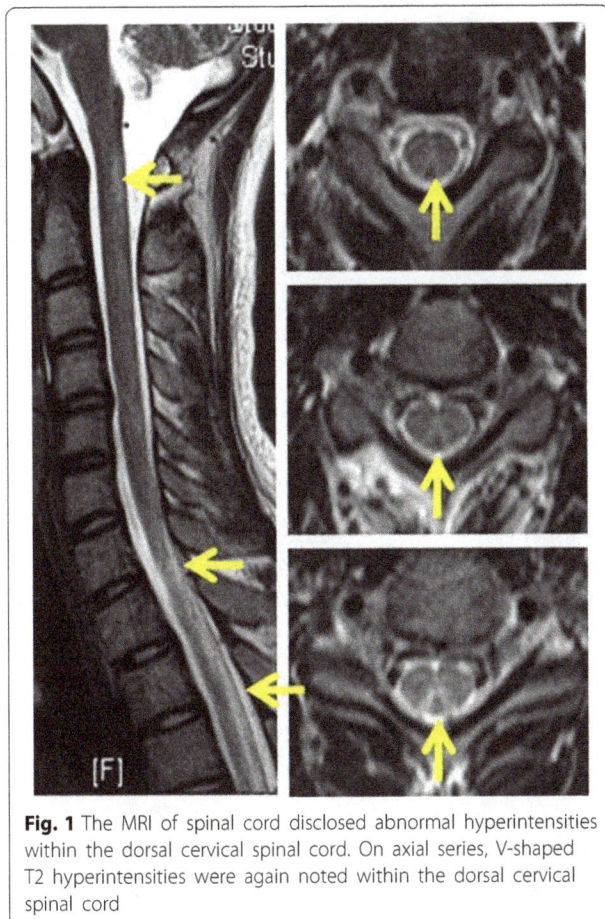

Fig. 1 The MRI of spinal cord disclosed abnormal hyperintensities within the dorsal cervical spinal cord. On axial series, V-shaped T2 hyperintensities were again noted within the dorsal cervical spinal cord

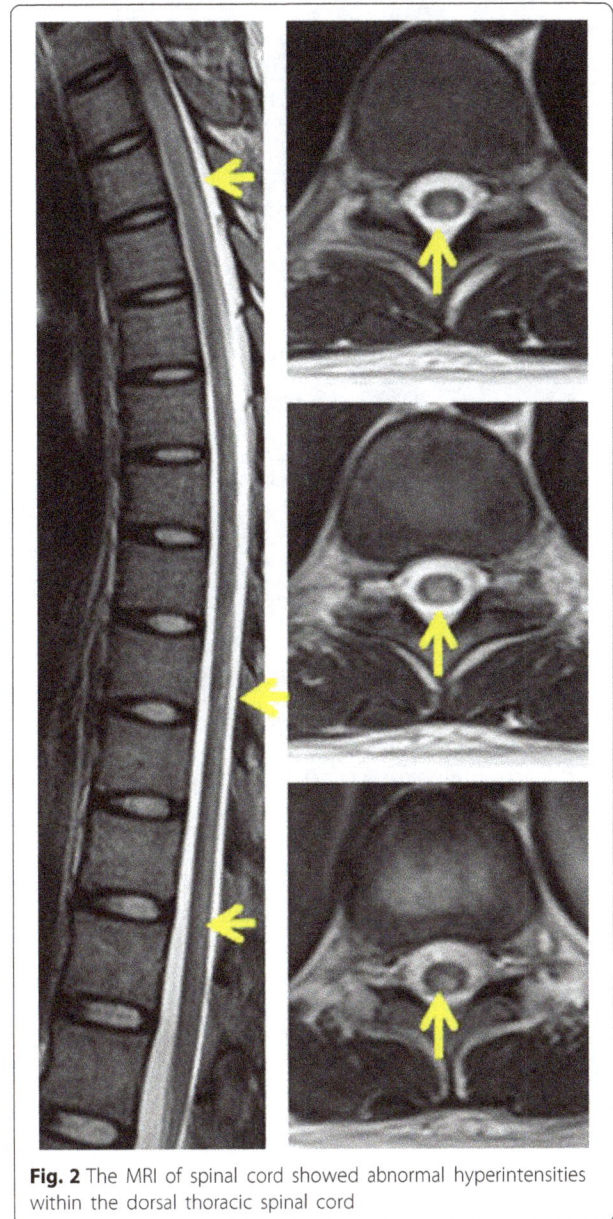

Fig. 2 The MRI of spinal cord showed abnormal hyperintensities within the dorsal thoracic spinal cord

Discussion and conclusions

N2O, a well-known anesthetic, has a long history for its recreational use, and its consumption is on the rise rapidly [2]. Several case studies have reported neurological and psychiatric complications of N2O use [1]. To date, there are only 18 cases describing SCD caused by N2O abuse. However, the exact mechanisms of SCD induced by N2O have not been well elucidated. N2O potentially interferes with methionine synthesis by inactivating methylcobalamin [3]. Except for the deficient methylation hypothesis, some other newly discovered functions of B12 in regulating cytokines and growth factors have also been raised [4].

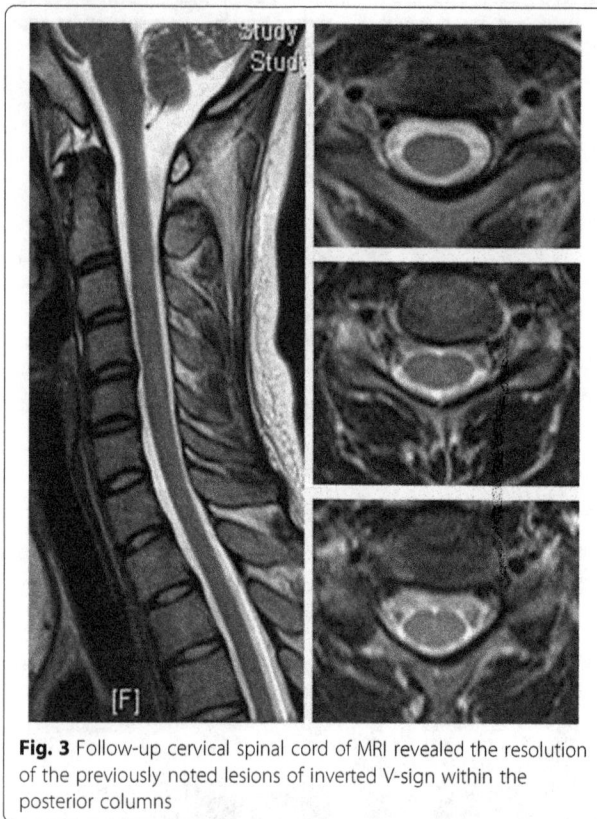

Fig. 3 Follow-up cervical spinal cord of MRI revealed the resolution of the previously noted lesions of inverted V-sign within the posterior columns

The strengths of our case were listed as follows. Firstly, our case revealed symmetric abnormal signal in the dorsal columns of the cervical and thoracic cord, especially with inverted V-sign on cervical spinal. To the best of our knowledge, only one case has been previously described of such longitudinally extensive myelopathy induced by N2O [5]. Our case also indicated symmetric, reversible changes in the posterior columns correlating well with patients' clinical symptoms after vitamin B12 supplementation. Secondly, to the best of our knowledge, this is the first report about the coexistence of mild cognitive impairment in patient with SCD by N2O abuse, in spite that the assessment of cognition was only measured by the MMSE. The underlying mechanism of cognitive decline may attributed to the neural toxicity of N2O or the metabolic disturbances from the lower level of metabolites such as folic acid and vitamin B12 or hyperhomocysteinemia [6]. Thirdly, abuse of N2O is common, but generally underestimated especially in developing countries. To date, this is also the first case reported in China (mainland).

In summary, the abuse of N2O has some potentially serious outcomes, especially in young patients presenting with myelopathic symptoms of unclear aetiology [7]. N2O induced SCD may be a very rare manifestation associated with N2O abuse. Early diagnosis and

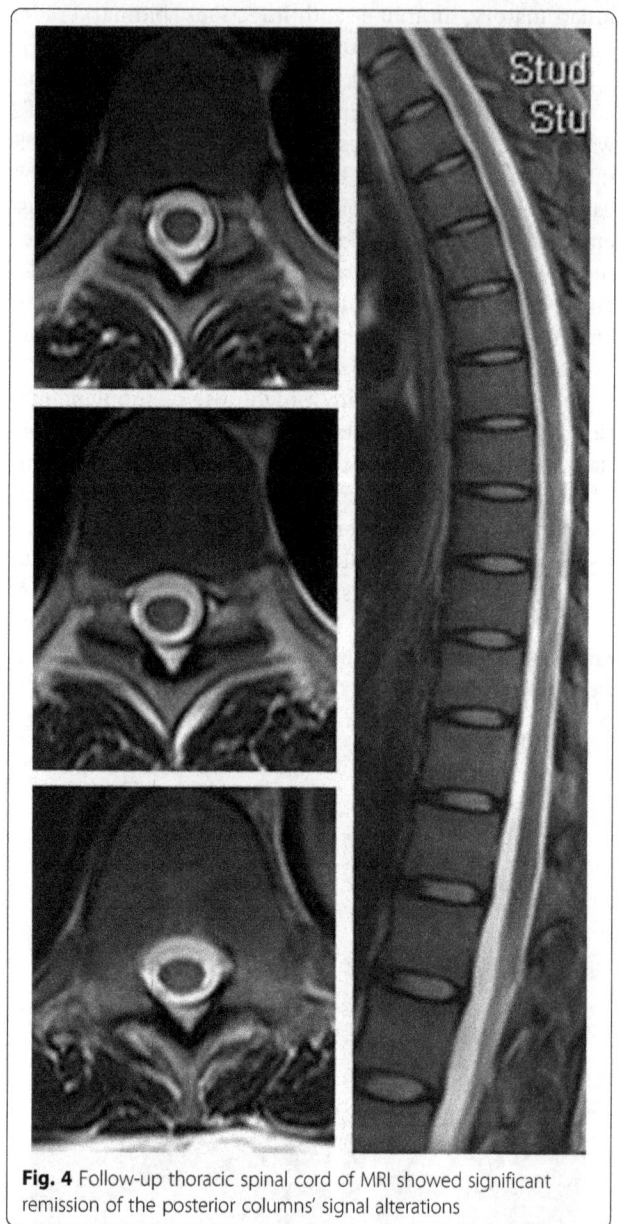

Fig. 4 Follow-up thoracic spinal cord of MRI showed significant remission of the posterior columns' signal alterations

treatment are crucial because it represents a treatable and potentially reversible cause of myelopathy with vitamin B12 [2]. Our case also raises awareness of an important complication of neural toxicity of N2O.

Abbreviations
CSF: Cerebrospinal fluid test; MMSE: Mini mental state examination; N2O: Nitrous oxide; SCD: Subacute combined degeneration

Acknowledgements
Not applicable

Funding
This work was supported by the National Natural Science Foundation of China (81301016) and the Beijing Municipal Administration of Hospitals' Youth Programme (QML20150303).

Nitrous oxide induced subacute combined degeneration with longitudinally extensive myelopathy...

83

Authors' contributions

JLY examined, evaluated the patient and drafted the manuscript. SKW performed and interpreted the MRI studies. TJ and WLH participated in the design of the case-report and helped to draft the manuscript. All authors read and approved the final manuscript.

Competing interests

The authors declare that they have no competing interests.

References

1. Garakani A, Jaffe RJ, Savla D, Welch AK, Protin CA, Bryson EO, et al. Neurologic, psychiatric, and other medical manifestations of nitrous oxide abuse: a systematic review of the case literature. Am J Addict. 2016;25:358–69.
2. Mancke F, Kaklauskaite G, Kollmer J, Weiler M. Psychiatric comorbidities in a young man with subacute myelopathy induced by abusive nitrous oxide consumption: a case report. Subst Abuse Rehabil. 2016;7:155–9.
3. Garakani A, Welch AK, Jaffe RJ, Protin CA, McDowell DM. Psychosis and low cyanocobalamin in a patient abusing nitrous oxide and cannabis. Psychosomatics. 2014;55:715–9.
4. Hathout L, El-Saden S. Nitrous oxide-induced B(1)(2) deficiency myelopathy: perspectives on the clinical biochemistry of vitamin B12. J Neurol Sci. 2011;301:1–8.
5. Ernst LD, Brock K, Barraza LH, Davis A, Nirenberg MJ. Longitudinally extensive nitrous oxide Myelopathy with novel radiographic features. JAMA Neurol. 2015;72:1370–1.
6. Smith AD, Refsum H. Homocysteine, B Vitamins, and cognitive impairment. Annu Rev Nutr. 2016;36:211–39.
7. Sotirchos ES, Saidha S, Becker D. Neurological picture. Nitrous oxide-induced myelopathy with inverted V-sign on spinal MRI. J Neurol Neurosurg Psychiatry. 2012;83:915–6.

13

Intracisternal tuberculoma: a refractory type of tuberculoma indicating surgical intervention

Fanfan Chen[1†], Lei Chen[2†], Yongfu Cao[1], Yongjun Yi[1], Jingwen Zhuang[1], Wuhua Le[1], Wei Xie[1], Lanbo Tu[1], Peng Li[1], Yimin Fang[3], Ling Li[4], Yuqing Kou[5], Kaikai Fu[5], Hua He[6*] and Hongbin Ju[7*]

Abstract

Background: Central nervous system (CNS) tuberculoma is a rare disease with severe neurological deficits. This retrospective research is to review the data of patients diagnosed as CNS tuberculoma. Surgeries were performed in all patients. The clinical features especially the neurological image and the anatomical characters of the tuberculomas were concerned.

Methods: Totally 11 patients diagnosed as CNS tuberculoma were admitted in Guangzhou First People's Hospital (7cases) and Changzheng Hospital (4 cases) during 2006–2015. The data including preoperative condition, neurological imaging, and surgical findings was collected and analyzed.

Results: The lesions of nine patients (9/11) were totally or subtotally excised and two (2/11) were partially excised. Neurological functions of all patients were improved after surgery without secondary infection. Lesions of nine (9/11) patients preoperatively progressed as a result of paradoxical reaction. Of the 9 patients demonstrated paradoxical progression, all lesions were partially or totally located at the cisterns or the subarachnoid space. Preoperative ATTs lasted 2 to 12 months and tuberculomas were not eliminated. The arachnoid was found thickened and tightly adhered to the lesions during surgeries. Of the 2 cases that paradoxical reaction were excluded, both patients (case 6, intramedullary tuberculoma; case 11, intradural extramedullary tuberculoma) were admitted at onset of the disease. ATTs were preoperatively given for 1 week as neurological deficits aggravated. The tuberculous lesions of CNS or other system showed no obvious change and paradoxical reaction could not be established in both cases.

Conclusions: Exudates of tuberculosis is usually accumulated in the cisterns and frequently results in the paradoxical formation of tuberculoma. Intracisternal tuberculoma is closely related to paradoxical reaction and refractory to anti-tuberculosis therapy. Micro-surgical excision is safe and effective. Early surgical intervention may be considered in the diagnosis of intracisternal tuberculoma especially when paradoxical reaction participates in the development of tuberculoma.

Keywords: Central nervous system, Paradoxical response, Tuberculosis, Spine, Tuberculoma

* Correspondence: hehua1624@smmu.edu.cn; bin7810@126.com
†Equal contributors
[6]Neurosurgery Department, Changzheng Hospital, The Second Military Medical University;State key Laboratory of Drug Research, Shanghai Institute of Material Medical, Chinese Academy of Sciences, 415# Fengyang Road, Shanghai 200003, China
[7]Spinal Surgery Department, Guangzhou First People's Hospital, Guangzhou Medical University, 1# Panfu Road, Guangzhou, Guangdong 510180, China
Full list of author information is available at the end of the article

Background

Tuberculosis (TB) with central nervous system (CNS) involvement occurs in approximately 1% of all TB patients and causes the highest morbidity and mortality [1]. CNS tuberculosis has various forms. Tuberculous meningitis (TM) is the most frequent form of CNS TB and CNS tuberculoma is the type next to TM [2, 3]. Spinal intradural tuberculomas including intramedullary and intradural extramedullary tuberculoma are exceptionally rare and account for approximate 2%–5% of all CNS tuberculoma [4]. Furthermore, Intradural extramedullary tuberculoma of the spinal cord is the most unusual type [5].

Although CNS tuberculoma is an uncommon disease, it usually presents with severe neurological deficits including altered mental status, hydrocephalus, cranial nerve palsies, hemiparesis and seizures et al. [6]. Anti-tuberculosis treatments (ATT) combined with surgeries in the treatment of CNS tuberculoma have been reported occasionally [7, 8]. However, most of the articles mainly described the rarity of this disease and clinical situation including diagnosis, medications and outcomes of surgeries [9–12]. The locations, possible pathogenesis and the relation between them were not mentioned in those reported cases, except for the optochiasmatic tuberculoma [13].

Of the patients in this study, we were aware of the characteristics that the subarachnoid space including cerebral cisterns and spinal subarachnoid space were susceptible regions for the formation of tuberculomas following TM and/or tuberculous arachnoiditis. This situation was also noticed by other doctors [4, 14]. Paradoxical reaction, defined as an phenomenon of effective medical treatment demonstrating opposite effect in certain lesions [15, 16], is prone to occur at the cisterns and frequently results in the formation of intracisternal tuberculoma [17, 18]. In most cases, ATT is effective in treating the CNS tuberculoma [19]. Unfortunately, when paradoxical reaction participates in the etiology of tuberculoma, the effectiveness of ATT is usually limited and additional corticosteroids is indicated [20]. Nevertheless, long period of medical therapy for resolving the lesion results in limited improvement or even deterioration of the impaired neurological function, especially for the spinal paradoxical tuberculoma [2]. From the above information, intracisternal tuberculoma, paradoxical reaction and their intimate relation result in the severity and difficulty of medicine treatment. Accordingly, rapid elimination of the tuberculoma by surgical intervention should be considered.

Methods

Patients' data

This retrospective research was approved by the ethics committee of Guangzhou First People's Hospital and Changzheng Hospital. From 2006 to 2015, 11 patients diagnosed as CNS tuberculoma requiring surgical intervention were admitted in the neurosurgery department of Guangzhou First People's Hospital, Guangdong, China and Changzheng Hospital, Shanghai. All patients underwent surgical excision of tuberculoma. Preoperative sputum smear was negative of tubercle bacillus of all patients. The diagnosis of tuberculosis of nine cases (pulmonary or CNS) was established in specialized hospital for tuberculosis. Two patients were diagnosed as spinal tuberculoma at onset of the disease and adequate ATT was administered for 1 week before sugeries. The age of patients ranged from 7 to 52 years old. Six patients were female and five were male. Of the nine patients with preoperative diagnosis of tuberculosis, effective ATT was applied. Effectiveness of ATT was evidenced by the improvement of the clinical symptom and radiological findings (including pulmonary or most part of the CNS lesions). However, new lesions or progression of one lesion was found in these nine patients in later period during the ATT. Paradoxical reactions were identified in these nine patients and additional corticosteroid was administered. Paradoxical reaction was not considered in the patient presenting intramedullary tuberculoma and the patient with intradural extramedullary tuberculoma of the fifth thoracic vertebra as both patients presented tuberculomas initially. For the two patients, surgeries were performed 1 week after ATT initiated as negative sputums for tubercle bacillus were confirmed. As shown in Table 1, the location of symptom related tuberculoma included the cerebral hemispheres (three cases), posterior fossa (three cases), and spinal (five cases, including one case of intramedullary tuberculoma and four cases of intradural extramedullary tuberculoma.).

Preoperative preparations

All patients were given routine examinations of blood, blood electrolyte, liver function and kidney function. Electrocardiography and chest radiography were performed to exclude cardiac or pulmonary contraindications for surgeries. Sputum smears were performed repetitively assuring negative result of tubercle bacillus. MRI was acquired for a preoperative evaluation. ATT based on the regimen of specialized hospital for treatment of tuberculosis and was continued during the entire hospital stay of the patient.

Surgical management

Two patients experienced two surgeries. One patient (patient 7) with tuberculoma locating at dorsal pons to cerebellum (cisterna ambiens) received external draininage of the tuberculoma at local hospital and relapsed after 2 months. A microsurgical excision was given by our team. Another patient (patient 3) with intradural extramedullary tuberculoma (co-existing with an intramedullary lesion situating at the ventral spinal cord

Table 1 Clinical data of patients

Patients	Range of age (years)	Site /related cistern	Outcome of Initial tuberculosis after ATT	ATT time before CNS progression	Paradoxical reaction (Y/N)
1	50–55	Right Cerebello -pontine Angle	Relieved (cough, subcutaneous tuberculous nodule)	12 months	Y
2	15–20	Right Cisterna Magna	Improved (Fever, multiple organ tuberculosis)	3 months	Y
3	25–30	T3-T10, Intradural extra-medullary/ intramedullary	Improved (Fever, pulmonary tuberculosis)	2 months	Y
4	15–20	Right Sylvian cistern	Improved (Fever, pulmonary tuberculosis)	10 months	Y
5	25–30	Left sylvian cistern	Improved (Fever) Progression (Headache)	6 months	Y
6	20–25	C5–6,intramedullary	Improved (Fever,pleural effussion), Progression (paraplegia)	1 week	N
7	10–15	Ambient cistern	Relieved (Pulmonary tuberculosis)	10 months	Y
8	40–45	T3–6 intradural extramedullary	Improved (Fever, pulmonary tuberculosis)	2 months	Y
9	15–20	T10–11 intradural extramedullary	Improved (Fever, pulmonary tuberculosis)	2 months	Y
10	5–10	T5 intradural extramedullary	Improved (Fever), Progression (paraplegia)	1 week	N
11	25–30	Left sylvian csitern	Improved (Fever) Progression (Headache)	6 months	Y

T thoracic, *C* cervical, *Y* yes, *N* no

without surgical intervention) underwent two surgeries for the intradural extramedullary tuberculoma. Other patients underwent operations once respectively. The symptom-inducing lesion was the surgical target in patient with multiple lesions. For example, patient 2 (Fig. 2c, d), the lesion locating at right cisterna magna (Fig. 2c, white arrow) was responsible for the hydrocephalus and hemiparesis. This lesion was the target of surgery. The lesion of left cerebellum was small and asymptomatic (Fig. 2c, d, red arrow). This lesion with other supratentorial lesions was resolved by the effective ATT. Precautions were taken to protect the surrounding

normal brain tissue from surgical contamination. For the spinal tuberculomas, pedicle screw fixation surgeries were performed if necessary. All patients were followed until the present time. Follow-ups were performed by telephone or at outpatient department in all patients.

Results

Preoperative MRI findings

For CNS tuberculoma, MRI is the most important examination for preoperative preparation. The lesions showed hypo- to iso-intense on T1WI (Fig. 1a) and mixed signal intensity on T2WI (Fig. 1b). Contrast-

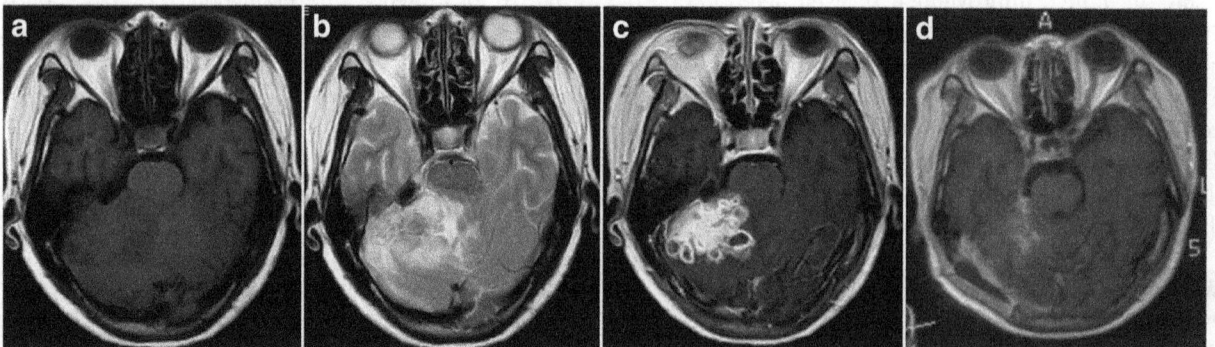

Fig. 1 Typical MRI of intracisternal tuberculoma. **a** The lesions showed iso- and hypo-intense on T1WI. **b** Mixed signal intensity on T2WI. **c** Contrast-enhanced T1WI sequence showed multiple ring enhancing lesions. **d** The postoperative MRI of the patient

enhanced T1WI sequence displayed isolated or conglomerated ring enhancing lesions accompanied with hypointense non-enhancing content inside in most situations (Fig. 1c, 2a, c).

This group of patients contained various locations of the CNS including temporal lobe, frontal lobe, cerebellopontine angle, cerebella and intravertebral canal. It is noteworthy that except one intramedullary tuberculoma case, all other cases were associated with the subarachnoid space, including the sylvian fissure (Fig. 2a), cerebellopontine angle (Fig. 1c), ambient cistern (Fig. 5a), cerebellomedullary cistern (Fig. 2c) and the subarachnoid space of the spinal cord (Fig. 3a).

Surgical findings

Patient 3 presented with coexisting intramedullary (Fig. 3a-d, red arrows) and intradural extramedullary lesions (Fig. 3,the continuous enhancing intradural extramedullary lesion from T3-T9). Preoperative evaluation identified that the lesions responsible for the symptoms were the multiple intradural extramedullary tuberculomas. Given that the intramedullary lesion was located at the ventral spinal cord, a direct excision of the intramedullary lesion might cause further spinal injury to the spinal function that was already seriously damaged, the intramedullary lesion was not resected. A laminectomy of T3-T4, T7-T9 or the excision of the corresponding extramedullary lesions was performed (Fig. 3b). However, the lesion of T9 was missed(Fig. 3b, white arrow). After 2 months of ATT, the following situations were displayed: extramedullary lesion of T9 enlarged (Fig. 3c, white arrow); the residual lesion of T5-T6 disappeared; the intramedullary lesion showed no change (Fig. 3a-c). A second time surgery was performed to remove the progressing extramedullary lesion of T9. At the same time, a pedicle screw fixation

was performed to maintain the stability of the spinal column (Fig. 3d).

The intramedullary tuberculoma was revealed to be well-defined lesions (Fig. 4a) which is totally different for the intradural extramedullary tuberculoma. As for the latter, the abscess extended on the surface of spinal cord (Fig. 4b). The irregular lesion adhere to surrounding tissues intimately. Similar situation was oberserved in the cerebral tuberculoma. Even for the same tuberculoma, the interface between the tuberculoma and parenchyma was relatively loose and easy to be separated (Fig. 5e, white arrow displayed the interface of the tuberculoma and the parenchyma of brain) while the adhesion of tuberculoma in the subarachnoid space was tight (Fig. 5f, white arrow displayed the adhesion of tuberculoma and arachnoid). This kind of close relation between subarachnoid space and the cisternal part of tuberculoma was due to the thickening arachnoid, the hyperplastic fibrous tissue closely surrounding the lesion. Coagulation and sharp dissection is necessary for separation. Furthermore, manipulation in the cisternal part of tuberculoma should be more careful as vital vessel may course in the cistern. Decisions of cutting or separation and reservation the vessel should be done based on clear identification (Fig. 5g, red arrow indicates the vessel after separation of arachnoid).

None of the patients experienced secondary infection following the surgical procedures. All of the patients were followed from the date of surgery until the present time. The outcomes of all patients were evaluated with Karnofsky Performance Scale in different neurological recovery periods. The recovery times of patients in this study were different. For the most severe case as case 3, 40 months had passed before the patient finally carried out daily activities (KPS was 90). For the other patient, it took about 2–6 months for recovery (KPS were 90–100).

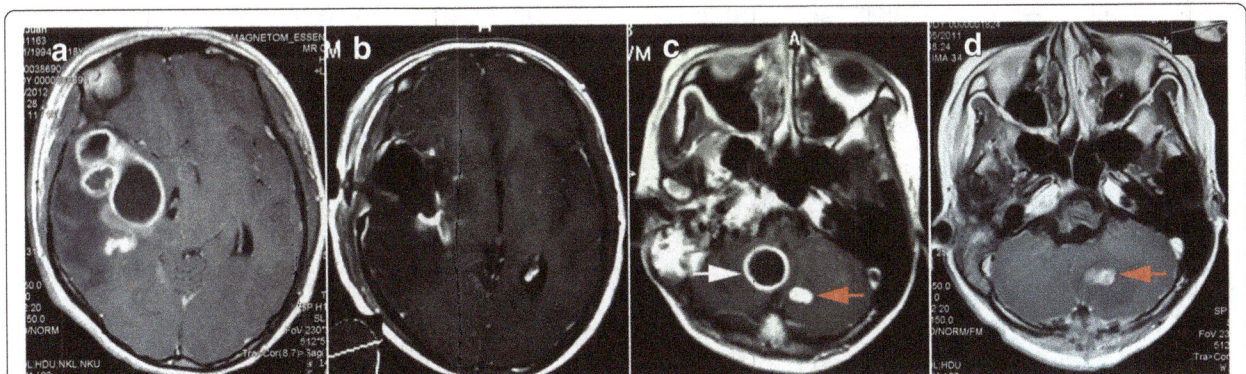

Fig. 2 Pre and post-surgical image of intracisternal tuberculoma. **a** Preoperative enhancing MRI of a tuberculoma locating at right sylvian fissure. **b** Postoperative enhancing MRI of a tuberculoma locating at right sylvian fissure. **c** Preoperative enhancing MRI showed a tuberculoma locating at right cisterna magna (white arrow). The tuberculoma of left cerebellum (red arrow) was resolved by ATT. **d** Postoperative enhancing MRI showed the tuberculoma locating at right cisterna magna was excised. The tuberculoma of left cerebellum (red arrow) was resolved by ATT in later period

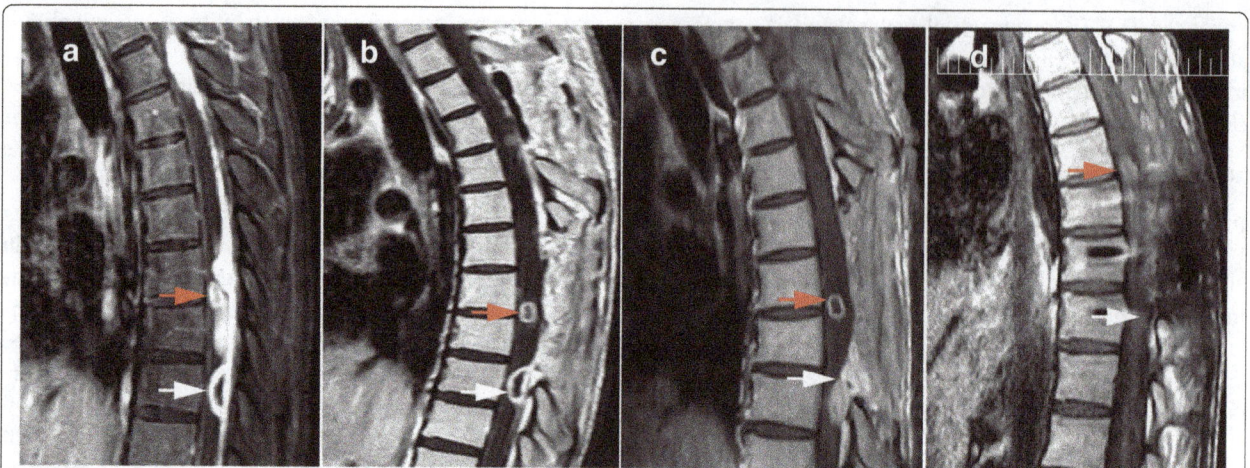

Fig. 3 MRI of a patient with intradural extramedullary tuberculoma and intramedullary tuberculoma (two operations). **a** Preoperative MRI of the first operation of the patient manifesting intradural extramedullary tuberculoma from T3 to T9 (the enhancing lesion from T3 to T9) and intramedullary tuberculoma (red arrow). **b** Postoperative MRI of the first operation of the patient manifesting intradural extramedullary tuberculoma from T3 to T9 and intramedullary tuberculoma (red arrow). The intramedullary tuberculoma of T7 was left untouched while the intradural extramedullary lesion of T9 was missed (white arrow). **c** Preoperative MRI of the second operation of the patient. The intradural extramedullary tuberculoma of T9 was the target of operation (white arrow). **d** Postoperative MRI of the second operation of the patient. The intradural extramedullary tuberculoma of T9 was excised (white arrow)

Pathology

All specimens were pathologically analyzed. The pathological characteristics including granulomas, necrosis, caseation, cell types (lymphocyte, Langerhans-type giant cell), and the result of acid-fast bacillus staining were recorded. Not all the pathological features were demonstrated in one case. Typical tuberculomas showed a granulomatous reaction consisting of epithelioid cells and giant cells mixed with mononuclear inflammatory cells (predominantly lymphocytes) that form a granuloma (Fig. 6b, c) [6, 21].

Discussion

CNS tuberculoma is a devastating disease with high morbidity and mortality. Although the outcome of the patients in this study was encouraging, the periods of preoperative ATT (for the paradoxical tuberculoma) were 2 to 12 months (average 5.9 ± 4.0 months). Neurological functions in most cases were aggravated during the ATT treatment as a result of a paradoxical reaction which limited the effect of ATT. Surgical excision of the lesion was a turning point for this group of patients. To our opinion, early surgical excision is an appropriate procedure when a paradoxical lesion formed. This is particularly critical for spinal tuberculoma [1, 22].

Although the clinical situations of the patients were different, for example the sites of the lesions and the response to treatment, we noticed that the tuberculoma of nine (9/11) patients who were considered paradoxical tuberculoma were correlated with the subarachnoid space. Furthermore, it was intriguing that the relapsed lesions of the two patients who

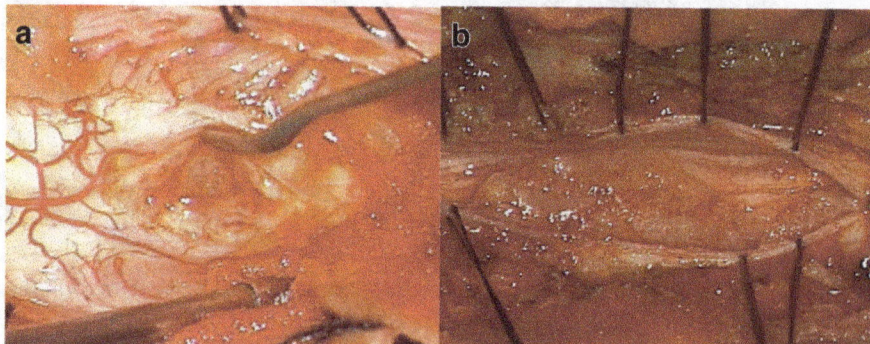

Fig. 4 Tuberculomas at different regions displayed different intraoperative situation. **a** Intramedullary tuberculoma displayed clear boundary and was easily separated. **b** Extramedullary tuberculoma displayed diffusive lesion with arachnoiditis which was tightly adhered to the spine and difficult for separation

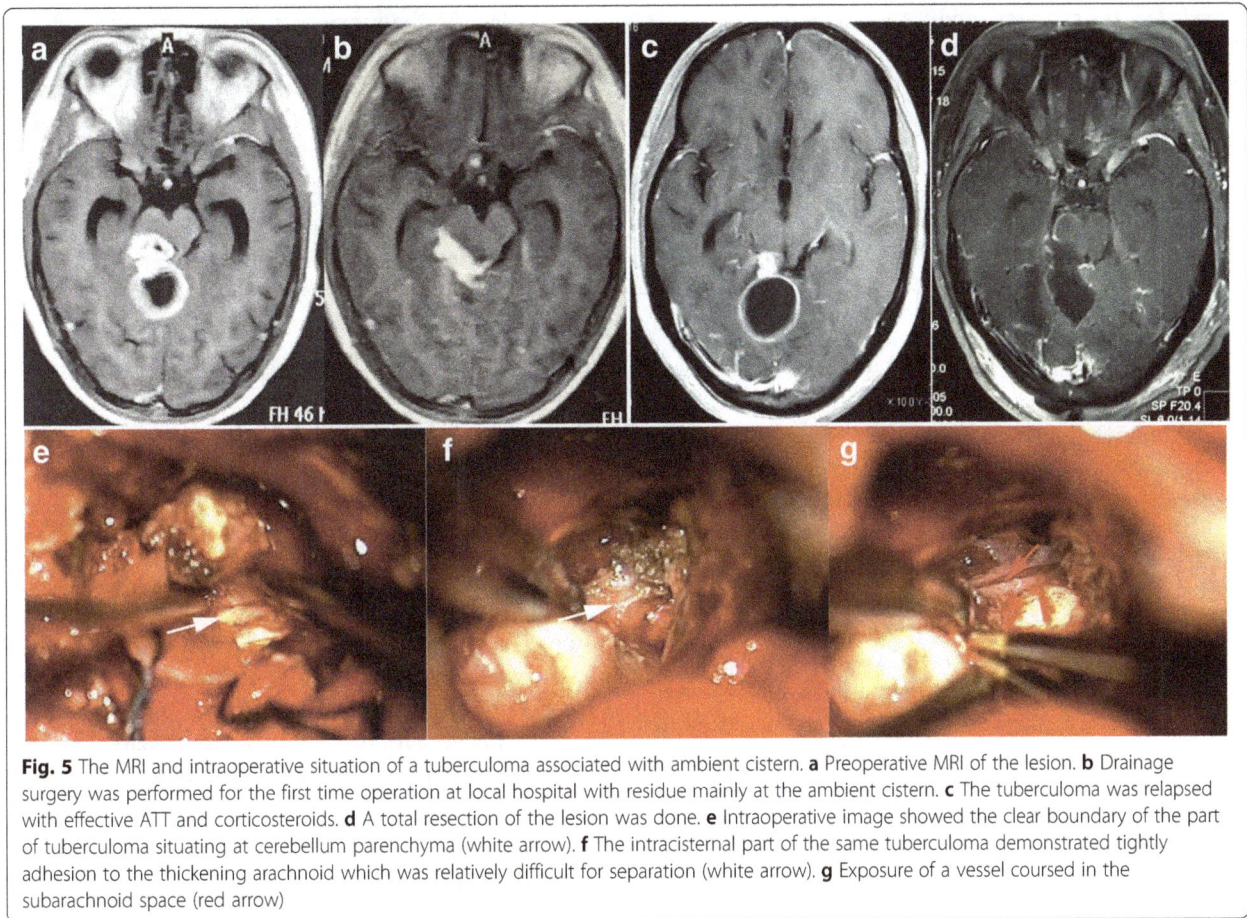

Fig. 5 The MRI and intraoperative situation of a tuberculoma associated with ambient cistern. **a** Preoperative MRI of the lesion. **b** Drainage surgery was performed for the first time operation at local hospital with residue mainly at the ambient cistern. **c** The tuberculoma was relapsed with effective ATT and corticosteroids. **d** A total resection of the lesion was done. **e** Intraoperative image showed the clear boundary of the part of tuberculoma situating at cerebellum parenchyma (white arrow). **f** The intracisternal part of the same tuberculoma demonstrated tightly adhesion to the thickening arachnoid which was relatively difficult for separation (white arrow). **g** Exposure of a vessel coursed in the subarachnoid space (red arrow)

experienced local recurrence were located at the dorsal ambient cistern or spinal subarachnoid space, respectively. We identified the thickening arachnoid adhered to the lesion during the surgery as described in previous literature [8]. The subarachnoid space involvement accompanied with the thickening arachnoid seems to be a potential risk factor for the occurrence and recurrence of tuberculoma. Meanwhile, frequent occurence of paradoxical reaction in the subarachnoid space furtherly proved the refractory nature of intracisternal tuberculoma.

Tuberculoma is frequently developed in subarachnoid space as a result of paradoxical reaction

The classical model of TM pathology suggests two steps of the pathological process of tuberculosis meningitis. Firstly, the mycobacteria begins to grow at the parenchyma or meninges of the brain or spinal cord, and then develops and matures into a tuberculous abscess. Secondly, the abscess breaks up and releases its contents into the subarachnoid space which causes TM [23]. TM may also be the result of the direct hematogenous spread of pulmonary tuberculosis [1]. Based on above

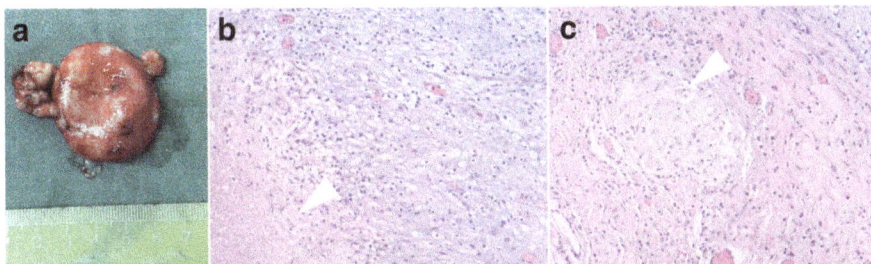

Fig. 6 The specimen of an intracisternal tuberculoma and the pathological examination. **a** The specimen of an intracisternal tuberculoma (patient 7). **b** Typical image showed the caseous necrosis of the specimen (arrow), epithelial cell and lymphocyte. **c** Typical image showed the tuberculous granuloma (arrow), epithelial cell and lymphocyte

knowledge, tuberculoma and TM may be considered as the initial manifestations of the CNS tuberculous pathology. More importantly, the subarachnoid space is a pathological and anatomical region where mycobacteria and its products frequently exist. The exudates of TM and the arachnoiditis usually accumulate at the subarachnoid space including the interpeduncular cisterns, optochiasmatic cistern, the ambient and the suprasellar cisterns, the sylvian fissures as well as the subarachnoid space of spine [17]. Spinal subarachnoid space is anatomically similar to the cerebral cisterns. This explained the facts that intradural extramedullary tuberculoma was closely related to the arachnoiditis as well [14]. Pathological progression following cisternal exudates includes arachnoiditis and tuberculoma [4, 11, 24]. This kind of cisternal tuberculoma displayed its own features other than the parenchymal tuberculoma. The gelatinous exudate is constrained by the hyperplastic thickened arachnoid whereas the exudate still could spread in the cistern. This illustrates multiple lobular tuberculoma is common in the images of published articles and in our cases which is different from the parenchymal tuberculoma (Fig. 1c, 2a) [8]. The adhesion of arachnoid led to the formation of the inter-septum of the tuberculoma. More importantly, the exudates in the cistern was considered a form of the paradoxical response [17]. Accordingly, tuberculoma secondary to the cisternal exudate was a product of paradoxical reaction too. It was reported the optochiasmatic region had a high propensity for accumulating a quantity of exudates, which was a frequent type of paradoxical reaction [25].

Intracisternal tuberculoma is refractory to ATT and an indication for surgical intervention

Based on the above information, because the cisternal tuberculoma shows a high rate of paradoxical development, the effectiveness of ATT is limited [23]. The immunological reaction based paradoxical reaction results in the progression of the lesion which calls for additional corticosteroids but no needs of change of ATT regimen [20]. Thus, prolonged therapeutic time is inevitable. At the same time, the paradoxical progression of the intracisternal lesion furtherly damages the neurological function which indicates surgery. Natarajan et al. believed that paradoxical intraduaral extramedullary tuberculoma was an indication for surgery [7]. According to our findings, the relatively enclosed space of a tuberculoma-occupying cistern which impedes the flow of CSF may result in a low concentration of medicine in the area. In the two relapsed cases reported in our study, the lesions were both situated in the subarachnoid space. As for the case of the tuberculoma locating at the ambient cistern to the cerebellum, even the drainage surgery had a limited effect and did not change the microenvironment of the intracisternal tuberculoma

(case 7). Finally, the safety of microsurgical excision had been proven as no secondary infection or dissemination was observed in literatures or our cases [9, 26]. All these factors ensure us that surgical resection should be early considered for the intracisternal tuberculoma.

Intracisternal tuberculoma is accompanied with serious neurological deficits requiring early resolving of the lesions

As mentioned above, Intracisternal tuberculoma is frequently progressed from paradoxical reaction and fast elimination of the lesions was usually difficult. It is worse that the exudates, arachnoiditis and/or tuberculoma developing in the cistern and adjacent parenchyma furtherly damage the neurological functions [23]. Tuberculoma in the cistern blocks the circulation of CSF resulting in hydrocephalus. The mass effect and surrounding edema may lead to the occurrence of hernia or the compression of vital structures of the CNS in certain areas. The exudates and tuberculoma can affect the blood vessels arranged in the area causing vasculitis and subsequently stroke [27]. In a univariate analysis, sylvian fissure exudates were predictors of stroke [28]. The critical site of the intracisternal tuberculoma also requires more attention especially surgical consideration.

Conclusions

Intracisternal and intradural extramedullary tuberculoma are specific forms of tuberculoma requiring particular attention. Exudates accumulation and arachnoiditis are the pathological changes occurring in these areas. Meanwhile, paradoxical reaction frequently participates in the formation of tuberculoma in these regions. This kind of intracisternal tuberculoma is refractory to ATT and corticosteroids which may take a long period to get the lesion resolved and potentially induce severe neurological injury. Surgical excision is an inevitable and necessary procedure for intracisternal tuberculoma for improving neurological function.

Abbreviations
ATT: Anti-tuberculosis treatment; CNS: Central nervous system; CSF: Cerebral spinal fluid; MRI: Magnetic resonance imaging; TB: Tuberculosis; TM: Tuberculous meningitis

Acknowledgements
We acknowledge Dr. Bing Luo, Jian Su, Hengchang Li and Zeng Yang for the clinical help; Dr. Xiangdong Xu for the MRI.

Funding
This work including the data collection, analysis and interpretation, manuscript revising was supported by National Natural Science Fund of China (81302187), PLA logistics research project (CWS14C063) and Fund of State Key Laboratory of Drug Research (SIMM1705KF-10).

Authors' contributions
HBJ, HH, FFC and LC participated in the design of this research. HH offered part of the data. FFC, LC wrote and revised the manuscript. WX, YYJ, YFC, WHL, JWZ, LBT, PL participated in the operation, treatment and data collection. YMF administered the ATT regimen. LL,YQ K, KKF carried out the data analysis. All authors have read and approved the final manuscript.

Competing interests
The authors declare that they have no competing interests.

Author details
[1]Neurosurgery Department, Guangzhou First People's Hospital, Guangzhou Medical University, 1# Panfu Road, Guangzhou, Guangdong 510180, China. [2]Neurosurgery Department, Shenzhen Second People's Hospital, Shenzhen University, 3002# Sungang Road, Shenzhen 518037, China. [3]Tuberculosis Department, Guangzhou Chest Hospital, 62# Hengzhi Gang Road, Guangzhou, Guangdong 510095, China. [4]Record Department, Guangzhou First People's Hospital, Guangzhou Medical University, 1# Panfu Road, Guangzhou, Guangdong 510180, China. [5]Department of Navy Medicine, The Second Military Medical University, 800# Xiangyin Road, Shanghai 200433, China. [6]Neurosurgery Department, Changzheng Hospital, The Second Military Medical University;State key Laboratory of Drug Research, Shanghai Institute of Material Medical, Chinese Academy of Sciences, 415# Fengyang Road, Shanghai 200003, China. [7]Spinal Surgery Department, Guangzhou First People's Hospital, Guangzhou Medical University, 1# Panfu Road, Guangzhou, Guangdong 510180, China.

References

1. DeLance AR, Safaee M, MC O, Clark AJ, Kaur G, Sun MZ, Bollen AW, Phillips JJ, Parsa AT. Tuberculoma of the central nervous system. J Clin Neurosci. 2013;20(10):1333–41.
2. Skendros P, Kamaria F, Kontopoulos V, Tsitouridis I, Sidiropoulos L. Intradural, eextramedullary tuberculoma of the spinal cord as a complication of tuberculous meningitis. Infection. 2003;31(2):115–7.
3. Das KK, Jaiswal S, Shukla M, Srivastava AK, Behari S, Kumar R. Concurrent cerebellar and cervical intramedullary tuberculoma: paradoxical response on antitubercular chemotherapy and need for surgery. J Pediatr Neurosci. 2014; 9(2):162–5.
4. Luo L, Pino J. An intradural extramedullary tuberculoma of the spinal cord in a non-HIV-infected patient: case report and review of the literature. Lung. 2006;184(3):187–93.
5. Dastur HM. Diagnosis and neurosurgical treatment of tuberculous disease of the CNS. Neurosurg Rev. 1983;6(3):111–7.
6. Thwaites GE, van Toorn R, Schoeman J. Tuberculous meningitis: more questions, still too few answers. The Lancet Neurology. 2013;12(10):999–1010.
7. Muthukumar N, Sureshkumar V, Ramesh VG. En plaque intradural extramedullary spinal tuberculoma and concurrent intracranial tuberculomas: paradoxical response to antituberculous therapy. Case report. Journal of neurosurgery Spine. 2007;6(2):169–73.
8. Rajshekhar V. Surgery for brain tuberculosis: a review. Acta Neurochir. 2015; 157(10):1665–78.
9. Li H, Liu W, You C. Central nervous system tuberculoma. J Clin Neurosci. 2012;19(5):691–5.
10. Botturi A, Prodi E, Silvani A, Gaviani P, Vanoli G, Carbone A, Salmaggi A. Brain tuberculoma (Mycobacterium Africanum): high index of suspicion helps in avoiding biopsy/surgery. Neurol Sci. 2012;33(2):363–5.
11. Roca B. Intradural extramedullary tuberculoma of the spinal cord: a review of reported cases. The Journal of infection. 2005;50(5):425–31.
12. Shingade RG, Prakashchandra SP. Role of advanced diagnostic imaging in intracranial Tuberculoma: MR spectroscopy. J Clin Diagn Res. 2015;9(8):TJ03–4.
13. Akhaddar A, El Hassani MY, Chakir N, Jiddane M. Optochiasmatic tuberculoma: complication of tuberculous meningitis. Report of a case and review of the literature. Journal of neuroradiology Journal de neuroradiologie. 2001;28(2):137–42.
14. Chang KH, Han MH, Choi YW, Kim IO, Han MC, Kim CW. Tuberculous arachnoiditis of the spine: findings on myelography, CT, and MR imaging. AJNR Am J Neuroradiol. 1989;10(6):1255–62.
15. Afghani B, Lieberman JM. Paradoxical enlargement or development of intracranial tuberculomas during therapy: case report and review. Clin Infect Dis. 1994;19(6):1092–9.
16. Nicolls DJ, King M, Holland D, Bala J, del Rio C. Intracranial tuberculomas developing while on therapy for pulmonary tuberculosis. Lancet Infect Dis. 2005;5(12):795–801.
17. Schoeman JF, Donald PR. Tuberculous meningitis. Handb Clin Neurol. 2013; 112:1135–8.
18. Verma R, Patil TB, Lalla R. Tuberculous optochiasmatic arachnoiditis. J Global Infect Dis. 2014;6(2):89.
19. Idris MN, Sokrab TE, Arbab MA, Ahmed AE, El Rasoul H, Ali S, Elzubair MA, Mirgani SM. Tuberculoma of the brain: a series of 16 cases treated with anti-tuberculosis drugs. The international journal of tuberculosis and lung disease. 2007;11(1):91–5.
20. Dheda K, Barry CE 3rd, Maartens G. Tuberculosis. Lancet. 2016;387(10024):1211–26.
21. Garg RK. Tuberculosis of the central nervous system. Postgrad Med J. 1999; 75(881):133–40.
22. Fox GJ, Mitnick CD, Benedetti A, Chan ED, Becerra M, Chiang CY, Keshavjee S, Koh WJ, Shiraishi Y, Viiklepp P, et al. Surgery as an adjunctive treatment for multidrug-resistant tuberculosis: an individual patient data Metaanalysis. Clin Infect Dis. 2016;62(7):887–95.
23. Garg RK, Malhotra HS, Kumar N. Paradoxical reaction in HIV negative tuberculous meningitis. J Neurol Sci. 2014;340(1–2):26–36.
24. Garg RK, Paliwal V, Malhotra HS. Tuberculous optochiasmatic arachnoiditis: a devastating form of tuberculous meningitis. Expert Rev Anti-Infect Ther. 2011;9(9):719–29.
25. Sinha MK, Garg RK, Anuradha HK, Agarwal A, Parihar A, Mandhani PA. Paradoxical vision loss associated with optochiasmatic tuberculoma in tuberculous meningitis: a report of 8 patients. The Journal of infection. 2010;60(6):458–66.
26. Jha D, Khatri P, Choudhary A, Sethi R, Kumar S. Endoscopic third ventriculostomy in prepontine-suprasellar tuberculoma with tuberculous meningitis hydrocephalus: a case report. Pediatr Neurosurg. 2007;43(1):42–6.
27. Schoeman JF, Van Zyl LE, Laubscher JA, Donald PR. Serial CT. Scanning in childhood tuberculous meningitis: prognostic features in 198 cases. J Child Neurol. 1995;10(4):320–9.
28. Cherian A, Thomas SV. Central nervous system tuberculosis. Afr Health Sci. 2011;11(1):116–27.

14

Widespread enlarged perivascular spaces associated with dementia and focal brain dysfunction

Daisuke Taniguchi[1], Hideki Shimura[1*] ⓘ, Masao Watanabe[1], Nobutaka Hattori[2] and Takao Urabe[1]

Abstract

Background: Enlarged perivascular spaces (PVS) are common magnetic resonance imaging (MRI) findings, whereas widespread enlarged PVS are extremely rare. Although most patients with widespread enlarged PVS remain asymptomatic, some develop neurological dysfunctions; however, it remains unclear whether these are the consequence of widespread enlarged PVS.

Case presentation: A 64-year-old female patient developed consciousness disturbance, cognitive dysfunctions, fluent aphasia, agraphia, acalculia, and left-right disorientation after suffering from bronchopneumonia. Brain MRI revealed unusually widespread enlarged PVS predominantly in the left cerebral hemisphere. Following bronchopneumonia treatment, her cognitive dysfunction, fluent aphasia, agraphia, acalculia, and left-right disorientation persisted despite improvement of her general condition. Furthermore, the hypoperfusion area on single photon emission computed tomography and slow wave sites on electroencephalography were consistent with the location of enlarged PVS, indicating that severe enlarged PVS impaired focal brain functions.

Conclusions: This case suggested that widespread enlarged PVS could be a potential cause of neurological deficits. We propose that impaired perivascular circulation due to enlarged PVS might lead to focal brain dysfunction.

Keywords: Perivascular space, Virchow-Robin space, Dementia, Magnetic resonance imaging

Background

Perivascular spaces (PVS), also known as Virchow-Robin spaces, surround the walls of brain parenchyma penetrating arteries, veins, and venules [1]. Overall, PVS are very common and considered normal findings on magnetic resonance imaging (MRI) of healthy individuals of all ages. These, however, can reach larger sizes, so-called enlarged PVS, especially in the elderly [1]. Widespread enlarged PVS are extremely rare and may signal brain abnormalities [2–13]. Although most patients with widespread enlarged PVS remain asymptomatic, some develop neurological deficits [2–4]. However, it is not clear whether enlarged PVS account for these deficits. Here, we report the case of a patient with widespread enlarged PVS, who has developed cognitive impairments

and higher cerebral dysfunction upon contracting bronchopneumonia.

Case presentation

A 64-year-old female patient was admitted to the emergency unit in our hospital due to progressive alterations of her mental status. Her medical history and that of her family were both unremarkable except that she was reported to have had several small brain cysts in the right posterior lobe while in her 30s. Three days prior to her admission, she developed a fever with upper respiratory tract symptoms, and complained of fatigue. On admission, her vital signs revealed a blood pressure of 180/100 mmHg, heart rate of 120 beats per minute, temperature of 38.0 °C, and oxygen saturation level of 98%. Her blood tests revealed elevated white-blood-cell counts (14,700 cells/μL) and C-reactive protein level (8.2 mg/dL). Her renal and liver functions as well as the levels of serum electrolytes were normal. The neurological examination revealed a Glasgow Coma Scale score of

* Correspondence: miurashimura@yahoo.co.jp
[1]Department of Neurology, Juntendo University Urayasu Hospital, 2-1-1 Tomioka, Urayasu, Chiba 279-0021, Japan
Full list of author information is available at the end of the article

E4V4M6, suggesting mental confusion. She showed temporal disorientation, and developed fluent aphasia, agraphia, acalculia, and left-right disorientation. However, she showed no weakness, ataxia, sensory disturbance, autonomic nervous dysfunction, or signs of meningeal irritation. Cerebrospinal-fluid (CSF) examination revealed normal opening pressure (120 mmH$_2$O), cell counts (2/μL, 100% monocytes), and protein levels (20 mg/dL). The CSF bacterial, fungal, and mycobacterium culture, CSF cytology, and cryptococcal antigen in serum tested all negative. Chest computed tomography (CT) revealed bronchopneumonia in the bilateral inferior lobes. We immediately started bronchopneumonia treatment with intravenous administration of ceftriaxone (2 g/day) for 5 days. Two days after admission, the fever subsided, the level of consciousness increased, and the patient became alert. However, her aphasia, agraphia, and acalculia persisted. Five days after admission, the patient was subjected to several neuropsychological examinations. Her Mini-Mental State Examination (MMSE) score was 18/30, suggesting recent memory loss, impaired attention, acalculia, and visual-constructive agnosia. Her total score on Frontal Assessment Battery was 5/18, suggesting frontal lobe dysfunction. Furthermore, the patient scored 14/36 on the Raven's colored progressive matrices test, which is a non-verbal evaluation of abstract reasoning. Electroencephalography (EEG) revealed slowing in the theta range predominantly in the left hemisphere, without epileptiform discharge. The patient's general condition continued to recover, and she was discharged 15 days after admission. However, the residual symptoms of recent memory loss, aphasia, agraphia, and acalculia persisted.

Brain MRI performed on the day of admission demonstrated multiple, confluent, well defined cystic lesions, predominantly in the left cerebral hemisphere (Fig. 1a–g). The cystic lesions were particularly found in the angular gyrus and the frontotemporal lobes (Fig. 1a–g). The Fluid Attenuated Inversion Recovery images revealed that the cystic lesions were isointense to CSF, and surrounded by rim of hyperintensities suggestive of perilesional gliosis (Fig. 1c). The cystic lesions were observed without gadolinium contrast enhancement (Fig. 1d, g). Furthermore, N-isopropyl-[123I] p-iodoamphetamine-single photon emission CT (123I-IMP SPECT) revealed extended areas of hypoperfusion in the entire left hemisphere and right frontal lobe, which may have resulted from the decrease of brain parenchyma volume (Fig. 2a). Magnetic resonance venography revealed no significant occlusive regions in the cerebral venous system (Fig. 2b). After excluding other causes of cystic conditions, a diagnosis of widespread enlarged PVS was made.

Through a two-year follow-up, brain MRI showed no remarkable changes compared with the initial MRI. The cognitive impairments and higher cerebral dysfunctions, such as aphasia, agraphia, and acalculia, did not deteriorate further, but were persistent as evidenced by an MMSE score of 18/30, which was evaluated every 6 months.

Discussion and conclusions

The MRI features of our patient were consistent with a widespread enlarged PVS [1]. The diagnostic work-up could exclude other causes of cystic condition, such as cystic neoplasm, cryptococcosis, neurocysticercosis, and mucopolysaccharidoses. There were no risk factors for cerebrovascular diseases. The patient was reported to have had several PVS almost 30 years before admission. Furthermore, the appearance of her PVS did not change after a 2-year follow-up. These findings suggested that a

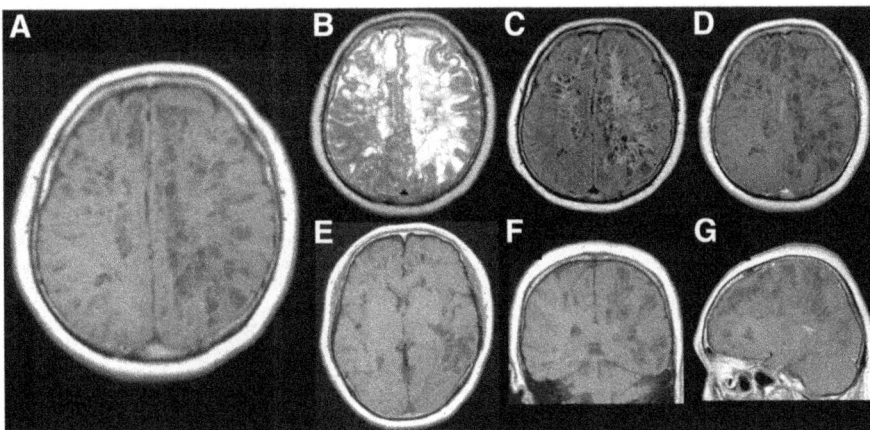

Fig. 1 Brain magnetic resonance imaging (MRI) showing multiple, confluent, and oval cystic lesions predominantly in the left cerebral hemisphere on T1 weighted imaging (**a**, **e**, **f**), T2 weighted imaging (**b**), Fluid Attenuated Inversion Recovery imaging (**c**), and gadolinium contrast enhancement imaging (**d**, **g**). Cystic lesions were found in particular in the angular gyrus and frontotemporal lobes (**a**, **e**). They are isointense to CSF (**c**), surrounded by rim of hyperintensities (**c**), and observed without gadolinium contrast enhancement (**d**, **g**)

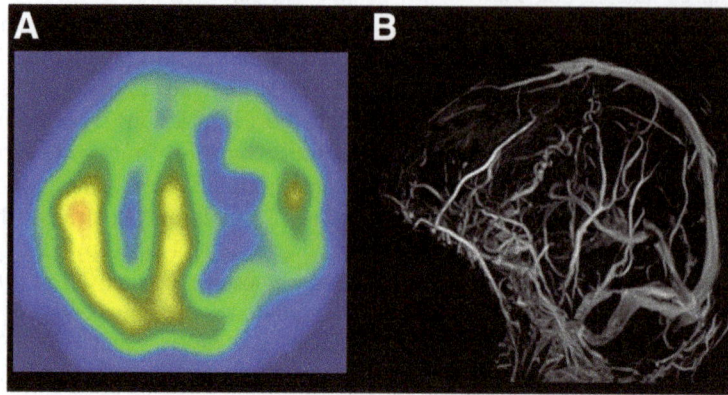

Fig. 2 Extended areas of hypoperfusion in the entire left hemisphere and right frontal lobe were observed by p-iodoamphetamine-single photon emission computed tomography (IMP-SPECT) (**a**). Magnetic resonance venography revealed no significant occlusive regions in the cerebral venous system (**b**)

widening of PVS might have progressed very slowly and asymptomatically in this case over the years before admission.

Indeed, most cases of widespread enlarged PVS show no neurological symptoms, and present with intact sensory and motor systems evidenced by normal sensory-evoked potentials and central motor conduction time [5]. In addition, functional MRI studies showed normal activation of the cortex adjacent to enlarged PVS [6–8]. Only three case studies of patients with widespread enlarged PVS in the cerebral white matter who developed neurological symptoms have been previously reported [2–4]. In one case, a patient with bilateral lesions of enlarged PVS developed dementia [2], while a second patient developed transient encephalopathy triggered by a mild respiratory infection [3]. The third case developed dementia and focal signs, where posterior and mediotemporal cerebral lesions were associated with hemiparesis and homonymous hemianopsia [4]. Enlarged PVS have been also correlated with poorer cognitive functions [9]. These findings are in line with our case report. Indeed, our patient initially showed no apparent neurological deficits. However, upon respiratory infection, she developed dementia and focal neurological deficits, including fluent aphasia, agraphia, acalculia, and left-right disorientation. Considering the broad perilesional gliosis, we assumed that there was a latent brain parenchymal damage caused by perivascular fluids pressure and inflammation due to enlarged PVS [14, 15]. Subsequently, the high fever triggered brain dysfunction, which consequently resulted in neurological symptoms. Fluent aphasia, agraphia, acalculia, and left-right disorientation might be associated with enlarged PVS in the left temporal hemisphere. The hypoperfusion and slow wave sites evidenced by SPECT and EEG, respectively, were associated with cystic lesions and indicated that widespread enlarged PVS impaired focal brain functions.

Although the underlying mechanisms of enlarged PVS have yet to be elucidated, recent studies revealed that the pulsatile components of blood pressure, namely the systolic blood pressure and pulse pressure, are associated with enlarged PVS [15]. However, previous studies have mainly focused on small-sized PVS (i.e., cerebral lacunae type III-a according to Poirier's classification [16]), and indicated that small PVS are biomarkers of vascular risk [15, 17–19]. In contrast, our case presented mainly multiple large PVS occupying the brain parenchyma (i.e.; cerebral lacunae type III-d according to Poirier's classification [16]), with no evidence of vascular risk factors. Thus, we considered that the enlarged PVS may have resulted from a dysfunctional drainage pathway through the PVS rather than from the continuous high pulsatility to penetrating arteries.

One of the central PVS functions is their contribution to the fluid movement and drainage in the brain. In particular, PVS are thought to be an important drainage pathway between the CSF and brain parenchyma [20–22]. Previous animal studies have demonstrated that the brain interstitial fluid is cleared into the CSF along the perivascular pathway. Therefore, decreased clearance of interstitial solutes occurs when the perivascular pathway is disrupted [20, 21]. Hence, widespread enlarged PVS may lead to brain dysfunction.

In conclusion, our case indicated that widespread enlarged PVS could be a potential cause of neurological deficits. We propose that the pathogenesis of widespread enlarged PVS might occur at the level of perivascular circulation.

Abbreviations
123I-IMP-SPECT: N-isopropyl-[123I] p-iodoamphetamine-single photon emission computed tomography; CSF: Cerebrospinal-fluid; CT: Computed tomography; EEG: Electroencephalography; MMSE: Mini-Mental State Examination; MRI: Magnetic resonance imaging; PVS: Perivascular spaces

Acknowledgements
None.

Funding
No funding was obtained for this study.

Authors' contributions
Acquisition of data: DT, HS, MW. Drafting of the manuscript: DT, HS. Critical revision of the manuscript for important intellectual content: MW, NH, TU. All authors read and approved the final manuscript.

Competing interests
The authors declare that they have no competing interests.

Author details
[1]Department of Neurology, Juntendo University Urayasu Hospital, 2-1-1 Tomioka, Urayasu, Chiba 279-0021, Japan. [2]Department of Neurology, Juntendo University School of Medicine, 2-1-1 Hongo, Bunkyo-ku, Tokyo 113-8421, Japan.

References

1. Kwee RM, Kwee TC. Virchow-Robin spaces at MR imaging. Radiographics. 2007;27(4):1071–86.
2. Vital C, Julien J. Widespread dilatation of perivascular spaces: a leukoencephalopathy causing dementia. Neurology. 1997;48(5):1310–3.
3. Cochrane TI, Nguyen TN. Swiss cheese brain. Neurology. 2007;68(2):140.
4. Buerge C, Steiger G, Kneifel S, Wetzel S, Wollmer MA, Probst A, Baumann TP. Lobar dementia due to extreme widening of Virchow-Robin spaces in one hemisphere. Case Rep Neurol. 2011;3(2):136–40.
5. Ugawa Y, Shirouzu I, Terao Y, Hanajima R, Machii K, Mochizuki H, Furubayashi T, Kanazawa I. Physiological analyses of a patient with extreme widening of Virchow-Robin spaces. J Neurol Sci. 1998;159(1):25–7.
6. Mathias J, Koessler L, Brissart H, Foscolo S, Schmitt E, Bracard S, Braun M, Kremer S. Giant cystic widening of Virchow-Robin spaces: an anatomofunctional study. AJNR Am J Neuroradiol. 2007;28(8):1523–5.
7. Ohta H, Kojima N, Ihara N, Ishigaki T, Todo G, Okamoto S. MR and Tc-99m HMPAO SPECT images in a case of unusual widening of perivascular spaces (Virchow-Robin spaces). Ann Nucl Med. 1999;13(6):437–9.
8. Young RJ, Lee V, Peck KK, Sierra T, Zhang Z, Jacks LM, Holodny AI. Diffusion tensor imaging and tractography of the corticospinal tract in the presence of enlarged Virchow-Robin spaces. J Neuroimaging. 2014;24(1):79–82.
9. Maclullich AM, Wardlaw JM, Ferguson KJ, Starr JM, Seckl JR, Deary IJ. Enlarged perivascular spaces are associated with cognitive function in healthy elderly men. J Neurol Neurosurg Psychiatry. 2004;75(11):1519–23.
10. Fumal A, de Noordhout AM, Collignon L. Neurological picture. Extreme unilateral widening of Virchow-Robin spaces mimicking stroke. J Neurol Neurosurg Psychiatry. 2009;80(1):64–5.
11. Molzer G, Robinson S. Case 202: extensive unilateral widening of Virchow-Robin spaces. Radiology. 2014;270(2):623–6.
12. Ogawa T, Okudera T, Fukasawa H, Hashimoto M, Inugami A, Fujita H, Hatazawa J, Shimosegawa E, Noguchi K, Uemura K. Unusual widening of Virchow-Robin spaces: MR appearance. AJNR Am J Neuroradiol. 1995;16(6): 1238–42.
13. Shiratori K, Mrowka M, Toussaint A, Spalke G, Bien S. Extreme, unilateral widening of Virchow-Robin spaces: case report. Neuroradiology. 2002;44(12): 990–2.
14. Wuerfel J, Haertle M, Waiczies H, Tysiak E, Bechmann I, Wernecke KD, Zipp F, Paul F. Perivascular spaces–MRI marker of inflammatory activity in the brain? Brain. 2008;131(Pt 9):2332–40.
15. Gutierrez J, Elkind MS, Cheung K, Rundek T, Sacco RL, Wright CB. Pulsatile and steady components of blood pressure and subclinical cerebrovascular disease: the northern Manhattan study. J Hypertens. 2015;33(10):2115–22.
16. Poirier J, Derouesne C. Cerebral lacunae. A proposed new classification. Clin Neuropathol. 1984;3(6):266.
17. Doubal FN, MacLullich AM, Ferguson KJ, Dennis MS, Wardlaw JM. Enlarged perivascular spaces on MRI are a feature of cerebral small vessel disease. Stroke. 2010;41(3):450–4.
18. Zhu YC, Tzourio C, Soumare A, Mazoyer B, Dufouil C, Chabriat H. Severity of dilated Virchow-Robin spaces is associated with age, blood pressure, and MRI markers of small vessel disease: a population-based study. Stroke. 2010; 41(11):2483 90.
19. Gutierrez J, Elkind MSV, Dong C, Di Tullio M, Rundek T, Sacco RL, Wright CB. Brain Perivascular spaces as biomarkers of vascular risk: results from the northern Manhattan study. AJNR Am J Neuroradiol. 2017;38(5):862–7.
20. Iliff JJ, Wang M, Liao Y, Plogg BA, Peng W, Gundersen GA, Benveniste H, Vates GE, Deane R, Goldman SA, et al. A paravascular pathway facilitates CSF flow through the brain parenchyma and the clearance of interstitial solutes, including amyloid beta. Sci Transl Med. 2012;4(147):147ra111.
21. Kress BT, Iliff JJ, Xia M, Wang M, Wei HS, Zeppenfeld D, Xie L, Kang H, Xu Q, Liew JA, et al. Impairment of paravascular clearance pathways in the aging brain. Ann Neurol. 2014;76(6):845–61.
22. Tarasoff-Conway JM, Carare RO, Osorio RS, Glodzik L, Butler T, Fieremans E, Axel L, Rusinek H, Nicholson C, Zlokovic BV, et al. Clearance systems in the brain-implications for Alzheimer disease. Nat Rev Neurol. 2015;11(8):457–70.

15

Effect of tendon vibration during wide-pulse neuromuscular electrical stimulation (NMES) on muscle force production in people with spinal cord injury (SCI)

Vanesa Bochkezanian[1,2,3]* [iD], Robert U. Newton[2,3,4], Gabriel S. Trajano[5], Amilton Vieira[6], Timothy S. Pulverenti[3] and Anthony J. Blazevich[3]

Abstract

Background: Neuromuscular electrical stimulation (NMES) is commonly used in skeletal muscles in people with spinal cord injury (SCI) with the aim of increasing muscle recruitment and thus muscle force production. NMES has been conventionally used in clinical practice as functional electrical stimulation (FES), using low levels of evoked force that cannot optimally stimulate muscular strength and mass improvements, and thus trigger musculoskeletal changes in paralysed muscles. The use of high intensity intermittent NMES training using wide-pulse width and moderate-intensity as a strength training tool could be a promising method to increase muscle force production in people with SCI. However, this type of protocol has not been clinically adopted because it may generate rapid muscle fatigue and thus prevent the performance of repeated high-intensity muscular contractions in paralysed muscles. Moreover, superimposing patellar tendon vibration onto the wide-pulse width NMES has been shown to elicit further increases in impulse or, at least, reduce the rate of fatigue in repeated contractions in able-bodied populations, but there is a lack of evidence to support this argument in people with SCI.

Methods: Nine people with SCI received two NMES protocols with and without superimposing patellar tendon vibration on different days (i.e. STIM and STIM+vib), which consisted of repeated 30 Hz trains of 58 wide-pulse width (1000 μs) symmetric biphasic pulses (0.033-s inter-pulse interval; 2 s stimulation train; 2-s inter-train interval) being delivered to the dominant quadriceps femoris. Starting torque was 20% of maximal doublet-twitch torque and stimulations continued until torque declined to 50% of the starting torque. Total knee extensor impulse was calculated as the primary outcome variable.

Results: Total knee extensor impulse increased in four subjects when patellar tendon vibration was imposed (59.2 ± 15.8%) but decreased in five subjects (− 31.3 ± 25.7%). However, there were no statistically significant differences between these sub-groups or between conditions when the data were pooled.

Conclusions: Based on the present results there is insufficient evidence to conclude that patellar tendon vibration provides a clear benefit to muscle force production or delays muscle fatigue during wide-pulse width, moderate-intensity NMES in people with SCI.

* Correspondence: v.bochkezanian@cqu.edu.au; vanesaboch@gmail.com
[1]Department of Exercise and Health Sciences, School of Health, Medical and Applied Sciences, Central Queensland University, Building 34.1.02, Bruce Highway, North Rockhampton, Qld 4702, Australia
[2]Exercise Medicine Research Clinic, Edith Cowan University, Perth, Australia
Full list of author information is available at the end of the article

Background

Spinal cord injury (SCI) is most commonly caused by trauma and interrupts the connection between supra-spinal and spinal regions of the CNS [1]. This leads to a reduction of the voluntary activation of muscles below the lesion level, reducing muscle force production, impairing physical function, and profoundly compromising physical health and quality of life (QoL) [1–3]. Furthermore, the reduction in muscle force production is a major predictor of mortality risk and seems to be partly attributable to the quantity (i.e. absolute muscle volume) and quality (i.e. muscle density) of muscle mass [4, 5].

A common method to increase muscular force production and muscle mass is the use of neuromuscular strength training. Particularly, high-intensity muscle contractions have been proven to enhance longevity and QoL in different clinical populations, such as diabetes type 2 and osteoporosis, as well as in older adults [6–9]. However, muscle strength training poses an increased challenge for people with a neurological condition, such as people with SCI. Alternatively, neuromuscular electrical stimulation (NMES) is a commonly used intervention in rehabilitation programs to increase muscle recruitment and thus muscle force production, especially in individuals with a complete loss of motor function [10–12]. NMES has been conventionally used in clinical practice as functional electrical stimulation (FES), i.e. a prolonged and low levels of evoked force NMES exercise paired simultaneously or intermittently with a functional task [12]. However, such interventions cannot optimally stimulate muscular strength and mass improvements, imposing a higher load to the muscle to obtain higher force output [13, 14] in accordance with the overload training principle [15], to obtain musculoskeletal changes in paralysed muscles.

The use of high intensity intermittent NMES training (hereafter referred to as near-maximal evoked muscle contractions) as a strength training tool has not been adopted clinically in people with SCI, probably due to the lack of evidence from long-term intervention trials documenting its physiological effects [16, 17] but mainly because these types of protocols generate rapid muscle fatigue and thus prevent the performance of repeated high-intensity muscular contractions [18–21]. This muscle fatigue is exacerbated in people with SCI due to the loss of fatigue-resistant motor units and their higher proportion of more fatigable motor units [22–26], making the rapid muscle fatigue induced by NMES a continuing issue [27, 28]. A clinical issue is therefore presented since higher volumes of strength training, in comparison to lower volumes, are known to promote greater health and functional adaptations, particularly in older adults and in clinical populations such as people with diabetes type 2 [29, 30]. For these reasons, early

muscle fatigue represents a problem and, if suboptimal stimulation parameters are used and NMES training elicits a rapid muscle fatigue, may prevent the delivery of the ideal dose of training to realise optimum musculoskeletal adaptations in paralysed muscles. Nonetheless, NMES as a strength training modality has previously been shown to stimulate quadriceps muscle hypertrophy [31–34], improved skeletal muscle oxidative capacity [35] and to improve lean muscle mass [33] and bone adaptations in people with SCI [36–38]. Yet, the use of NMES as high-intensity strength training mode has not been extensively investigated and, due to the limited evidence supporting its use for increasing muscle strength [39, 40] is not commonly used in clinical practice.

One promising method to enhance force production whilst minimising muscle fatigue is the application of tendon vibration [41, 42]. Tendon vibration may generate trains of Ia-afferent signals to the spinal cord that induce a progressive excitation of homonymous motor neurones and promote the development of persistent inward calcium (Ca^{2+}) or sodium (Na^+) currents at their dendritic trees [43–45]. Thus, this method could amplify and prolong the synaptic input and create a sustained depolarisation leading to an increased recruitment of motor units (i.e. self-sustained firing) and increase muscle force production, especially when coupled with wide-pulse width (e.g. 1000 μs) NMES [46, 47]. Importantly, however, vibration tends to preferentially excite low-threshold (i.e. fatigue resistant) motor units [48], which exhibit significant endurance and are therefore likely to contribute to a great total muscular work before fatigue is induced. In previous studies the positive effects of vibration were observed in able-bodied populations during wide-pulse width NMES applied both at relatively low (~ 5% MVC force) [46] and high (~ 20% MVC force) [47] levels of muscle force production, suggesting that vibration may augment muscle contraction force and allow a greater total muscular effort before fatigue during wide-pulse width NMES even when relatively high contraction intensities are used, such as those required for strength training. However, it is unknown whether the imposition of tendon vibration onto wide-pulse width NMES promotes such benefits in people with SCI. In fact, it is also not known whether tendon vibration might elicit an additional excitation of the motor neuron pool through the same (central) pathways as wide-pulse width NMES [43–45, 49] and therefore instead promote a greater muscle fatigue in partially or completely paralysed muscles.

In a previous study [50], patellar tendon vibration during wide-pulse width NMES in able-bodied individuals resulted in an increased total muscle work performed in "positive responders" only, but a reduced total work in others. Nonetheless, within the whole study cohort the application of patellar tendon vibration tended to minimise voluntary muscle fatigue caused by the NMES [50], and would thus have allowed the study participants to immediately perform other physical activities without a notable negative impact on performance. Thus, it is of great interest to determine whether similar effects would be obtained in people with SCI. The purpose of the present study, therefore, was to determine whether patellar tendon vibration superimposed onto wide-pulse width NMES under standard clinical conditions elicits a greater peak muscle force with less muscle fatigue (i.e. a greater total impulse) when compared to NMES applied without patellar tendon vibration in people with SCI. We hypothesised that patellar tendon vibration superimposed onto wide-pulse width NMES would elicit a greater peak muscle force with less muscle fatigue (i.e. a greater total impulse) that NMES applied without patellar tendon vibration in people with SCI.

Methods

Subjects

Nine subjects with SCI (3 females, 6 males) were recruited from the Spinal Cord Injuries Australia (SCIA) Activity-based therapy exercise program "NeuroMoves" and the Perth community (mean ± SD, age: 39.4 ± 10.6 y; height: 176.2 ± 9.7 cm; body mass 80.6 ± 9.6 kg). Four subjects were classified as complete spinal cord injury (AIS A) and five were classified as incomplete (AIS B-D). All subjects were recruited by word of mouth or email and had a SCI of more than 6 months. Prior to the study, subjects were given detailed information about the procedures and the risks of participating in the study, and they all signed a written consent form. Subjects completed the Physical Activity Readiness Questionnaire (PAR-Q) to ensure safe exercise participation and refrained from vigorous exercise (48 h) and alcohol (24 h) and stimulant consumption (e.g. caffeine, energy drinks for 6 h) prior to testing.

Participants included in this study had medical clearance and were fit and medically stable to participate in this study. Participants were asked to replicate the same physical routine for each session. Sessions were completed at the same time of the day and under the same experimental conditions. This research study was approved by the Edith Cowan University Human Ethics Committee (reference number: 11,623). Subject characteristics are detailed in Table 1.

Procedures

The procedures used in this study followed the methodology described in a previous study in healthy individuals [50], but was adapted to people with SCI accordingly. All subjects attended the Neuromuscular Physiology Laboratory at Edith Cowan University on three occasions on different days (1 day per week for the duration of 4 weeks) with a minimum of 7 days between sessions. One week before starting data collection, the subjects attended a full familiarisation session where the NMES protocol was applied to the dominant quadriceps femoris with and without simultaneous patellar tendon vibration. Each subject received 1 min of tendon vibration and 3 min of NMES to ensure they could tolerate the intervention; all subjects tolerated the NMES and tendon vibration protocols well. The subsequent two sessions were used to complete the following two experimental protocols in a random order without replication: 1) NMES only (STIM); and 2) NMES superimposed onto tendon vibration (STIM+Vib).

In familiarisation and experimental sessions, the subjects were asked to produce a voluntary knee extension contraction of approximately 50% of perceived maximal voluntary exertion while seated on an isokinetic dynamometer. If any voluntary contractions were visualised and recorded, then a standardised warm-up protocol was performed, consisting of isometric knee extensions

Table 1 Subject characteristics. Subject levels of injury, completeness of lesion, time since injury, AIS scale score, medication type and response to tendon vibration (i.e. whether a tendon vibration reflex response is detectable). Complete (C) lesion means no voluntary muscle contraction below the level of injury. Incomplete (I) lesion means some voluntary muscle contraction below the level of injury [71]

Subject	Level of injury	Complete (C)/Incomplete (I)	Time since injury (y)	AIS	Medication	Positive responder to tendon vibration	Negative responder to tendon vibration
A	T_7	I	3	B	Baclofen		x
B	T_6	C	6	A	Oxybutin		x
C	T_6	C	5	A	Baclofen		x
D	C_6-C_7	C	4	A	Baclofen		x
E	T_{12}	I	2	D	Baclofen		x
F	C_7	C	1	A	Baclofen	x	
G	T_5	I	20	D	Baclofen	x	
H	T_3	I	2	B	Baclofen	x	
I	L_3	I	4	D	N/A	x	

at 30%, 50%, 70% and 90% of perceived maximal effort before performing a series of three knee extension MVICs. However, if no voluntary contraction was recorded then three attempts of maximal voluntary contractions (MVICs) were instructed without warm-up efforts. The subjects were seated with hip and knee joint angles of 85° and 90°, respectively (0 ° = full knee extension), with the thigh and trunk secured to the dynamometer chair and the knee joint aligned with the center of rotation of the dynamometer. All subjects were instructed to produce a force against the dynamometer arm by extending the knee as fast and hard as possible for 3 s, and verbal encouragement and visual feedback were provided during all MVICs irrespective of the subject's ability to voluntarily activate their lower limbs. This method was implemented to be consistent with the procedures among all subjects.

Electrical stimulation and tendon vibration protocols

NMES was delivered by a high-voltage constant-current electrical stimulator (400 V, DS7A, Digitimer Ltd., Welwyn Garden City, UK) through four self-adhesive stimulation electrodes (Axelgaard, PALS, USA) placed over the rectus femoris (RF), vastus lateralis (VL), and vastus medialis (VM); two 5×10 cm electrodes were placed over RF and one 5×5 cm electrode was placed on each of the VM and VL, approximately at their motor points. The electrodes were then moved if necessary to elicit the greatest twitch response with low stimulation intensity in every session [51]. The electrode positions were marked on a plastic sheet for each subject and indelible ink was used to mark these positions on the skin to ensure identical electrode placement at subsequent sessions.

To habituate the subjects to the electrical stimulations- and after the attempts of MVCIs, two electrical square-wave stimuli (1000 µs square-wave pulses separated by 5 ms) were delivered to the dominant leg (determined in familiarisation session using NMES) every 20 s while the stimulation current was increased from 30 to 99 mA in 10-mA increments until a plateau in the maximum peak twitch torque was observed. This was defined as maximal peak twitch torque ($\tau_{tw,p}$) and was used as the "target torque". A second, submaximal peak twitch torque ($\tau_{tw,sub}$) recording was obtained at 40 mA and retained for analysis of changes in submaximal torque, to assess the ability of the muscle to contract under submaximal conditions, which are often used in a clinical context. Subsequently, a maximum of three trains of NMES (described below) were performed at different stimulation current intensities until reaching the closest value to the target torque. This procedure was replicated in all participants regardless of their response to the imposed current. All participants in this study showed an increase in evoked torque when increasing the current from 30 to 99 mA (maximum output allowed by the electrical stimulator) and the level of evoked torque was set equal or close to the maximal peak twitch torque ($\tau_{tw,p}$).

The NMES protocol consisted of repeated 30-Hz trains of 58 wide-pulse width (1000 µs) symmetric biphasic pulses (0.033-s inter-pulse interval), where a single train duration was 2 s and the inter-train interval was 2 s (i.e. 2-s on and 2-s off). The level of evoked torque was set equal or close to the maximal peak twitch torque ($\tau_{tw,p}$), which should be equivalent to ~ 20% of MVIC.

Patellar tendon vibration was applied using a vibration device (Deep Muscle Stimulator, Las Vegas, NV, USA), which mechanically vibrated the tendon at 55 Ha and amplitude of 7 mm (confirmed through direct measurement of high-speed video). The two test conditions were:

STIM: Electrically-evoked muscle contractions produced by delivering the NMES protocol until torque was reduced to ≤50% of the target torque (i.e. $\tau_{tw,p}$) in one electrically-evoked contraction, which was defined as "target fatigue".

STIM + Vib: Electrically-evoked contractions delivered as in STIM, but superimposed with patellar tendon vibration which was applied for at least 5 s before NMES and after target fatigue was reached.

For a graphical representation of the STIM and STIM +Vib protocols please refer to Fig. 1.

Data collection and analysis
Peak evoked torque, torque-time integral and number of contractions

Two measures of peak-twitch evoked torque were analysed: one submaximal ($\tau_{tw,sub}$) evoked at a 40-mA current, and one maximal ($\tau_{tw,p}$) obtained from the peak of the torque-current relationship. These were obtained both before and after the NMES protocols were delivered. The total torque-time integral (TTI) was used to provide a measure of the total exercise stimulus received by the muscle in each condition. TTI was calculated as the product of torque and time calculated from the onset of the first stimulation train (STIM) or vibration onset (STIM+Vib) to the end of the final evoked contraction when "target fatigue" was reached (as defined in Procedures). Peak evoked torque was defined as the highest torque value obtained after the onset of the first stimulation train for both STIM and STIM+Vib. TTI and peak evoked torque were compared between STIM and STIM+Vib. The post-study data analysis revealed that some subjects responded with a greater TTI

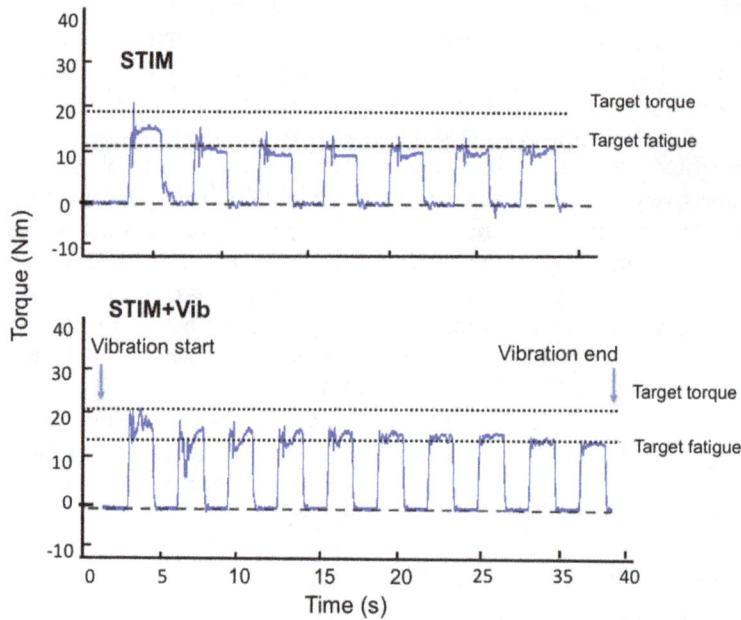

Fig. 1 Graphical representation of the STIM and STIM+Vib. STIM and STIM+Vib protocols in one of the participants can be observed in this graph. Blue traces refer to the torque forces evoked by the NMES protocols

after STIM+Vib than STIM (i.e. positive responders to patellar tendon vibration) whilst others showed no difference or a lower TTI after STIM+Vib than STIM (i.e. negative responders to patellar tendon vibration), as described in Results. Therefore, a second analysis was performed after separating subjects into positive and negative responders to patellar tendon vibration (described in Procedures). Positive and negative responders were identified not only during the training sessions but also during pilot testing sessions where different NMES protocols with superimposed patellar tendon vibration were utilised. Although the pilot data are not presented in the present article, this information reinforced the identification of positive and negative responders to patellar tendon vibration during at least one pilot session and provided confidence in the interpretation of results. The total number of contractions was measured as the number of contractions from the beginning of the first evoked contraction reaching the target torque until the last contraction when reaching 50% of the target torque ("target fatigue").

Statistical analysis

Two-way repeated measures analysis of variance (ANOVA) was used to compare changes in all variables between conditions (STIM, STIM+Vib) over time (PRE, POST). A Wilcoxon test was conducted to compare STIM, STIM+Vib between PRE-and POST in positive and negative responders to patellar tendon vibration whilst using assessments at PRE as the covariates. Pairwise t-tests were performed when significant interaction

effects were found. A chi- square test for independence was used to assess whether an association existed between subjects with complete and incomplete SCI and the likelihood of being a positive or negative responders. Statistical significance was set at an alpha level of $p \leq 0.05$ and values are reported as mean ± SD.

Results

Peak evoked torque, torque-time integral (TTI) and total number of contractions

No statistical differences in peak evoked torque ($p = 0.43$; Fig. 2a), torque-time integral (TTI; $p = 0.39$; Fig. 2b) or total number of contractions ($p = 0.78$) were observed between STIM and STIM+Vib. Nonetheless, the response to STIM+Vib (based on TTI) was clearly greater than in STIM in some subjects (40% of sample) but lesser (or negative) in others. Thus, an additional comparative analysis of positive versus negative responders to patellar tendon vibration was undertaken, where positive responders to patellar tendon vibration were defined as those subjects who responded with a greater TTI in STIM+Vib when compared to STIM. This analysis revealed no statistical difference in TTI between STIM and STIM+Vib for positive or negative responders (Fig. 3), or a difference between STIM and STIM+Vib for the whole cohort collectively. However, the between-condition difference was dissimilar between the responder groups when using $\tau_{tw,p}$ at PRE for both conditions as a covariate ($p = 0.02$); TTI was 59.2 ± 15.8% greater in STIM+Vib than STIM in positive responders to patellar tendon vibration ($p = 0.13$) but 31.3

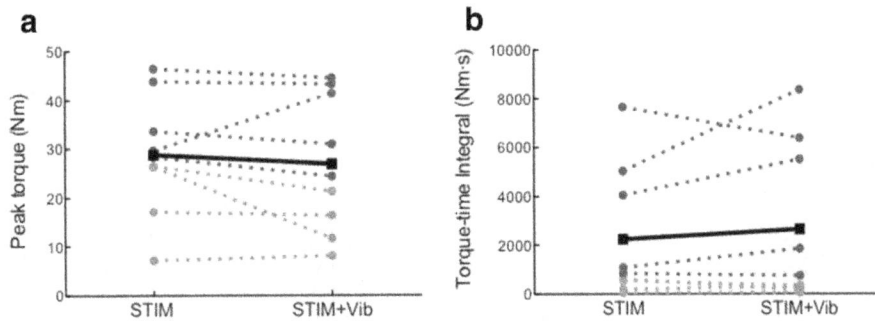

Fig. 2 Peak torque and Torque-Time Integral (TTI) in STIM and STIM+Vib conditions. **a** Peak torque production (Nm) in STIM and STIM+Vib conditions for all subjects. No statistically significant differences were found between the two conditions **b** Torque-time integral (TTI; Nm·s) in STIM and STIM+Vib conditions for all subjects. No statistically significant differences were found between the two conditions. Grey dashed lines represent individual subjects and the black solid line represents the group mean. Darker grey dots indicate subjects with incomplete spinal cord injury (SCI) and light grey dots indicate subjects with complete SCI

± 25.7% less in STIM+Vib than STIM in negative responders ($p = 0.14$), as shown in Fig. 3. There was also no clear effect of completeness of lesion (complete or incomplete SCI) on the likelihood of being a positive or negative responder to tendon vibration (χ^2 (1, $n = 9$) = 1.10, $p = 0.70$). Also, no significant differences were found between the conditions (STIM and STIM+Vib) for total number of contractions, despite a trend being observed; the mean total number of contractions for positive responders to tendon vibration for STIM was 56.5 ± 60.5 and for STIM+Vib was 70.2 ± 68.9, whilst the means for negative responders to tendon vibration were

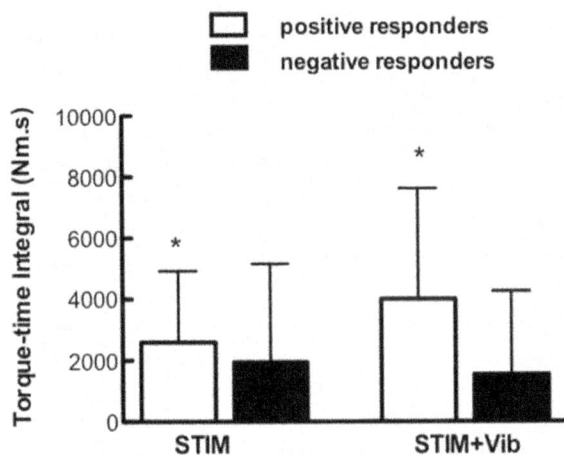

Fig. 3 Torque-Time Integral (TTI; Nm·s) in STIM and STIM+Vib. TTI recorded in STIM and STIM+Vib conditions for positive and negative responders to tendon vibration. Significant increases of 59.2 ± 15.8% in TTI in STIM+Vib compared to STIM for positive responders to tendon vibration ($p = 0.13$) and decreases of − 31.3 ± 25.7% in STIM +Vib for negative responders to tendon vibration ($p = 0.14$) were observed, when using $\tau_{tw,p}$ at PRE for both conditions as a covariate ($p = 0.02$), however TTI was not statistically different between conditions. * Significantly different between positive and negative responders ($p < 0.05$)

41.6 ± 37.4 for STIM and 33.8 ± 30.9 for STIM+Vib (figure not shown).

Muscle force measures: Maximal evoked force ($\tau_{tw,p}$) and submaximal evoked force ($\tau_{tw,sub}$)

There was a significant effect of time, as the relative maximal force ($\tau_{tw,p}$; $p = 0.00$) and submaximal force ($\tau_{tw,sub}$; $p = 0.00$) decreased from PRE to POST in both conditions (STIM and STIM+Vib). However, a similar pattern was observed in STIM+Vib and STIM conditions, as there were no significant effects of condition ($\tau_{tw,p}$: $p = 0.21$; $\tau_{tw,sub}$: $p = 0.13$) and no significant condition × time interaction ($\tau_{tw,p}$: $p = 0.98$; $\tau_{tw,sub}$: $p = 0.77$). Submaximal twitch torque ($\tau_{tw,sub}$) declined by 40.4 ± 4.7% and maximal force ($\tau_{tw,p}$) declined by 27.0 ± 5.0% of baseline in STIM, whilst $\tau_{tw,sub}$ declined by 45.0 ± 4.2% and $\tau_{tw,p}$ declined by 30.6 ± 5.0% of baseline on STIM +Vib (Fig. 4).

Discussion

The purpose of this study was to determine whether patellar tendon vibration superimposed onto wide-pulse width NMES would elicit greater peak muscle force production and/or induce less muscle fatigue (i.e. increase the total impulse before fatigue) than NMES alone in people with spinal cord injury (SCI). The main finding was that the torque-time integral (TTI) measured at the point of fatigue (i.e. 50% of initial evoked torque) was not statistically different between STIM and STIM+Vib conditions, although a significantly greater TTI was found in four (of nine) "positive" responders to patellar tendon vibration (59.2 ± 15.8%). Thus, in four of the present participants, the addition of the patellar tendon vibration allowed for a greater total muscular work to be performed, but a lower total muscular work was completed in the other five subjects (− 31.3 ± 25.7%). However, these changes were not statistically different

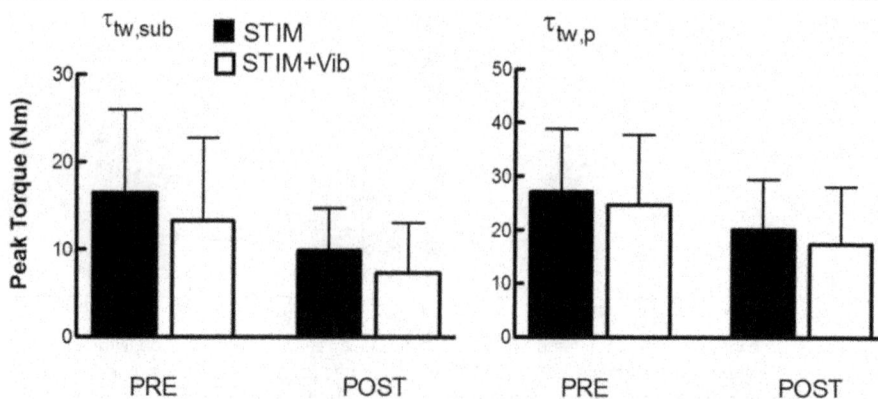

Fig. 4 Submaximal ($\tau_{tw,sub}$) and maximal ($\tau_{tw,p}$) peak twitch torque recorded before (PRE) and after (POST) STIM and STIM+Vib. Submaximal ($\tau_{tw,sub}$: 40 mA) and maximal ($\tau_{tw,p}$) electrical stimulation peak twitch torques recorded before (PRE) and after (POST) STIM and STIM + Vib. Submaximal twitch torque ($\tau_{tw,sub}$; top panel) declined $40.4 \pm 4.7\%$ and maximal force ($\tau_{tw,p}$; bottom panel) declined $27.0 \pm 5.0\%$ of baseline in STIM, whilst $\tau_{tw,sub}$ declined $45.0 \pm 4.2\%$ and $\tau_{tw,p}$ declined $30.6 \pm 5.0\%$ of baseline in STIM+Vib. However, no statistically significant differences were found between the two conditions

between conditions. Moreover, as observed from Fig. 2, there was no evidence that completeness of lesion (complete vs. incomplete SCI) was a factor influencing the likelihood of being a responder to patellar tendon vibration. Therefore, whilst the imposition of patellar tendon vibration during wide-pulse width NMES may allow for a greater impulse to be provided before fatigue in some individuals, it is not apparently clear who might benefit from the application of patellar tendon vibration in people with SCI based on our results.

The use of patellar tendon vibration superimposed onto wide-pulse width NMES was hypothesised to allow for a greater training impulse prior to fatigue, which might be of practical significance since it might evoke greater chronic increases in muscle strength and mass as well as improve muscle performance after a period of training [36, 52]. However, this appears to be the case only in some individuals who show a positive response to patellar tendon vibration. The ability to produce greater forces after a period of training may allow for higher volumes of muscle work to be performed during a physical rehabilitation session and thus generate early improvements in physical performance and physical health benefits in people with SCI; this hypothesis should thus be tested using a longitudinal study design. A reflex response induced by patellar tendon vibration may facilitate the initiation, maintenance and strength of any residual voluntary contraction in people with incomplete SCI. The use of patellar tendon vibration in those with a complete lesion can help to regulate the reflex response, which is highly altered after a complete SCI, by stimulating reflex pathways. Previous research has shown that somatosensory information continues to flow in a modified manner after a complete SCI and that there is a potential to generate motor patterns if this somatosensory input is stimulated by the use of methods

such as NMES and tendon vibration [53, 54]. The mechanisms of action of tendon vibration relate to the tonic vibration reflex (TVR), elicited by the application of tendon vibration, which may potentially help recruit more motor units and thus increase muscle force production when used in combination with NMES [46]. Greater muscular forces elicited by the tendon vibration when superimposed to NMES were found in previous studies in able-bodied people [46] and were attributed to the generation of persistent inward currents, recruiting higher-threshold motor units through reflexive pathways and increasing muscle force production [55, 56]. On the other hand, the reduced training impulse prior to fatigue observed in the negative responders to patellar tendon vibration suggested that patellar tendon vibration may be detrimental for some people and that in these people the use of (wide-pulse width) NMES alone may be more beneficial. This response observed in negative responders to patellar tendon vibration may speculatively be caused by the low-to-moderate frequency (55 Hz) vibration resulting in a stimulation of Golgi tendon organs, which can cause autogenic inhibition and potentially decrease the motor output [57]. Therefore, the present, individual-specific results cannot confirm the hypothesis that superimposing patellar tendon vibration onto wide-pulse width NMES would elicit an additional greater peak muscle force with less muscle fatigue (i.e. a greater total impulse) when compared to NMES applied without patellar tendon vibration in most people with a SCI.

These variable responses to patellar tendon vibration may also be explained by the highly individual functional deficits found between individuals with incomplete SCI, where the transmission of the sensory-motor information is altered at the synaptic level [58, 59] and there is a muscle spindle afferent dysfunction in both complete and incomplete lesions to the spinal cord [58, 59]. A similar inter-individual variability in response to wide-pulse width NMES has also been suggested to originate from a difference in monoamine levels between individuals [43] and could be one reason for the different response to patellar tendon vibration superimposed onto wide-pulse width NMES observed in the current study. This difference in monoamine levels could be exacerbated by the altered neuromuscular system in people with spinal cord injuries [60], such as changes in the excitability of the motor neurone [61], fibre type transformation towards fast-fatigable [60] and high levels of muscle atrophy [62]. Another factor that could have decreased the stretch reflex and thus prevented the formation of PICs is the use of antispasmodic medications, such as Baclofen [63]. On the other hand, the increased TTI in positive responders to patellar tendon vibration might be attributable to the development of tonic vibration reflexes (TVR) which increase muscle force contributions between the evoked muscular contractions [47, 64]. However, the activation of already hyper-excitable sensory pathways by the use of patellar tendon vibration in people suffering from a spinal cord injury may have either triggered episodes of intrinsic phasic spasticity in some participants [65], whilst attenuated spasticity symptoms in others [66], and thus may have increased the variability in the response to wide-pulse width NMES and patellar tendon vibration observed in the present study. These hypotheses will need to be explored in further studies investigating explicitly the pathophysiological responses (i.e. spasticity) of paralysed muscles to tendon vibration superimposed onto wide-pulse width NMES.

Another important finding of the current study was that the decline in evoked muscle force was not attenuated by the application of patellar tendon vibration. Muscle fatigue experienced after both STIM and STIM+Vib could be attributed to the "peripheral fatigue" (i.e. contractile alterations) induced by NMES, due to the repeated activation of the same muscle fibres, especially due to the missing sensory feedback from the muscles to the spinal cord to prevent failure after a SCI [67–69]. It may also be possible that patellar tendon vibration activated not only excitatory but also inhibitory interneurons and thus negated the possible positive effects of patellar tendon vibration on muscle fatigue [70]. Accordingly, results from this study are inconclusive regarding the effects of superimposing patellar tendon vibration onto wide-pulse width NMES in people with SCI and future research studies are needed to investigate the mechanisms of action of tendon vibration in chronically paralysed muscles. Moreover, the present results remain to be verified in future studies in a larger cohort of people with SCI, whilst also considering the potentially-confounding factors of age, level of injury, AIS classification (complete vs. incomplete), time since injury, spasticity and medication use, which may impact in the measured outcomes.

Conclusion

The imposition of patellar tendon vibration onto moderate-frequency, wide-pulse width NMES may allow for a greater amount of muscular work (muscle force production) to be completed before fatigue in a proportion of participants (i.e. positive responders to tendon vibration) with SCI. However, a lesser response may also be elicited in participants who respond negatively to patellar tendon vibration (60% in the current study) and thus, for those cases, wide-pulse width NMES alone may provide greater benefits. The use of patellar tendon vibration superimposed onto wide-pulse width NMES did not minimise the (peripheral) fatigue elicited by the training session. Based on the present results there is insufficient evidence to conclude that patellar tendon vibration improves muscle force production during the use of wide-pulse width NMES in people with SCI. In the clinic, it is suggested that people with SCI are assessed for their response to patellar tendon vibration in order that the appropriate protocol is implemented. Nonetheless, replication of these findings is required before clear decisions as to whether to implement the strategy in clinical practice can be made.

Abbreviations

$\tau_{tw,p}$: Maximal evoked torque (peak twitch torque); $\tau_{tw,sub}$: Submaximal evoked torque (peak twitch torque); AIS: American Spinal Injury Association Impairment Scale; FES: Functional electrical stimulation; MVC: Maximal voluntary contraction; MVIC: Maximal voluntary isometric contraction; NMES: Neuromuscular electrical stimulation; QoL: Quality of life; RF: Rectus femoris; SCI: Spinal cord injury; STIM: Neuromuscular electrical stimulation protocol; STIM+Vib: Neuromuscular electrical stimulation superimposed onto tendon vibration protocol; TTI: Torque-time integral; VL: Vastus lateralis; VM: Vastus medialis

Acknowledgements

Not applicable.

Funding

Spinal Cord Injuries Australia (SCIA) Collaborative Research Program grant to Robert Newton.

Authors' contributions

VB, AB, RN, GT made substantial contributions to conception and design of this study. VB, AB, AV, GT, TP made substantial contributions to acquisition of data, analysis and interpretation of data. All authors participated in drafting the article or revising it critically for important intellectual content. All authors gave final approval of the version to be submitted and any revised version.

Competing interests

The authors declare that they have no competing interests.

Author details

[1]Department of Exercise and Health Sciences, School of Health, Medical and

Applied Sciences, Central Queensland University, Building 34.1.02, Bruce Highway, North Rockhampton, Qld 4702, Australia. [2]Exercise Medicine Research Clinic, Edith Cowan University, Perth, Australia. [3]Centre for Sports and Exercise Science, School of Medical and Health Sciences, Edith Cowan University, Joondalup, Australia. [4]UQ Centre for Clinical Research, The University of Queensland, Brisbane, Australia. [5]School of Exercise and Nutrition Sciences, Institute of Health and Biomedical Innovation, Queensland University of Technology (QUT), Brisbane, Australia. [6]UDF-University Centre, Brasilia, Brazil.

References

1. Tewarie RDS, Hurtado A, Bartels RHMA, Grotenhuis JA, Oudega M. A clinical perspective of spinal cord injury. Neurorehabil. 2010;27(2):129–39.

2. Oyster ML, Karmarkar AM, Patrick M, Read MS, Nicolini L, Boninger ML. Investigation of factors associated with manual wheelchair mobility in persons with spinal cord injury. Arch of Phys Med and Rehab. 2011;92(3):484–90.

3. Hosseini SM, Oyster ML, Kirby RL, Harrington AL, Boninger ML. Manual wheelchair skills capacity predicts quality of life and community integration in persons with spinal cord injury. Arch of Phys Med and Rehab. 2012; 93(12):2237–43.

4. Schaap LA, Pluijm SM, Deeg DJ, Harris TB, Kritchevsky SB, Newman AB, et al. Higher inflammatory marker levels in older persons: associations with 5-year change in muscle mass and muscle strength. J Gerontol A Biol Sci Med Sci. 2009;64((11):1183–9.

5. Srikanthan P, Karlamangla AS. Muscle mass index as a predictor of longevity in older adults. Am J Med. 2014;127(6):547–53.

6. Orlando G, Balducci S, Bazzucchi I, Pugliese G, Sacchetti M. Neuromuscular dysfunction in type 2 diabetes: underlying mechanisms and effect of resistance training. Diabetes-Metab Res Rev. 2016;32(1):40–50.

7. Andrade SD, da Silva JN. The effects of resistance training in osteoporosis: a systematic review. RBNE. 2015;9(50):144–9.

8. Clark JE, Goon DT. The role of resistance training for treatment of obesity related health issues and for changing health status of the individual who is overfat or obese: a review. J Sports Med Phys Fitness. 2015;55(3):205–22.

9. Caserotti P, Aagaard P, Larsen JB, Puggaard L. Explosive heavy-resistance training in old and very old adults: changes in rapid muscle force, strength and power. Scand J Med Sci Sports. 2008;18(6):773–82.

10. Barbeau H, Ladouceur M, Mirbagheri MM, Kearney RE. The effect of locomotor training combined with functional electrical stimulation in chronic spinal cord injured subjects: walking and reflex studies. Brain Res. 2002;40(1–3):274–91.

11. Harvey LA, Fornusek C, Bowden JL, Pontifex N, Glinsky J, Middleton JW, et al. Electrical stimulation plus progressive resistance training for leg strength in spinal cord injury: a randomized controlled trial. Spinal Cord. 2010;48(7):570–5.

12. Thrasher TA, Ward JS, Fisher S. Strength and endurance adaptations to functional electrical stimulation leg cycle ergometry in spinal cord injury. Neurorehabil. 2013;33(1):133–8.

13. American College of Sports Medicine. Progression models in resistance training for healthy adults. Med Sci Sports Exerc. 2009;41(3):687–708.

14. Ahtiainen JP, Pakarinen A, Alen M, Kraemer WJ, Hakkinen K. Muscle hypertrophy, hormonal adaptations and strength development during strength training in strength-trained and untrained men. Eur J Appl Physiol. 2003;89(6):555–63.

15. Enoka R. Neuromechanics of human movement 2002.

16. Hortobagyi T, Maffiuletti NA. Neural adaptations to electrical stimulation strength training. Eur J Appl Physiol. 2011;111(10):2439–49.

17. Alon G. Guest editorial - Use of neuromuscular electrical stimulation in neureorehabilitation: A challenge to all. J Rehabil Res Dev. 2003;40(6):IX–XII.

18. Hillegass EA, Dudley GA. Surface electrical stimulation of skeletal muscle after spinal cord injury. Spinal Cord. 1999;37(4):251–7.

19. Gregory CM, Recruitment BCS. Patterns in human skeletal muscle during electrical stimulation. Phys Ther. 2005;85(4):358–64.

20. Gorgey AS, Mahoney E, Kendall T, Dudley GA. Effects of neuromuscular electrical stimulation parameters on specific tension. Eur J Appl Physiol. 2006;97(6):737–44.

21. Ibitoye MO, Hamzaid NA, Hasnan N, Abdul Wahab AK, Davis GM. Strategies for rapid muscle fatigue reduction during fes exercise in individuals with spinal cord injury: a systematic review. PLoS One. 2016;11(2):e0149024.

22. Bickel CS, Gregory CM, Dean JC. Motor unit recruitment during neuromuscular electrical stimulation: a critical appraisal. Eur J Appl Physiol. 2011;111(10):2399–407.

23. Bickel CS, Slade JM, VanHiel LR, Warren GL, Dudley GA. Variable-frequency-train stimulation of skeletal muscle after spinal cord injury. J Rehabil Res Dev. 2004;41(1):33–40.

24. Adams GR, Harris RT, Woodard D, Dudley GA. Mapping of electrical muscle stimulation using MRI. J Appl Physiol. 1993;74(2):532–7.

25. Burnham R, Martin T, Stein R, Bell G, MacLean I, Steadward R. Skeletal muscle fibre type transformation following spinal cord injury. Spinal Cord. 1997;35(2):86–91.

26. Pelletier CA, Hicks AL. Muscle fatigue characteristics in paralyzed muscle after spinal cord injury. Spinal Cord. 2011;49(1):125–30.

27. Karu ZZ, Durfee WK, Barzilai AM. Reducing muscle fatigue in fes applications by stimulating with N-let pulse trains. IEEE Trans Biomed Eng. 1995;42(8):809–17.

28. Gorgey AS, Poarch HJ, Dolbow DR, Castillo T, Gater DR. Effect of adjusting pulse durations of functional electrical stimulation cycling on energy expenditure and fatigue after spinal cord injury. J Rehab Res Dev. 2014;51(9):1455–68.

29. Borde R, Hortobagyi T, Granacher U. Dose-response relationships of resistance training in healthy old adults: a systematic review and meta-analysis. Sports Med. 2015;45(12):1693–720.

30. Schoenfeld BJ, Ogborn D, Krieger JW. Dose-response relationship between weekly resistance training volume and increases in muscle mass: a systematic review and meta-analysis. J Sports Sci. 2017;35(11):1073–82.

31. Bickel CS, Yarar-Fisher C, Mahoney ET, McCully KK. Neuromuscular electrical stimulation–induced resistance training after SCI: a review of the Dudley protocol. Top Spinal Cord Inj Rehabil. 2015;21(4):294–302.

32. Dudley GA, Castro MJ, Rogers S, Apple DF. A simple means of increasing muscle size after spinal cord injury: a pilot study. Eur J Appl Physiol Occup Physiol. 1999;80(4):394–6.

33. Gorgey AS, Mather KJ, Cupp HR, Gater DR. Effects of resistance training on adiposity and metabolism after spinal cord injury. Med Sci Sports Exerc. 2012; 44(1):165–74.

34. Mahoney ET, Bickel CS, Elder C, Black C, Slade JM, Apple D, et al. Changes in skeletal muscle size and glucose tolerance with electrically stimulated resistance training in subjects with chronic spinal cord injury. Arch Phys Med Rehabil. 2005;86(7):1502–4.

35. Erickson ML, Ryan TE, Backus D, McCully KK. Endurance neuromuscular electrical stimulation training improves skeletal muscle oxidative capacity in individuals with motor-complete spinal cord injury. Muscle Nerve. 2017;55(5):669–75.

36. Dudley-Javoroski S. Muscle and bone plasticity after spinal cord injury: review of adaptations to disuse and to electrical muscle stimulation. J Rehabil Res Dev. 2008;45(2):283–96.

37. Hangartner TN, Rodgers MM, Glaser RM, Barre PS. Tibial bone density loss in spinal cord injured patients: effects of FES exercise. J Rehabil Res Dev. 1994; 31(1):50–61.

38. Shields RK, Dudley-Javoroski S, Law LA. Electrically induced muscle contractions influence bone density decline after spinal cord injury. Spine. 2006;31(5):548–53.

39. Glinsky J, Harvey L, Van Es P. Efficacy of electrical stimulation to increase muscle strength in people with neurological conditions: a systematic review. Physiother Res Int. 2007;12(3):175–94.

40. Harvey LA. Physiotherapy rehabilitation for people with spinal cord injuries. J Physiother. 2016;62(1):4–11.

41. Ribot-Ciscar E, Butler JE, Thomas CK. Facilitation of triceps brachii muscle contraction by tendon vibration after chronic cervical spinal cord injury. J Appl Physiol. 2003;94(6):2358–67.

42. Cotey D, Hornby TG, Gordon KE, Schmit BD. Increases in muscle activity produced by vibration of the thigh muscles during locomotion in chronic human spinal cord injury. Exp Brain Res. 2009;196(3):361–74.

43. Collins DF. Central contributions to contractions evoked by tetanic neuromuscular electrical stimulation. Exerc Sport Sci Rev. 2007;35(3):102–9.

44. Gondin J, Giannesini B, Vilmen C, Dalmasso C, le Fur Y, Cozzone PJ, et al. Effects of stimulation frequency and pulse duration on fatigue and metabolic cost during a single bout of neuromuscular electrical stimulation.

Muscle Nerve. 2010;41(5):667–78.

45. Wegrzyk J, Foure A, Vilmen C, Ghattas B, Maffiuletti NA, Mattei JP, et al. Extra forces induced by wide-pulse, high-frequency electrical stimulation: occurrence, magnitude, variability and underlying mechanisms. Clin Neurophysiol. 2015;126(7):1400–12.

46. Magalhaes FH, Kohn AF. Vibration-induced extra torque during electrically-evoked contractions of the human calf muscles. J NeuroEng Rehabil. 2010;7

47. Trajano GS, Seitz LB, Nosaka K, Blazevich AJ. Can passive stretch inhibit motoneuron facilitation in the human plantar flexors? J Appl Physiol. 2014;117(12):1486–92.

48. Bongiovanni LG, Hagbarth KE. Tonic vibration reflexes elicited during fatigue from maximal voluntary contractions in man. J Physiol-London. 1990;423:1–14.

49. Neyroud D, Armand S, De Coulon G, Da Silva SRD, Wegrzyk J, Gondin J, et al. Wide-pulse-high-frequency neuromuscular electrical stimulation in cerebral palsy. Clin Neurophysiol. 2016;127(2):1530–9.

50. Bochkezanian V, Newton RU, Trajano GS, Vieira A, Pulverenti TS, Blazevich AJ. Effect of tendon vibration during wide-pulse neuromuscular electrical stimulation (NMES) on the decline and recovery of muscle force. BMC Neurol. 2017;17(1):82.

51. Bergquist AJ, Wiest MJ, Collins DF. Motor unit recruitment when neuromuscular electrical stimulation is applied over a nerve trunk compared with a muscle belly: quadriceps femoris. J Appl Physiol. 2012;113(1):78–89.

52. Bax L, Staes F, Verhagen A. Does neuromuscular electrical stimulation strengthen the quadriceps femoris? Syst Rev Random Controlled Trials Sports Med. 2005;35(3):191–212.

53. Edgerton VR, Roy RR. Activity-dependent plasticity of spinal locomotion: implications for sensory processing. Exerc Sport Sci Rev. 2009;37(4):171–8.

54. Edgerton VR, Tillakaratne NJ, Bigbee AJ, de Leon RD, Roy RR. Plasticity of the spinal neural circuitry after injury. Annu Rev Neurosci. 2004;27:145–67.

55. Bergquist AJ, Clair JM, Lagerquist O, Mang CS, Okuma Y, Collins DF. Neuromuscular electrical stimulation: implications of the electrically evoked sensory volley. Eur J Appl Physiol. 2011;111(10):2409–26.

56. Collins DF, Burke D, Gandevia SC. Large involuntary forces consistent with plateau-like behavior of human motoneurons. J Neurosci. 2001;21(11):4059–65.

57. Fallon JB, Macefield VG. Vibration sensitivity of human muscle spindles and Golgi tendon organs. Muscle Nerve. 2007;36(1):21–9.

58. Rehabilitation LJS. Following brain damage: some neurophysiological mechanisms. Physiological correlates of clinically observed changes in posture and tone following lesions of the central nervous system. Int Rehabil Med. 1981;4(4):195–9.

59. Xia R, Rymer WZ. Reflex reciprocal facilitation of antagonist muscles in spinal cord injury. Spinal Cord. 2005;43(1):14–21.

60. Biering-Sorensen B, Kristensen IB, Kjaer M, Biering-Sorensen F. Muscle after spinal cord injury. Muscle Nerve. 2009;40(4):499–519.

61. Kim HE, Corcos DM, Hornby TG. Increased spinal reflex excitability is associated with enhanced central activation during voluntary lengthening contractions in human spinal cord injury. J Neurophysiol. 2015;114(1):427–39.

62. Gordon T, Mao J. Muscle atrophy and procedures for training after spinal-cord injury. Phys Ther. 1994;74(1):50–60.

63. Li Y, Li X, Harvey P, Bennett D. Effects of baclofen on spinal reflexes and persistent inward currents in motoneurons of chronic spinal rats with spasticity. J Neurophysiol. 2004;92(5):2694–703.

64. Magalhaes FH, de Toledo DR, Kohn AF. Plantar flexion force induced by amplitude-modulated tendon vibration and associated soleus V/F-waves as an evidence of a centrally-mediated mechanism contributing to extra torque generation in humans. J NeuroEng Rehabil. 2013;10:32.

65. Adams MM, Hicks AL. Spasticity after spinal cord injury. Spinal Cord. 2005;43(10):577–86.

66. D'Amico JM, Condliffe EG, Martins KJB, Bennett DJ, Gorassini MA. Recovery of neuronal and network excitability after spinal cord injury and implications for spasticity. Front Integr Neurosci. 2014;8:36.

67. Mizrahi J. Fatigue in functional electrical stimulation in spinal cord injury. J Electromyogr Kinesiol. 1997;7(1):1–2.

68. Binder-Macleod SA, Snyder-Mackler L. Muscle fatigue: clinical implications for fatigue assessment and neuromuscular electrical stimulation. Phys Ther. 1993;73(12):902–10.

69. Kent-Braun JA. Central and peripheral contributions to muscle fatigue in humans during sustained maximal effort. Eur J Appl Physiol Occup Physiol. 1999;80(1):57–63.

70. Eklund G, Hagbarth KE, Hagglund JV, Wallin EU. The late reflex responses to muscle stretch - the resonance hypothesis versus the long-loop hypothesis. J Physiol-London. 1982;326(5):79–90.

71. Kirshblum SC, Burns SP, Biering-Sorensen F, Donovan W, Graves DE, Jha A, et al. International standards for neurological classification of spinal cord injury (revised 2011). J Spinal Cord Med. 2011;34(6):535–46.

16

Does burst-suppression achieve seizure control in refractory status epilepticus?

Kanitpong Phabphal[1*], Suparat Chisurajinda[1], Thapanee Somboon[2], Kanjana Unwongse[2] and Alan Geater[3]

Abstract

Background: The general principles in the administration of anesthetic drugs entail not only the suppression of seizure activity but also the achievement of electroencephalography burst suppression (BS). However, previous studies have reported conflicting results, possibly owing to the inclusion of various anesthetic agents, not all patients undergoing continuous electroencephalography (cEEG), and the inclusion of anoxic encephalopathy. This study aimed to analyze the effects of midazolam-induced BS on the occurrence outcomes in refractory status epilepticus patients.

Methods: Based on a prospective database of patients who had been diagnosed with status epilepticus via cEEG, multivariate Poisson regression modules were used to estimate the effect of midazolam-induced BS on breakthrough seizure, withdrawal seizure, intra-hospital complications, functional outcome at 3 months, and mortality. Modules were based on a pre-compiled directed acyclic graph (DAG).

Results: We included 51 non-anoxic encephalopathy, refractory status epilepticus patients. Burst suppression was achieved in 26 patients (51%); 25 patients (49%) had non-burst suppression on their cEEG. Breakthrough seizure was less often seen in the burst suppression group than in the non-burst suppression group. The incidence risk ratio [IRR] was 0.30 (95% confidence interval = 0.13–0.74). There was weak evidence of an association between BS and increased withdrawal seizure, but no association between BS and intra-hospital complications, mortality or functional outcomes was observed.

Conclusion: This study provides evidence that BS is safe and associated with less breakthrough seizures. Additionally, it was not associated with an increased rate of intra-hospital complications or long-term outcomes.

Keywords: Burst suppression, Refractory status epilepticus, Midazolam, Outcome

Background

Refractory status epilepticus (RSE) is defined as status epilepticus that cannot be controlled with an adequate dose of first-line and second-line antiepileptic drugs [1]. Refractory status epilepticus develops in approximately 30–40% of patients with status epilepticus [1].

This condition is associated with progressively increasing intrahospital mortality ranging between 19 and 67% depending on the study [1, 2]. Also, RSE patients experience functional impairment at discharge and long-term morbidity [1, 2]. The best management of refractory status epilepticus remains unclear. However, current guidelines recommend treatment with a continuous infusion

of an anesthetic drug [1]. Available anesthetic drugs for continuous infusion include midazolam, propofol and pentobarbital. The major concerns of an anesthetic drug infusion are prolonged duration of mechanical ventilation, immobilization, hypotension, cardiac complications as well as propofol-infusion syndrome [2]. Midazolam has been shown to have a wide margin of safety and broad /therapeutic index, and be easy to use [1, 3].

A previous systematic review found that patients receiving pentobarbital had a lower frequency of breakthrough seizure as well as a lower rate of treatment failure [2]. However, these results were biased because of a lack of continuous electroencephalogram (cEEG) in the pentobarbital group and in those patients commonly experiencing subtle or non-convulsive seizures [2]. A recent guideline has recommended the initiation of an

---

* Correspondence: pkanitpo@medicine.psu.ac.th
[1]Neurology Unit, Department of Medicine, Faculty of Medicine, Prince of Songkla University, Hat Yai, Songkhla 90110, Thailand
Full list of author information is available at the end of the article

anesthetic infusion with cEEG to suppress seizure activity or burst suppression [1]. There are limited studies with conflicting results reporting on the effect of anesthetic drug-induced BS and its related clinical outcomes [1, 4–7]. However, different anesthetic agents have been used in the groups being evaluated. There is a scarcity of studies assessing the effects of EEG-BS in midazolam-treated RSE patients. The current study, therefore was conducted to examine the associations between midazolam-induced burst suppression and 1) the occurrence of breakthrough seizure, and 2) the occurrence of withdrawal seizure. Secondary outcomes were 1) intrahospital complications, 2) functional outcome at 3 months, and 3) mortality at 3 months.

Methods

We compiled a systematic database of patients who had been diagnosed with status epilepticus by means of cEEG between from June 2005 and April 2016 at Songklanagarind Hospital, Thailand. Patients' characteristics throughout treatment and follow up were collected from the clinical records by the first author. However, the treatment strategies were decided by attending neurologist and/or intensivist. Patients who continued to experience either clinical or electrographic seizure after receiving adequate dose of an initial benzodiazepine followed by some second acceptable antiepileptic drugs were considered to be RSE [1].

Treatment protocol in our institution

The initial treatment of all status epilepticus patients consisted of intravenous diazepam (lorazepam is not available in our country) plus phenytoin (loading dose 20 mg/kg) or valproate (loading dose 20–30 mg/kg) or phenobarbital (loading dose 20 mg/kg) or levetiracetam (30–40 mg/kg). All patients treated with midazolam were on a mechanical ventilator (endotracheal tube insertion) and transferred to the intensive care unit. The midazolam dose was adjusted by the neurologist and/or intensivist base on the clinical observation of seizures and EEG monitoring. In our institution, midazolam is considered the first-line anesthetic drug for refractory status epilepticus as intensivists are familiar with its use in the management of agitated patients who are on a mechanical ventilator. Once the patient was seizure-free for 24 h, midazolam was tapered off over 6–24 h. The reduction rate was adjusted by the attending physician under cEEG monitoring to assess seizure recurrence. The causes of status epilepticus were categorized as central nervous system infection, metabolic disease, static brain lesion and antiepileptic drugs withdrawal. Patients were classified as having breakthrough seizure if any seizure occurred after 12 h of intravenous midazolam therapy or withdrawal seizure if any seizure occurred during the tapering off or within 12 h after the discontinuation of intravenous midazolam [8]. A good outcome was determined if, at 3 months, the patient's condition returned to the clinical baseline or if the modified Rankin scale score was 0–2. A bad outcome was deemed if, at 3 months, the patient's condition was evaluated to have a modified Rankin scale score of 3–6. Complications were categorized into: 1) respiratory complications (defined as the presence of hypoxemia, pulmonary edema, acute respiratory distress syndrome, and/or tracheostomy); 2) cardiac complications (defined as the presence of hypotension—mean arterial pressure < 70 mmHg or systemic blood pressure < 90 mmHg requiring a new administration of or an increase in the dose of vasopressor—new-onset arrhythmias, myocardial infarction or heart failure); 3) fever/infection (defined as the presence of a temperature of > 38.3°C or a positive culture needing antibiotics); 4) thromboembolic complications (deep vein thrombosis demonstrated by an ultrasound and/or pulmonary embolism demonstrated by lung CT-angiography); 5) gastrointestinal complications like ileus (defined as the absence of bowel movements in the absence of evidence of mechanical obstruction), intestinal ischemia (confirmed by surgical exploration), and gastrointestinal bleeding (both overt and covert demonstrated by an occult bleeding test), 6) hepatobiliary complications such as hepatitis (elevation of transaminases 3 times the upper limit of the normal values), pancreatitis (elevation of lipase > 3 times the upper limit of the normal values); and 7) acute kidney injury requiring renal replacement therapy. An electrographic seizure was diagnosed when paroxysmal EEG patterns with a discrete onset and evolution were present; periodic lateralized or generalized epileptiform discharges alone were not considered electrographic seizures.

The inclusion criteria were: 1) patients aged 15 years or older experiencing focal-onset seizures with a secondarily generalized seizure that cannot be controlled with an adequate dose of first-line and second-line antiepileptic drugs; 2) patients receiving midazolam for the treatment of RSE; and 3) patients undergoing cEEG. We excluded patients: 1) receiving an anesthetic drug other than midazolam and diagnosed with 2) epileptic syndrome; 3) psychogenic SE; 4) anoxic encephalopathy; or 5) complex partial SE.

The approval of our institution's review board was obtained for the study.

Statistical analysis

The basic patient characteristics and outcomes of BS and non-BS were compared using either the Pearson chi-squared or Fisher exact test. Prior to analysis, a Directed Acyclic Graph (DAG) was compiled to depict explicitly the potential relationships among predictors and outcomes. The associations between exposure and each outcome coded as yes/no were estimated using the Poisson regression adjusting for confounding variables (total effect) or confounding and intermediate variables (direct effect), as indicated by the DAG using the software DAGitty, version 2.3 [9].

The following variables were included in the DAG: EEG (BS), age, withdrawal seizure, breakthrough seizure, dose of midazolam, complications, etiology, status epilepticus severity score (SESS), time between SE diagnosis and start of midazolam, and outcome. The relationships between each of the variables were assigned by KP and AG based on knowledge regarding these associations from the literature review. Stata statistical software Version 14.1 (Stata Corp, College Station, TX) was used to analyze the data.

Results

We recorded 112 patients with SE over the study period. Fifty-one non-anoxic encephalopathy RSE patients met the criteria and were included in the analysis. We excluded 61 patients who responded to initial antiepileptic drugs, had SE of an anoxic encephalopathy origin or received an anesthetic other than midazolam (Fig. 1). The median age was 49 years. Twenty-three patients (45.1%) were classified as having an acute encephalitis etiology. Eighteen patients (35.3%) had metabolic and 6 (11.7%) static lesions in the brain. There was a high variation in the time from the onset of SE to the treatment with midazolam ranging from 5 to 75 h (median 24 h). Ten patients had both breakthrough seizure and withdrawal seizure. Forty percent of patients had at least one breakthrough seizure and 33 % had at least on withdrawal seizure. Burst suppression was achieved in 26 (51%) patients; 25 (49%) patients had non-burst suppression on cEEG. The median maximum dose was 0.91 mg/kg. Seventy-two percent of all patients received a midazolam dose of ≥ 0.4 mg/kg. The median SESS was 4. In 84% of cases, seizure termination occurred within 60 min of initial midazolam infusion. Thirty-one (60.78%) patients

had breakthrough seizure and 21 cases (41.18%) suffered withdrawal seizure. The mean hospital length of stay was 16 days (range 5 to 32 days). The average SESS was 4 (Table 1). Mortality among patients with RSE was 39.2%.

Comparison between burst- vs non-burst suppression groups

The demographic and clinical characteristics of our participants are summarized in Table 1. There was no difference in baseline characteristics between the two groups. Regarding the disease etiologies of the patients who experienced successful burst suppression, they were: encephalitis (50%), metabolic (38.4%), static lesion (3.8%) and drug withdrawal (7.7%). In the non-burst suppression group, 48% of patients received midazolam within 24 h compared with 54% in the burst suppression group.

Treatment outcome

The mean dose of midazolam in the burst suppression group was 0.9 mg/kg (range 0.21 to 2.5 mg/kg), and that of the non-burst suppression group was 1.23 mg/kg (range 0.3 mg/kg to 3.1 mg/kg); however, the difference was not statistically significant ($p = 0.12$). Breakthrough seizure was less often seen in the BS group than in the non-BS group. Its incidence risk ratio [IRR] was 0.30 (95% confidence interval 0.13–0.74). There was a tendency toward higher withdrawal seizure in the BS group as a direct effect of BS (IRR 2.04, 95% CI 0.76–5.47).

The incidence of in-hospital complications was comparable between the two groups. The common complications were pulmonary complications, cardiac complications and infection (43.1% vs. 21.6 vs. 39.2%, respectively). Interestingly, in the non-burst suppression group, hypotension and infection were less frequent than in the burst suppression group but without statistical significance. After adjusting for confounding factors, the achievement of BS was not associated with intra-hospital mortality, pulmonary complications, cardiac complications, fever/infection,

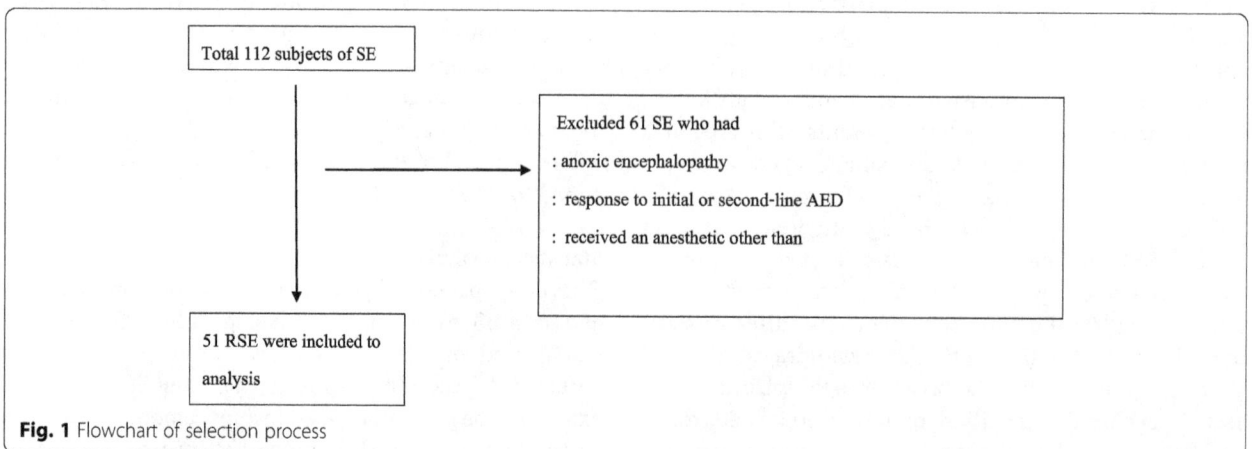

Fig. 1 Flowchart of selection process

Table 1 Characteristics of patients in burst suppression and non-burst suppression groups

Variable	Burst suppression group	Non-burst suppression group	P-value[b]
	n (%)	n (%)	
Age (years)			0.136
< 30	5 (19.2)	8 (32.0)	
30–60	9 (34.6)	12 (48.0)	
> 60	12 (46.2)	5 (20.0)	
Sex			0.068
male	16 (61.5)	9 (36.0)	
female	10 (38.5)	16 (64.0)	
Etiology			0.353
encephalitis	13 (50)	10 (40.0)	
metabolic	10 (38.5)	8 (32.0)	
static lesion	1 (3.8)	5 (20.0)	
drug withdrawal	2 (7.7)	2 (8.0)	
History of epilepsy			0.067
yes	7 (26.9)	13 (52.0)	
no	19 (73.1)	12 (48.0)	
Number of antiepileptic drugs (before midazolam therapy)			0.35
2	10 (38.5)	5 (20.0)	
3	11 (42.3)	14 (56.0)	
4	5 (19.2)	6 (24.0)	
Status epilepticus severity score			0.27
3	7 (29.9)	12 (48.0)	
4	15 (57.7)	11 (44.0)	
> 4	4 (15.4)	2 (8.0)	
Dose of midazolam (mg/kg/day)			0.350
< 0.6	10 (38.5)	5 (20.0)	
0.6–1.2	11 (42.3)	14 (56.0)	
> 1.2	5 (19.2)	6 (24.0)	
Time to midazolam therapy (hours)			0.676
≤ 24	14 (53.8)	12 (48.0)	
> 24	12 (46.2)	13 (52.0)	
Length of hospital stay (days)			0.747
< 14	11 (42.3)	8 (32.0)	
14–21	9 (34.6)	10 (40.0)	
> 21	6 (23.1)	7 (28.0)	
Breakthrough seizure			< 0.001
no	19 (73.1)	1 (4.0)	
yes	7 (26.9)	24 (96.0)	
Withdrawal seizure			0.061
no	12 (46.2)	18 (72.0)	

Table 1 Characteristics of patients in burst suppression and non-burst suppression groups (Continued)

Variable	Burst suppression group	Non-burst suppression group	P-value[b]
	n (%)	n (%)	
yes	14 (53.8)	7 (28.0)	
Pulmonary complication			0.657
no	14 (53.8)	15 (60.0)	
yes	12 (46.2)	10 (40.0)	
Cardiac complication			0.789
no	20 (76.9)	20 (80.0)	
yes	6 (23.1)	5 (20.0)	
Fever/infection			0.301
no	14 (53.8%)	17 (68%)	
yes	12 (46.2%)	8 (32%)	
In-hospital mortality			0.029
alive	12 (46.2)	19 (76.0)	
dead	14 (53.8)	6 (24.0)	
Functional outcome at 3 months[a]			0.379
good	7 (58.3)	8 (42.1)	
poor	5 (41.7)	11 (57.9)	

[a]excluding dead patients
[b]Chi-square test

thromboembolic complications, gastrointestinal complications, hepatobiliary complications or acute renal injury.

Concerning functional outcome at 3 months, according to the univariate analysis, a higher proportion of death in hospital occurred in the burst suppression than in the non-burst suppression group ($p = 0.029$, Table 1). However, this result was not confirmed after the adjustment for confounding factors (Table 2). The burst suppression or non-burst suppression was not statistically significant in terms of functional outcome (Table 2).

Discussion

In this historical follow-up study of non-anoxic encephalopathy, refractory status epilepticus patients treated with midazolam, we found that breakthrough seizure was less often seen in the burst suppression group than the non-burst suppression group. The incidence risk ratio [IRR] was 0.30 (95% confidence interval 0.13–0.74). There was weak evidence of an association between BS and increased withdrawal seizure, but no association between BS and intra-hospital complications was observed. We also found a higher mortality in BS compared with non-BS patients (53.8% vs. 24.0%), but this difference was not confirmed to be statistically meaningful after controlling for confounding factors. Moreover, among surviving patients, no difference in functional outcome was seen at 3 months.

Table 2 Estimated adjusted incidence risk ratio (and 95% confidence interval) for the effect of burst suppression on various outcomes for which unbiased estimates could be made according to the conceptual causal diagram

Outcome	Effect	Controlled variable	Burst suppression	Incidence risk ratio[a] (95% confidence interval)	P-value
Breakthrough seizure	Total = Direct	Etiology Status epilepticus severity score Dose of midazolam	Yes	0.30 (0.13–0.74)	0.009
Withdrawal seizure	Total	Etiology Status epilepticus severity score Dose of midazolam	Yes	2.04 (0.76–5.47)	0.157
	Direct	Breakthrough seizure Dose of midazolam	Yes	2.71 (0.89–8.25)	0.080
In-hospital mortality	Total	Etiology Status epilepticus severity score Dose of midazolam Time to midazolam therapy	Yes	2.02 (0.74–5.54)	0.170
	Direct	Breakthrough seizure Cardiac complication Dose of midazolam Etiology Pulmonary complication Fever/infection Status epilepticus severity score Time to midazolam therapy	Yes	3.25 (0.70–15.02)	0.131
Poor functional outcome at 3 months	Total	Etiology Dose of midazolam Time to midazolam therapy Status epilepticus severity score	Yes	0.75 (0.22–2.57)	0.646
Poor functional outcome at 3 months	Direct	Breakthrough seizure Withdrawal seizure Dose of midazolam Etiology Status epilepticus severity score Cardiac complication Pulmonary complication Fever/infection Time to midazolam therapy	Yes	0.13 (0.01–1.67)	0.116
Pulmonary complication	Total = Direct	Dose of midazolam Status epilepticus severity score	Yes	1.13 (0.46–2.82)	0.785
Cardiac complication	Total = Direct	Dose of midazolam Status epilepticus severity score	Yes	0.90 (0.25–3.27)	0.872
Fever/infection	Total = Direct	Status epilepticus severity score	Yes	1.38 (0.55–3.46)	0.498

[a]Adjusted for confounding and/or intermediate as required by the DAG

Burst suppression is defined as an electroencephalography finding consisting of a continuous alternation between of high-voltage slow waves (burst) and periods of depressed electrical activity [10]. Only sparse information is available with respect to the pathophysiological cellular mechanism of its pattern. It is, however, known that EEG bursts are associated with phasic synaptic depolarizing cellular potentials, occasionally crowned by action potential. A previous study has shown that suppression periods are due to the absence of synaptic activity among cortical neurons [11]. Medication, especially anesthetic agents titrated to attain burst suppression was associated with a significantly lower incidence of breakthrough seizure [4]. Nevertheless, whether EEG burst suppression is more effective than no electrographic seizure per se as an endpoint therapy

for RSE remains unknown. Recently, Hernandez et al. conducted a retrospective study of 80 RSE patients in a neurological intensive care unit who were associated using video EEG. These authors also preferred general anesthesia and burst suppression was achieved in 78%. [12] The association between BS and seizure control in RSE has only been studied in small retrospective studies [2, 4]. In a retrospective study of pentobarbital-treated patients, the frequency of seizure relapse was 50% (6 in 12 patients) when BS was achieved compared with 15% (3 in 20 patients) in patients with a flat record ($p = 0.049$) [4] . However, this study suffered from differences in basic clinical characteristics of the population between the two groups, and a lack of continuous EEG monitoring performed throughout the barbiturate infusion as well as a multivariate analysis [4]. Claassen et al.

conducted a systematic review of 28 articles (involving patients treated with different anesthetic drugs) and found that BS on EEG was associated with a lower frequency of breakthrough seizure, but it was not associated with the outcome. Interestingly, none of the patients who received midazolam achieved BS on cEEG in this review [2]. Our study was conducted to evaluate the effect of midazolam-induced BS. We found that BS on cEEG was associated with a lower frequency of breakthrough seizure; incidence risk ratio [IRR] 0.30 (95% CI 0.13–0.74, $p < 0.01$).

Overall, withdrawal seizure occurred in 21% of cases in our study compared with 40% of patients treated with midazolam [13–15], 20% of patients treated with pentobarbital [4, 16], and 10% of patients treated with propofol [17] reported in other studies. Fernandez et al. conducted a study to compare the effect of low dose versus high dose in patients with refractory status epilepticus and found that withdrawal seizure was less often seen in the high dose group [18]. Our study found that patients with BS were not statistically significant different compared with those of the non-BS group in this regard; IRR 2.04 (95% CI 0.76–5.47, $p = 0.157$) after controlling for confounding variables (total effect).

There were no differences between complications such as hypotension, cardiac complications and infection among the burst suppression and non-burst suppression patients [8]. In general, high doses of anesthetic drug infusion are associated with hypotension [18]. The use of pentobarbital to induce burst suppression has been associated with a higher incidence of hypotension compared with other anesthetics [4], but this finding was not supported by our study. We found no evidence that midazolam-induced BS was associated with pulmonary complications, cardiac complications, hepatobiliary complications, gastrointestinal complications, fever/infection, thromboembolism or acute renal injury.

Mortality in our study was 39% at discharge. At 3 months, 29.4% of patients had a good outcome. Other studies have found no association between therapy with intravenous anesthetic drugs and increased mortality. The systematic review by Claassen et al. reported a mortality rate of 46% in the midazolam group [4]. Previously reported mortality rates among RSE patients treated with low-dose midazolam and high-dose midazolam were 61 and 45%, respectively [4–6]. A recent retrospective study explored the association between different anesthetic agent-induced BS and their outcomes and found no association with poor outcome, including mortality, and poor functional outcome at discharge [6]. Our study was conducted to investigate the effect of midazolam on intra-hospital mortality, complication rate and functional outcome at 3 months. We found a higher mortality in BS compared with non-BS patients (53.8%

vs. 24.0%, respectively), but this difference was not confirmed after controlling for confounding factors. Furthermore, among surviving patients, no difference in functional outcome was seen at 3 months.

The main limitations of our study were its small sample size, its being conducted in a single department, and its retrospective analysis. Few studies have investigated the association between BS and seizure outcome. They have included fewer than 35 RSE cases with cEEG [4, 6] and have not focused on a single anesthetic agent [5, 7]. Our investigation included more patients than previous studies, but it also has the limitation of being a retrospective study. However, a prospective study would be unethical due to the guidelines that recommend the endpoint of anesthetic induced-BS [1]. In fact, our data were collected prospectively and include many parameters. Due to the retrospective nature of our study, we did not control either the initial dose of midazolam or the time to the commencement of midazolam therapy after diagnosis. Finally, our study was conducted in a single department and did not focus on the characteristics of BS such as high epileptiform bursts. Future research should address these issues.

The strengths of our study consist in, firstly, its focus on a single anesthetic drug. Midazolam has been shown to have a wide margin of safety and a broad therapeutic index and is easy to use. Secondly, we based the statistical analysis on an explicit causal framework to ensure an appropriate co-variate adjustment in the regression analysis. The results of our study will be applied in the future management of RSE.

Conclusion

In this historical follow-up study of the effect of the treatment with midazolam to induce BS in refractory status epilepticus using historical prospectively-collected data revealed that (1) burst suppression on cEEG was associated with a lower rate of breakthrough seizure but not with withdrawal seizure, mortality or functional outcome; and (2) burst suppression was not associated with hypotension, cardiac complications or infection.

Abbreviations

BS: Burst suppression; cEEG: Continuous electroencephalography; DAG: Directed Acyclic Graph; EEG: Electroencephalography; EEG-BS: Electroencephalography- burst suppression; IRR: Incidence risk ratio; RSE: Refractory status epilepticus; SE: Status epilepticus; SESS: Status epilepticus severity score

Acknowledgements

The authors wish to thank Mrs. Edmond Subashi from International Affairs Division, Faculty of Medicine, Prince of Songkla University for English language review and Miss. Walailuk Jitpiboon, who gave us the assistance with statistical analysis.

Funding

This work was supported by grants Faculty of Medicine, Prince of Songkla University. The funders had no role in designing the study, or in collection, analysis, and interpretation of the data, or in writing the manuscript.

Authors' contributions
KP participated in the conception, the design of the study, acquisition of raw data, the analysis of the clinical data, drafting the manuscript and the critical revision of the manuscript for scientific validity. SC, TS and KU participated in the conception, acquisition of raw data, drafting the manuscript and the critical revision of the manuscript for scientific validity. AG participated in the design of the study, the analysis of the clinical data, drafting the manuscript and the critical revision of the manuscript for scientific validity. All authors read and approved the final manuscript.

Competing interests
The authors declare that they have no competing interest.

Author details
[1]Neurology Unit, Department of Medicine, Faculty of Medicine, Prince of Songkla University, Hat Yai, Songkhla 90110, Thailand. [2]Prasat Neurological Institute, Bangkok 10400, Thailand. [3]Epidemiology Unit, Department of Epidemiology, Faculty of Medicine, Prince of Songkla University, Hat Yai, Songkhla 90110, Thailand.

References
1. Brophy GM, Bell R, Claassen J, Alldredge B, Bleck TP, Glauser T, et al. Guideline for the evaluation and management of status epilepticus. Neurocrit Care. 2012;17:3–23.
2. Claassen J, Hirsch LJ, Emerson RG, Mayer SA. Treatment of refractory status epilepticus with pentobarbital, propofol, or midazolam: a systematic review. Epilepsia. 2002;42:146–53.
3. Bellante F, Legros B, Depondt C, Créteur J, Taccone FS, Gaspard N. Midazolam and thiopental for the treatment of refractory status epilepticus: a retrospective comparison of efficacy and safety. J Neurol. 2016;263:799–806.
4. Krishnammurthy KB, Drishalane FW. Depth of EEG suppression and outcome in barbiturate anesthetic treatment of status epilepticus. Epilepsia. 1999;40:759–62.
5. Johnson EL, Carballido N, Ritzl EK. EEG characteristics of successful burst suppression for refractory status epilepticus. Neurocrit Care. 2016;25:407–14.
6. Kang BU, Jung KH, Shin JW, Moon JS, Byun JI, Lim JA, et al. Induction of burst suppression or coma using intravenous anesthetic in refractory status epilepticus. J Clin Neurosci. 2015;22:854–8.
7. Rossetti AO, Logroscino G, Bromfield EB. Refractory status epilepticus: effect of treatment aggressiveness on prognosis. Arch Neurol. 2005;62:1698–702.
8. Hocker SE, Britton JW, Mandrekar JN, Wijdicks EF, Rabinstein AA. Predictors of outcome in refractory status epilepticus. JAMA Neurol. 2003;70:72–7.
9. Textor J, Hardt J, Knüppel S. DAGitty: a graphical tool for analyzing causal diagrams. Epidemiology. 2011;5:745.
10. Amzica F. What does burst suppression really mean? Epilepsy Behav. 2015;49:234–7.
11. Steriade M, Amzica F, Contreras D. Cortical and Thalamic cellular correlates of electroencephalographic burst-suppression. Electroen-cephalogr. Clin Neurophysiol. 1994;90:1–16.
12. Hernandez OH, Zapata JE, Jimenez M, Massaro M, Guerra A, Arango JC, et al. Refractory status epilepticus: experience in a neurological intensive care unit. J Clin Care Med. 2014; https://doi.org/10.1155/2014/821462.
13. Kumar A, Bleck TP. Intravenous midazolam for the treatment of refractory status epilepticus. Crit Care Med. 1992;20:483–8.
14. Parent JM, Lowenstein DH. Treatment of refractory generaized status epilepticus with continuous infusion of midazolam. Neurology. 1994;44:1837–40.
15. Naritoku DK, Sinha S. Prolongation of midazolam half-life after sustained infusion for status epilepticus. Neurology. 2000;54:1366–8.
16. Yaffe K, Lowenstein DH. Prognostic factors of pentobarbital therapy for refractory generalized status epilepticus. Neurology. 1993;43:895–900.
17. Brown LA, Levin GM. Role of propofol in refractory status epilepticus. Ann Pharmacother. 1998;32:1053–9.
18. Fernandez A, Lantigua H, Lesch C, Shao B, Foreman B, Schmidt JM, et al. High-dose midazolam infusion for refractory status epilepticus. Neurology. 2014;82:359–65.

Axonal chronic injury in treatment-naïve HIV+ adults with asymptomatic neurocognitive impairment and its relationship with clinical variables and cognitive status

Rui-li Li[1†], Jun Sun[1†], Zhen-chao Tang[2], Jing-ji Zhang[3*] and Hong-jun Li[1*] ⓘD

Abstract

Background: HIV is a neurotropic virus, and it can bring about neurodegeneration and may even result in cognitive impairments. The precise mechanism of HIV-associated white matter (WM) injury is unknown. The effects of multiple clinical contributors on WM impairments and the relationship between the WM alterations and cognitive performance merit further investigation.

Methods: Diffusion tensor imaging (DTI) was performed in 20 antiretroviral-naïve HIV-positive asymptomatic neurocognitive impairment (ANI) adults and 20 healthy volunteers. Whole-brain analysis of DTI metrics between groups was conducted by employing tract-based spatial statistics (TBSS), including fractional anisotropy (FA), mean diffusivity (MD), axial diffusivity (AD) and radial diffusivity (RD). DTI parameters were correlated with clinical variables (age, CD4[+] cell count, CD4[+]/CD8[+] ratio, plasma viral load and duration of HIV infection) and multiple cognitive tests by using multilinear regression analyses.

Results: DTI quantified diffusion alterations in the corpus callosum and corona radiata (MD increased significantly, $P < 0.05$) and chronic axonal injury in the corpus callosum, corona radiata, internal capsule, external capsule, posterior thalamic radiation, sagittal stratum, and superior longitudinal fasciculus (AD increased significantly, $P < 0.05$). The impairments in the corona radiata had significant correlations with the current CD4[+]/CD8[+] ratios. Increased MD or AD values in multiple white matter structures showed significant associations with many cognitive domain tests.

Conclusions: WM impairments are present in neurologically asymptomatic HIV+ adults, periventricular WM (corpus callosum and corona radiata) are preferential occult injuries, which is associated with axonal chronic damage rather than demyelination. Axonopathy may exist before myelin injury. DTI-TBSS is helpful to explore the WM microstructure abnormalities and provide a new perspective for the investigation of the pathomechanism of HIV-associated WM injury.

Keywords: HIV, Asymptomatic neurocognitive impairment, White matter, Diffusion tensor imaging

* Correspondence: jingjizhang2013@aliyun.com; lihongjun00113@126.com
†Equal contributors
3STD and AIDS clinical treatment center, Beijing YouAn Hospital, Capital Medical University, No.8, Xi Tou Tiao, Youanmen Wai, Feng Tai District, Beijing 100069, China
1Department of Radiology, Beijing YouAn Hospital, Capital Medical University, No.8, Xi Tou Tiao, Youanmen Wai, Feng Tai District, Beijing 100069, China
Full list of author information is available at the end of the article

Background

HIV can enter the central nervous system (CNS) soon after seroconversion and cause persistent CNS inflammation [1]. With ongoing injury to the brain, it may lead to cognitive, behavioural and motor abnormalities, which are called HIV-associated neurocognitive disorders (HAND) [2]. HAND can be clinically subdivided into three categories: asymptomatic neurocognitive impairment (ANI), mild neurocognitive disorder (MND) and HIV-associated dementia (HAD) [3]. ANI is the mildest and most common type of HAND (accounting for 70%), which is characterized by mild cognitive impairment on neuropsychological performance tests without obvious accompanying difficulties in daily functioning [4]. HAD is the most severe form. These definitions are mainly based upon an individual's performance on multiple cognitive domains and a brief self-report of cognitive difficulties in daily life. These neuropsychological tests are time consuming (~ 3 h) and are usually performed in specific research institutions [3], so patients in ANI stages are rarely diagnosed in traditional outpatient visits (15–30 min).

Conventional structural magnetic resonance imaging (MRI) scans are unable to detect early HIV-associated brain white matter (WM) abnormalities [5]. As a noninvasive and rapidly evolving MRI technique, diffusion tensor imaging (DTI) can measure the diffusion of water molecules in WM, and more recently, it has become a popular method for studying HIV-induced WM microstructural integrity [6–12]. So far, tract-based spatial statistics (TBSS) is the most frequently recommended and employed method of analysis for DTI [13], which overcomes the limitations of conventional methods (region of interest, ROI; voxel-based analysis, VBA). There are four parameters for DTI, including fractional anisotropy (FA), mean diffusivity (MD), axial diffusivity (AD), and radial diffusivity (RD). As a marker of the diffusion directionality of water molecules, FA can reflect the deviation of water motion and provide information about the microstructural integrity of highly oriented microstructures [14]. MD is a marker of the molecular motion speed and can reflect the average diffusion in all three directions [15]. AD is assumed to reflect diffusivity parallel to the WM tract, and RD represents diffusion perpendicular to the tract [16]. Generally, FA and MD are influenced by AD and RD. Decreased FA and increased MD are measures of neuronal injury, increased AD is a measure of axonal chronic damage, and increased RD is a measure of myelin damage [7, 17].

Though many DTI studies on HIV have reported a loss of WM integrity [6–12], few studies have focused on the WM microstructure in neuroasymptomatic HIV+ individuals without treatment. Zhu T et al. found that WM injuries in neurologically asymptomatic HIV patients are mainly located in the posterior part of both hemispheres (MD, AD, RD increased significantly) [7]. Wang B et al. observed a decrease in FA in the corpus callosum and anterior corona radiata and an increase in MD, RD, and AD in most skeleton locations [8]. In both studies, the neuropsychological tests were assessed by AIDS Dementia Complex (ADC) staging according to the Memorial Sloan Kettering (MSK) staging system, and an ADC score of 0 or 0.5 was considered neurocognitive asymptomatic. Zhuang Y et al. investigated WM changes in ANI patients diagnosed according to the Frascati criteria [3] and found no significant WM microstructural differences between HIV-infected and healthy controls [18]. Cysique LA et al. reported that the location of WM injury in ANI cases was the anterior limb of the internal capsule [19]. The above findings still exhibit differences.

HIV-associated WM damage includes demyelination and axonal injury; however, the relationship between them and the neuropathology of HIV-related WM impairment is still unclear. The primary oligodendrocyte and myelin damage leading to secondary axonal damage (outside-in) or primary axonopathy triggering oligodendrocyte injury and demyelination (inside-out) are indistinguishable [20]. WM alterations may contribute to cognitive deficits in HIV-infected patients [7, 18, 21]. It is worth noting that the relationship between WM abnormalities and cognitive status has not been well characterized or systematically assessed.

Moreover, the effects of multiple clinical contributors on cerebral WM integrity merit further investigation. The various potential clinical influencing variables include factors that are directly related to HIV disease (i.e., $CD4^+$ level, $CD4^+/CD8^+$ ratio, plasma viral load and duration of HIV infection) and factors that can affect the CNS, such as ageing. Recent studies have identified that HIV duration was significantly correlated with DTI parameters [7, 22]. FA values in the corpus callosum were negatively correlated with the duration of infection in antiretroviral-naïve primary HIV infection patients [23]. Cohen RA et al. reported that the CD4 nadir and the duration of HIV infection may be risk factors for cerebral injury [24]. However, other studies showed dissenting results that age can exacerbate HIV-associated WM abnormalities [11, 25]. Regrettably, there were discrepancies in previous findings.

In the present study, we aimed to investigate the WM microstructural changes in treatment-naïve HIV patients with ANI through DTI-TBSS technology. In particular, the current study was confined to treatment-naïve patients to rule out the possibility of antiretroviral therapy (ART) erosion on WM integrity. We also wanted to quantify the relationships between WM damage and age, $CD4^+$ counts, $CD4^+/CD8^+$ ratio, plasma viral load, duration of HIV infection and cognitive status.

Methods

Subjects

The protocol was approved by the ethics committee. HIV participants were recruited from infectious disease outpatient clinic of Beijing YouAn Hospital, Capital Medical University. The inclusion criteria for patients were as follows: age ≥ 18 years, naïve to ART prior to enrolment, and HAND stage of ANI. According to the inclusion criteria, we enrolled twenty patients from June 2014 to July 2016. Twenty seronegative healthy volunteers matched for age, gender and education level were recruited from the same community by advertisements. All subjects provided written informed consent prior to enrolment. The exclusion criteria for both HIV-infected and HIV-negative participants were as follows: 1) age < 18 years; 2) neurological disorders: epilepsy, stroke, an active or known past opportunistic infection of the CNS; 3) alcohol or drug abuse within the last 6 months; 4) stable anxiety or depression, including those managed by stable anti-anxiety or antidepressant therapy; 5) contraindication to MR; 6) trauma, tumours, infection (except HIV), vascular diseases and other visible brain lesions on standard MRI (T_1WI and T_2-fluid attenuated inversion recovery (FLAIR)).

In the HIV-infected individuals, HIV was confirmed by an enzyme-linked immunosorbent assay and western blot analysis. The duration of HIV infection was determined according to patients' self-reports on their risk behaviours. The recent $CD4^+$ counts were performed within 2 weeks of neuroimaging. HIV RNA levels were measured from blood plasma. The mode of HIV infection was sexual contact (male homosexual contact for 14 patients, heterosexual contact for 6 patients). The years of education ranged from 13 to 19 years (mean: 16.5 ± 1.8 years).

Two to three hours prior to the MRI scanning, each patient underwent a comprehensive neuropsychological assessment, including 6 cognitive domains and a report of cognitive difficulties in daily life. Self-questionnaires of daily functioning were assessed with a short Activity of Daily Living scale [26]. The neurocognitive evaluation surveys the following abilities: verbal fluency (Animal Verbal Fluency Test, AFT), attention/working memory (Continuous Performance Test-Identical Pair, CPT-IP; Wechsler Memory Scale, WMS-III; Paced Auditory Serial Addition Test, PASAT), executive function (Wisconsin Card Sorting Tests, WCST-64), memory (learning and delayed recall) (Hopking Verbal Learning Test, HVLT-R; Brief Visuospatial Memory Test, BVMT-R), speed of information processing (Trail Marking Test A, TMT- A) and fine motor skills (Grooved Pegboard, dominant and non-dominant Hands) [4, 27]. Raw scores for each test were transformed into T-scores and adjusted for age, gender, and education level. T-scores across more tests for one cognitive domain were averaged to calculate domain-specific T-scores. Patients whose cognitive impairment involved two or more cognitive abilities (performance of at least one standard deviation below the mean for norms on neuropsychological tests) and presented no cognitive difficulties in everyday life were diagnosed with ANI [3]. All patients were diagnosed with ANI according to the Frascati criteria [3].

Twenty patients and twenty healthy controls received MRIs. All scans were reviewed by an experienced neuroradiologist for motion artefacts and evidence of unknown brain lesion, which could have affected DTI indices. The image quality of one patient was poor. After communicating with the patient, we immediately reacquired data and obtained good image quality. No MRI scans were required to be excluded from DTI analysis. Thus, we presented data for 20 patients and 20 controls.

MRI protocols

All MRI scans were performed on a Siemens Trio 3.0 Tesla imager. Standard structural images were acquired using axial T_1WI (repetition time (TR) = 250 ms, echo time (TE) = 2.46 ms) and T_2-FLAIR combined fat saturation (TR = 8000 ms, TE = 2370.9 ms, inversion time = 97 ms) sequences to check whether there were visible intracranial lesions. For DTI data, a single-shot echo-planar imaging sequence was used for acquisition. The parameters for DTI were: TR = 3300 ms, TE = 90 ms, slice thickness = 4 mm with 1.2 mm gap, number of slices = 63, matrix size = 128 × 128, field of view = 230 × 230 mm, number of excitations = 3, space resolution = 1.8 mm × 1.8 mm × 1.8 mm, total acquisition time = 3.39 min. Diffusion sensitizing gradients were applied along 20 non-collinear directions with b = 1000 s/mm^2, and one b = 0 s/mm^2.

DTI datasets were performed and analysed using FSL5.0 (FMRIB Image Analysis Group, Oxford, UK, http://www.fmrib.ox.ac.uk/fsl) [28]. Details of the DTI processing steps, including pre-processing and TBSS processing, have been described previously [8, 29]. There were three steps for pre-processing. The raw DTI images were first corrected for the effects of eddy currents and head movements and deformations using eddy current correction within FDT. Then, brain mask extraction was performed on one of the no-diffusion-weighting (b = 0) images by running the Brain Extraction Tool in FSL. Finally, the diffusion tensor model was computed using DTIFIT within FDT for whole brain volumes to generate tensor-derived maps, including FA, MD, AD, and RD. TBSS-processing includes four steps. The first is image registration. Using the FA map as a target template for registration, more accurate results can be achieved, as FA is a normalized measure of eigenvalue standard deviation and represents the degree of diffusion directionality. A common registration target brain image template (FMRIB58_FA) was identified, and all subjects' FA images were aligned to this target using FMRIB's non-linear image registration tool, through which all the FA volumes were aligned to a $1.0 \times 1.0 \times 1.0$ mm³ Montreal Neurological Institute standard space. Second, the mean of all aligned FA images was skeletonized, and a mean FA skeleton image (threshold = 0.2) was generated. Third, the aligned FA image for each subject was projected onto the mean FA skeleton by filling the skeleton with maximum FA values from the nearest relevant tract centre to generate a skeletonized FA map. Corresponding skeletonized maps for the other diffusion measures (MD, AD and RD) were also similarly generated. Lastly, voxelwise statistical analyses of DTI metrics were carried out on the skeleton space.

Statistical analysis

Demographic characteristics of the HIV+ participants and healthy controls were analysed with IBM SPSS Statistics (version 22.0). Chi-squared analysis was used to evaluate the sex distribution between HIV+ patients and healthy controls. Independent t-test analysis was used to calculate the differences in age and education level between the two groups. Significance was defined as $p < 0.05$.

For TBSS analysis, voxel-wised statistics of the DTI parameters (FA, MD, AD, RD) for the two group differences were tested in the general linear model framework using the FSL randomize tool with a non-parametric permutation testing (5000 random permutations) [30]. The threshold-free cluster enhancement (TFCE) method with a threshold set at 0.95 was used to obtain correction for multiple comparisons [31], and statistical maps were obtained with family-wise error (FWE) correction at the $p < 0.05$ level. The significant group differences in tracts were located with the Johns Hopkins University (JHU)-ICBM-DTI-81 WM Label Atlas.

To investigate the relationships between DTI metrics and clinical variables and cognitive performance for HIV-positive patients, multiple linear regression analysis between DTI indices and age, CD4+ counts, CD4+/CD8+ ratio, plasma viral load, duration of HIV infection and scores of cognitive performance was performed. A significance level of 0.05 was obtained using IBM SPSS Statistics (version 22.0).

Results
Demographic information
The demographic and clinical information for HIV+ patients and healthy controls are listed in Table 1. There were no significant differences in age, sex, or education level (in years) between the HIV+ patients and healthy controls.

Table 1 Clinical and demographic data of study participants

Items	Patient group (N = 20)	Control Group (N = 20)	p-value
Age	30.6 ± 9.6	31.5 ± 7.6	0.325[b]
Sex (M/F)	19:1	19:1	1.000[a]
Education level (year)	16.5 ± 1.8	16.1 ± 0.8	0.372[b]
Duration of infection (year)	3.1 ± 0.9	N/A	N/A
CD4 (cells/ml)	254.6 ± 168.8	N/A	N/A
Viral load (log) (copies/ml)	4.26 ± 1.1	N/A	N/A

N number of subjects, M male, F female, N/A not applicable or available, a Chi-squared analysis, b Independent t test, Significance level P < 0.05

White matter abnormalities in ART-naïve HIV+ patients at ANI stage

Voxel-based TBSS demonstrated significant differences in DTI parameters (MD and AD values) of HIV-infected individuals compared to controls. The FA map and RD map revealed no significant differences between the two groups. The results were illustrated in Fig. 1 and Table 2. Compared with healthy controls, HIV-positive patients exhibited significantly higher MD in the genu, body and splenium of corpus callosum, bilateral anterior and superior corona radiate. Increased AD was observed in extensive brain regions, including the genu, body and splenium of the corpus callosum; bilateral anterior and superior corona radiata, anterior limb of the internal capsule, external capsule; left retrolenticular part of the internal capsule, posterior corona radiata, posterior thalamic radiation, sagittal stratum, superior longitudinal fasciculus (all $P < 0.05$). Regions of increased AD were much more prevalent than those of MD.

Correlations between DTI metrics and clinical variables for HIV-infected patients

Fig. 2 shows the regression coefficients and significance for clinical clinics on MD and AD values in the regions of white matter impairment. The increased MD values in the right anterior corona radiate were negatively correlated with CD4+/CD8+ ratios ($r = -0.437$, $P = 0.05$) (Table 3). Similar analyses showed that the increased AD values in the left posterior corona radiata were negatively correlated with CD4+/CD8+ ratios ($r = -0.488$, $P = 0.029$) (Table 4). The increased AD values in the right anterior limb of the internal capsule were positively correlated with viral load ($r = -0.848$, $P = 0.019$) and CD4+/CD8+ ratios ($r = -0.717$, $P = 0.003$) (Table 4).

Correlations between DTI metrics and cognitive performance for HIV-infected patients

Reduced cognitive scores were significantly correlated with either increased MD or AD in multiple white matter structures (Fig. 3, Table 3 and Table 4). Verbal

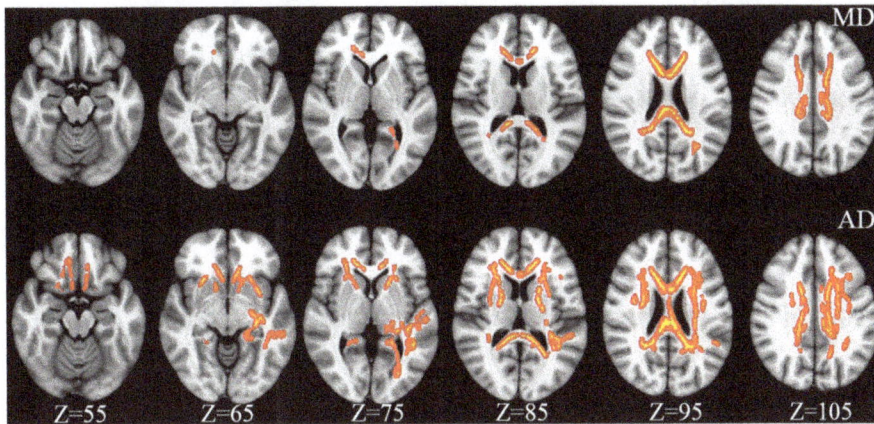

Fig. 1 TBSS analysis of DTI indices between HIV+ and control groups (Transverse section). Areas in red-yellow are regions where MD and AD were significantly increased (P < 0.05, corrected by TFCE) in HIV-infected individuals compared with controls. The number below each brain image indicates the Z coordinate in the Montreal Neurological Institute (MNI) space. MD, mean diffusivity; AD, axial diffusivity

fluency scores were negatively correlated with AD values in the left anterior corona radiata, anterior limb of the internal capsule and right superior corona radiata. Attention/working memory scores were positively correlated with AD values in the left anterior limb of the internal capsule and right superior corona radiate. Memory (learning and delayed recall) test scores were negatively correlated with MD values in the genu of the corpus callosum, anterior corona radiata (bilateral) and superior corona radiata (right). A positive correlation was observed between the speed of information processing scores and MD values in the genu of the corpus

callosum, anterior corona radiata (bilateral) and superior corona radiata (right), AD values in the genu of the corpus callosum, anterior limb of the internal capsule (bilateral) and posterior thalamic radiation (left). Fine motor scores were negatively correlated with MD values in the genu of the corpus callosum, anterior and superior corona radiata (right), and AD values in the superior corona radiata (right).

Discussion

This study not only supports but also further extends previous DTI findings in neuroasymptomatic HIV-positive

Table 2 Location and cluster size of abnormal WM tracts between HIV patients and healthy controls

WM structures (JHU-WM Atlas)	Side	HIV patients vs. controls cluster size	
		MD	AD
Genu of corpus callosum	–	587	973
Body of corpus callosum	–	1299	1901
Splenium of corpus callosum	–	962	1615
Anterior corona radiata	R	256	918
Anterior corona radiata	L	236	716
Superior corona radiata	R	121	448
Superior corona radiata	L	255	845
Anterior limb of internal capsule	R	–	306
Anterior limb of internal capsule	L	–	363
External capsule	R	–	186
External capsule	L	–	279
Retrolenticular part of internal capsule	L	–	215
Posterior corona radiata	L	–	332
Posterior thalamic radiation	L	–	287
Sagittal stratum	L	–	105
Superior longitudinal fasciculus	L	–	358

WM white matter, *MD* mean diffusivity, *AD* axial diffusivity, *L* left, *R* right, *JHU-WM Atlas* the ICBM-DTI-81 White Matter Atlas

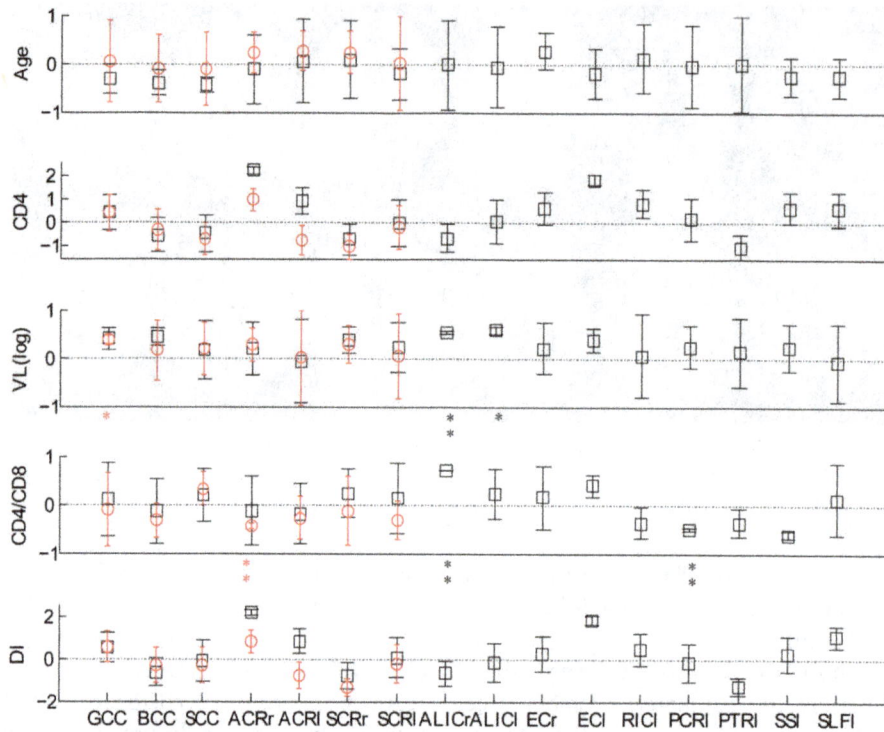

Fig. 2 Regression coefficients and significance for clinical variables and white matter impairments. The increased MD values in the right ACR negatively correlated with CD4+/CD8+ ratios. The increased AD values in the left PCR negatively correlated with CD4+/CD8+ ratios. The increased AD values in the right ALIC positively correlated with viral load and CD4+/CD8+ ratiosNote: bar: P value; *: p < 0.1; **: p < 0.05; red circle: regression coefficients of MD; black square: regression coefficients of AD.MD, mean diffusivity; AD, axial diffusivity; GCC, genu of corpus callosum; BCC, body of corpus callosum; SCC, splenium of corpus callosum; ACR, anterior corona radiata; SCR, superior corona radiata; ALIC, anterior limb of internal capsule; EC, external capsule; RIC, retrolenticular part of internal capsule; PCR, posterior corona radiata; PTR, posterior thalamic radiation; SS, sagittal stratum; SLF, superior longitudinal fasciculus. l, left; r, right; VL, viral load; DI, duration of infection.

Table 3 Regression coefficients and significance for MD values and clinical variables and cognitive status scores

		MD values of HIV-associated white matter impairment						
		GCC	BCC	SCC	ACR_R	ACR_L	SCR_R	SCR_L
Clinical Variables	Age	0.057	− 0.118	−0.096	0.221	0.26	0.239	0.016
	CD4	0.433	−0.282	− 0.637	0.986	− 0.724	−1.001	− 0.142
	CD4/CD8	− 0.101	− 0.331	0.331	− 0.437**	− 0.274	− 0.127	− 0.307
	VL(log)	0.381*	0.162	0.207	0.277	0.006	0.287	0.055
	DI	0.564	−0.281	−0.326	0.815	−0.8	−1.319	− 0.224
Cognitive Status	VF	−0.053	0.012	−0.169	−0.114	− 0.135	−0.293	− 0.459*
	A/WM	0.021	−0.004	−0.238	0.21	−0.001	0.424	0.141
	EF	−0.272	−0.226	− 0.2	−0.172	− 0.133	−0.194	− 0.218
	M(LDR)	−0.417**	−0.338	0.159	−0.511**	− 0.559**	−0.501**	− 0.281
	SIP	0.684**	0.427*	0.155	0.559**	0.583**	0.444**	0.239
	FM	−0.417**	−0.259	−0.403*	− 0.391**	− 0.321*	− 0.474**	−0.443*

The regression coefficients and significance results were calculated by the multiple linear analysis method. *MD* mean diffusivity, *GCC* genu of corpus callosum, *BCC* body of corpus callosum, *SCC* splenium of corpus callosum, *ACR* anterior corona radiata, *SCR* superior corona radiata, *L* left, *R* right, *VL* viral load, *DI* duration of infection, *VF* Verbal Fluency, *A/WM* Attention/Working Memory, *EF* Executive Functioning, *SIP* Speed of Information Processing, *MS* Motor Skills, * P < 0.1, ** P < 0.05

Table 4 Regression coefficients and significance for AD values and clinical variables and cognitive status scores

		AD values of HIV-infected in different brain regions															
		GCC	BCC	SCC	ACR_R	ACR_L	SCR_R	SCR_L	ALIC_R	ALIC_L	EC_R	EC_L	RIC_L	PCR_L	PTR_L	SS_L	SLF_L
Clinical Variables	Age	−0.321	−0.395	−0.446	−0.111	0.053	0.078	−0.202	−0.025	−0.065	0.27	−0.19	0.115	−0.051	−0.006	−0.251	−0.264
	CD4	0.475	−0.521	−0.416	2.242	0.978	−0.68	0.008	−0.644	0.082	0.645	1.852	0.841	0.18	−1.02	0.673	0.613
	CD4/CD8	0.108	−0.139	0.2	−0.125	−0.185	0.242	0.126	0.717**	0.224	0.153	0.394	−0.366	−0.488**	−0.372	−0.613	0.12
	VL(log)	0.404	0.445	0.164	0.201	−0.061	0.379	0.228	0.533**	0.579*	0.211	0.376	0.059	0.242	0.124	0.22	−0.083
	DI	0.547	−0.64	−0.088	2.21	0.848	−0.782	0.082	−0.672	−0.143	0.276	1.876	0.484	−0.167	−1.267	0.265	1.071
Cognitive Status	VF	−0.256	−0.333	−0.194	−0.411	−0.507**	−0.67**	−0.502	0.196	−0.671**	0.059	−0.16	0.396	−0.057	0.102	0.126	−0.437
	A/WM	0.237	0.238	−0.219	0.474	0.147	0.619**	0.461	0.201	0.566**	0.091	0.062	−0.078	0.245	−0.243	−0.219	0.115
	EF	−0.278	−0.406*	−0.385*	−0.305	0.045	−0.227	−0.183	−0.394*	0.099	−0.406	−0.251	−0.249	−0.408*	−0.339*	−0.24	0.394
	M(LDR)	0.011	−0.028	0.334	−0.148	−0.272	−0.307	−0.132	0.245	0.079	0.067	0.134	−0.038	−0.272	−0.074	0.116	0.068
	SIP	0.589**	0.382*	0.178	−0.049	0.206	0.136	0.176	0.631**	0.544**	0.082	−0.125	0.435	0.17	0.529**	0.362	0.123
	FM	−0.329	−0.447*	−0.241	−0.179	−0.268	−0.622**	−0.441	0.081	−0.232	−0.281	−0.469	0.026	−0.172	0.143	0.092	−0.406

The regression coefficients and significance results were calculated by the multiple linear analysis method. AD axial diffusivity, GCC genu of corpus callosum, BCC body of corpus callosum, SCC splenium of corpus callosum, ACR anterior corona radiata, SCR superior corona radiata, L left, R right, ALIC anterior limb of internal capsule, EC external capsule, RIC retrolenticular part of internal capsule, PCR posterior corona radiata, PTR posterior thalamic radiation, SS sagittal stratum, SLF superior longitudinal fasciculus, VL viral load, DI duration of infection, VF Verbal Fluency, A/WM Attention/Working Memory, EF Executive Functioning, SIP Speed of Information Processing, MS Motor Skills, * $P < 0.1$, ** $P < 0.05$

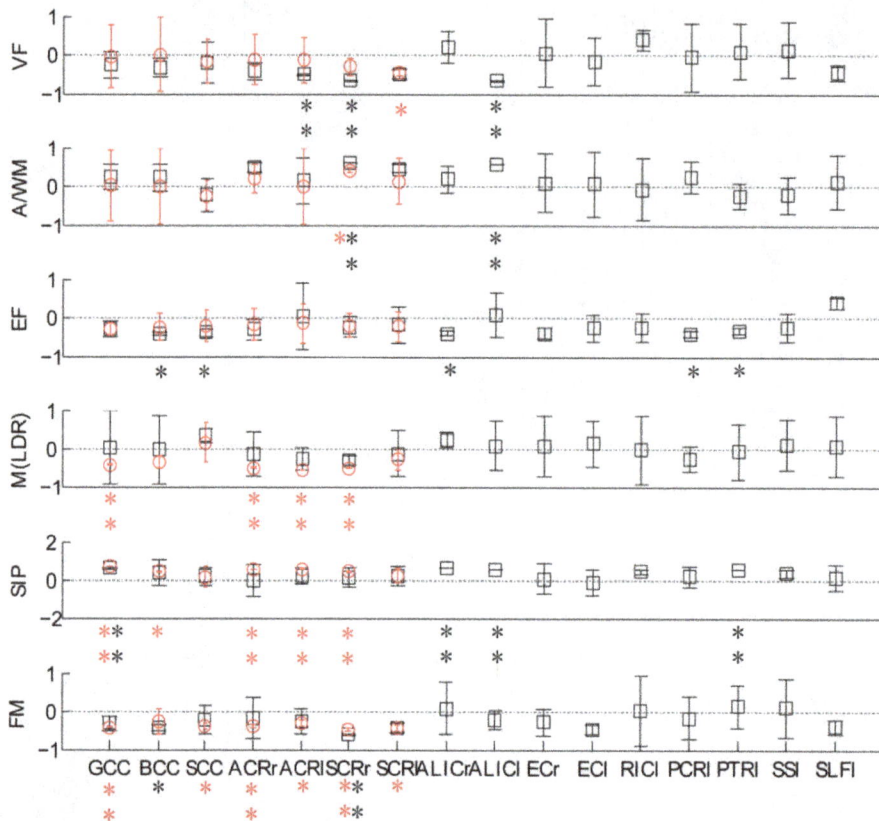

Fig. 3 Regression coefficients and significance for white matter alterations and cognitive performance. Verbal fluency scores were negatively correlated with AD values in the left ACR, ALIC and right SCR. Attention/working memory scores were positively correlated with AD values in the left ALIC and right SCR. Memory (learning and delayed recall) test scores were negatively correlated with MD values in the GCC, ACR (bilateral) and SCR (right). A positive correlation was observed between speed of information processing scores and MD values in the GCC, ACR (bilateral) and SCR (right), AD values in the GCC, ALIC (bilateral) and PTR (left). Fine motor scores were negatively correlated with MD values in the GCC, ACR (right) and SCR (right), AD values in the SCR (right)Note: bar: P value; *: p < 0.1; **: p < 0.05; red circle: regression coefficients of MD; black square: regression coefficients of AD.MD, mean diffusivity; AD, axial diffusivity; GCC, genu of corpus callosum; BCC, body of corpus callosum; SCC, splenium of corpus callosum; ACR, anterior corona radiata; SCR, superior corona radiata; ALIC, anterior limb of internal capsule; EC, external capsule; RIC, retrolenticular part of internal capsule; PCR, posterior corona radiata; PTR, posterior thalamic radiation; SS, sagittal stratum; SLF, superior longitudinal fasciculus. l, left; r, right; VF, Verbal Fluency; A/WM, Attention/ Working Memory; EF, Executive Functioning; M(LDR), memory (learning and delayed recall); SIP, Speed of Information Processing; FM, fine motor.

individuals. One purpose of this study is to explore the microstructure changes of WM in treatment-naïve ANI patients employing the DTI-TBSS method. Compared with healthy controls, ANI patients exhibited significantly increased MD and AD in the corpus callosum and anterior and superior corona radiate. The corpus callosum and corona radiata were distributed around the lateral ventricle. The anterior limb of internal capsule, external capsule, retrolenticular part of the internal capsule, posterior corona radiata, posterior thalamic radiation, sagittal stratum, and superior longitudinal fasciculus presented significantly increased AD, and we found that most of them were also close to the ventricles. It is speculated that HIV-associated WM involvement is selective rather than random. Periventricular WM, especially the corpus callosum and corona radiata, are more vulnerable to viral invasion and neuroinflammation in early HIV infection in

adults, which are consistent with previous studies [6–8, 32, 33]. Ragin et al. even found a loss of WM integrity in the corpus callosum within 100 days of HIV infection [33]. It is not clear why these regions were vulnerable to viral invasion and neuroinflammation. One possible explanation is that the choroid plexus is the blood-cerebrospinal fluid (CSF) barrier, and HIV can accumulate in the CSF when it is destroyed. Studies have shown that HIV can infiltrate the CSF as early as 8 days after exposure [34], and CSF serves as a proxy for the brain parenchyma and the reservoir for monocytes linked to HIV neuropathogenesis [35]. Early neuroinvasion was identified by measurable markers of CSF inflammation [34], and the WM tracts around the ventricle might be affected gradually. The interpretation of these results requires caution, and future investigation will be needed to better characterize them.

WM tracts with increased AD are more extensive than those of increased MD. The overlap and differences of the two DTI parameters (MD and AD) in significantly altered cerebral regions reflect differences in the nature and degree of WM injury. Increased MD indicates an increase of the water molecules' diffusion speed, which is caused by cell degeneration and a decrease of membrane density. Increased MD may reflect inflammation or increased glial activation, a measure of neuronal injury. Increased AD is a marker of axonal chronic damage [7, 36]. Increased RD is associated with the destruction of myelin integrity and is used as a marker for demyelination [16, 17, 37]. RD abnormalities were not found in the current ANI study. It was concluded that MD changes in ANI subjects were mainly attributable to increased AD, suggesting chronic axonal injury rather than the disruption integrity of myelin in early HIV infection. A similar study found elevated CSF neurofilament light chain concentration and its correlation with MRS-based metabolites in primary HIV infection [32], and the neurofilament light chain is a sensitive marker of axonal injury. These findings demonstrate that axonopathy may exist before myelin injury, and this may be a novel observation. However, whether can axonal injury trigger demyelination (inside-out) is not yet clear. In recent DTI studies on ultra-early HIV infection, the authors focused only on FA and MD, and AD and RD were not calculated [23, 33]. AD and RD are also important, as they provide information on the nature of the WM microstructure alterations observed in HIV patients. Researching on multiple metrics of DTI may help us to comprehend the pathophysiology of HIV-related WM injury. The relationship of axonal and myelin injury needs to be better characterized in future HAND pathology studies.

FA abnormalities were also not found in ANI patients, which implies that RD maybe the predominant factor that contributes to decreased FA. Similar findings also have been reported, which showed that FA changes were attributable to increased RD [14, 38]. In addition, several DTI studies noted that significant alterations in FA were found mainly in cognitively impaired HIV-infected patients [7, 39]. Thus, MD may be a more sensitive biomarker than FA in evaluating WM injury in early HIV infection.

Our previous DTI study in early HIV infection showed significant differences in MD, AD, and RD values between a therapy naïve HIV+ group and healthy control group [29]. One resemblance between the two studies is the distribution of white matter abnormalities. Another similarity is that white matter abnormalities are all reflected in the changes of MD and AD values, rather than FA values. The difference is that the previous study has a wider range of WM injury. Additionally, changes of RD values can be seen in a few WM tracts (genu of corpus callosum and superior corona radiate), which indicates myelin damage. A possible reason is that HIV-infected patients in the previous study were classified into ADC stage 0 according to the MSK classification. While MSK is a decent scale to globally express the state of cognitive functioning, it is not very sensitive to changes in less affected patients. The Frascati scale used in the current study may be more sensitive to identify and classify individuals with subclinical impairment. More detailed neuropsychological assessment for earlier HIV-infected patients is the novel element of the current study relative to the previous study. Corrêa et al. found that HIV patients with planning deficits had significantly decreased FA, increased MD and RD values, predominantly in frontal lobes, genu and splenium of the corpus callosum, and much less widespread abnormalities were seen in the AD values compared with normal controls. HIV+ patients with planning deficits also had significantly decreased FA values and increased MD and RD values in some white matter regions compared to those without planning deficits [40]. No significant abnormalities AD values were seen between the two groups. These results indicated that RD abnormal values predominated in the areas of decreased FA compared to AD values, suggesting that demyelination could play a role in the physiopathology of HIV-related WM injury, which is not completely consistent with our results. The possible reason for the difference between the two results was that participants in the previous article all received ART, and with longer known infection. Antiretroviral drugs may be injurious to brain cell elements. The influence of treatment on brain structure and function are less clear [41]. HIV+ patients on low CNS penetration ART had a significantly greater fMRI response amplitude compared to the HIV+ patients on high CNS penetration ART or normal controls [42]. To the best of our knowledge, no studies have detected the effects of ART regimen CNS penetration effectiveness on WM microstructure. Effects of treatment should be explored in future studies.

The MD values in the right anterior corona radiata and AD values in the left posterior corona radiata have a significantly negative correlation with $CD4^+/CD8^+$ ratios, and the regression coefficient is 0.437 and 0.488, respectively; in other words, WM microstructure changes (43.7% in the anterior corona radiata, 48.8% in the posterior corona radiate) can be influenced by $CD4^+/CD8^+$ ratios. The abnormality of AD values was related to axonal chronic injury. Clinically, the lower $CD4^+/CD8^+$ ratios were related to immunosenescence [43]. This might imply that immunosenescence among the ANI patients would accelerate the axonal chronic injury in the corona radiata, and the lower $CD4^+/CD8^+$ ratio might be an important predictor of WM injury in the corona radiata. Furthermore, we found that plasma viral load remained independently associated with AD values in the right anterior limb of the internal capsule, and the regression coefficient was 0.533. The higher the plasma viral load, the higher are the AD values in the right anterior limb of the internal capsule. The higher plasma viral load represents the activity and replication of HIV in the human internal environment. The positive correlation indicates that the WM microstructure in the anterior limb of the internal capsule was susceptible to viral replication in HIV infection. The current findings were not fully consistent with previous studies [7, 11, 22–25], and the results of previous studies also varied. This may be due to the difference and heterogeneity in participants with diverse treatments, sample size, cognitive status, and disease durations. Further studies are needed to resolve this incongruity and reliability.

Associations between WM microstructure alterations and cognitive impairment were observed in the current study. Several other studies have reported that WM changes were related to HIV-associated cognitive difficulties [44–46]. WM microstructure changes in the anterior and superior corona radiata and anterior limb of the internal capsule were significantly correlated with poorer verbal fluency. WM damage in the genu of the corpus callosum and anterior and superior corona radiata were significantly correlated with poorer memory (learning and delayed recall) and slower fine motor speed. The corona radiata is the radiated projection fibre connecting the internal capsule to the cerebral cortex. The corona radiata and internal capsule are important WM nodes that promote the transfer of sensorimotor information between the brain stem, thalamus and frontostriatal circuit [47]. The anterior corona radiate connects the anterior and medial nuclei of the thalamus to the prefrontal cortex. The superior corona radiate involves corticospinal tracts and the posterior frontal part of the anterior thalamic radiation [7]. The corpus callosum is the largest and most prominent WM tract, which is responsible for the communication of interhemispheric information. The genu of the corpus callosum contains the posterior frontal part of callosal fibres [7]. The corpus callosum and corona radiate are pivotal in extensive cognitive function, such as verbal fluency, attention, memory, psychomotor speed and executive functioning. The significant correlation between neurocognitive performance and MD and AD values from multiple WM microstructures suggests that WM abnormalities have functional consequences. HIV-related cognitive impairment may be associated with cortical and subcortical track loss caused by WM fibre bundle damage, and the WM microstructure may serve as an indicator to objectively predict cognitive deficits and

progression. However, a multivariate model also showed that the WM microstructure alterations in the superior corona radiate and anterior limb of the internal capsule better predicted sustained attention/working memory. WM injury in the genu of the corpus callosum, anterior and superior corona radiata, anterior limb of the internal capsule and posterior thalamic radiation were significantly correlated with faster speed of information processing. A potential explanation for this may be some sort of compensatory mechanism, and it needs to be further verified in future multimodal studies (DTI combined functional MRI).

There were several limitations in the current study. First, the study was limited to a small sample size. A larger sample size would be more helpful to improve the power of the statistical analysis. Second, the participants were almost exclusively male, which may prevent the generalization of these results to HIV-infected women. Certainly, given that the gender gap is narrowing with rates of infection increasing in women, we are trying our best to extend our studies to include female patients in the future. Third, a cognitively intact HIV-positive group will be studied in further work. Fourth, a longitudinal follow-up study is imperative to observe the dynamic changes of WM after ART.

Conclusions

The observations of the current study strengthen the possibility that HIV-infected individuals at the ANI stage have underlying WM fibre abnormalities, which could be measured by increased MD, and the pathogenesis of this damage is likely to be predominantly the axonal chronic injury associated with increased AD. DTI has the potential to promote a better understanding of the pathogenesis of brain WM changes. Specific brain regions around the ventricle, especially the corpus callosum and corona radiata, are susceptible to be involved. Relationship exists between WM damage, HIV-related clinical factors, and cognitive status. HIV patients with a history of advanced immune suppression and higher viral load may be at high risk of WM injury. WM damage and disconnection to the cortex probably contribute to cognitive impairments.

Abbreviations
AD: Axial diffusivity; ADC: AIDS Dementia Complex; ANI: Asymptomatic neurocognitive impairment; ART: Antiretroviral therapy; CNS: Central nervous system; CSF: Cerebrospinal fluid; DTI: Diffusion tensor imaging; FLAIR: Fluid attenuated inversion recovery; HAND: HIV-associated neurocognitive disorders; MD: Mean diffusivity; MRI: Magnetic resonance imaging; MSK: Memorial Sloan Kettering; RD: Radial diffusivity; TBSS: Tract-based spatial statistics; WM: White matter

Funding
This work was supported by the Beijing Municipal Administration of Hospitals Incubating Program (PX2016036), The Beijing Municipal Administration of Hospitals Clinical Medicine Development of Special

Funding (ZYLX201511), The National Nature Science Foundation of China (81571634, 81771806), The capital medical university research and incubation funding (PYZ2017124).

Authors' contributions

Research design: RLL, JS, JJZ and HJL. Data collection: RLL and JJZ. Data processing and analysis of DTI-TBSS: RLL and ZCT; Multiple regression analysis: RLL and JS. Writing and revising the manuscript: RLL, JS, ZCT, JJZ and HJL. All authors have read and approved the final manuscript.

Competing interests

HJL, the corresponding author of this article, is a member of the editorial board (Associate Editor) of BMC Neurology. The authors declare that they have no competing interests.

Author details

[1]Department of Radiology, Beijing YouAn Hospital, Capital Medical University, No.8, Xi Tou Tiao, Youanmen Wai, Feng Tai District, Beijing 100069, China. [2]School of Mechanical, Electrical & Information Engineering, Shandong University, No.180, West Wenhua Road, Weihai 264209, Shandong Province, China. [3]STD and AIDS clinical treatment center, Beijing YouAn Hospital, Capital Medical University, No.8, Xi Tou Tiao, Youanmen Wai, Feng Tai District, Beijing 100069, China.

References

1. Ances BM, Ellis RJ. Dementia and neurocognitive disorders due to HIV-1 infection. Semin Neurol. 2007;27(1):86–92.
2. Heaton RK, Franklin DR, Ellis RJ, McCutchan JA, Letendre SL, Leblanc S, Corkran SH, Duarte NA, Clifford DB, Woods SP, et al. HIV-associated neurocognitive disorders before and during the era of combination antiretroviral therapy: differences in rates, nature, and predictors. J Neuro-Oncol. 2011;17(1):3–16.
3. Antinori A, Arendt G, Becker JT, Brew BJ, Byrd DA, Cherner M, Clifford DB, Cinque P, Epstein LG, Goodkin K, et al. Updated research nosology for HIV-associated neurocognitive disorders. Neurology. 2007;69(18):1789–99.
4. Heaton RK, Clifford DB, Franklin DR Jr, Woods SP, Ake C, Vaida F, Ellis RJ, Letendre SL, Marcotte TD, Atkinson JH, et al. HIV-associated neurocognitive disorders persist in the era of potent antiretroviral therapy: CHARTER study. Neurology. 2010;75(23):2087–96.
5. Tucker KA, Robertson KR, Lin W, Smith JK, An H, Chen Y, Aylward SR, Hall CD. Neuroimaging in human immunodeficiency virus infection. J Neuroimmunol. 2004;157(1–2):153–62.
6. Tang Z, Liu Z, Li R, Yang X, Cui X, Wang S, Yu D, Li H, Dong E, Tian J. Identifying the white matter impairments among ART-naïve HIV patients: a multivariate pattern analysis of DTI data. Eur Radiol. 2017;27(10):4153–62.
7. Zhu T, Zhong J, Hu R, Tivarus M, Ekholm S, Harezlak J, Ombao H, Navia B, Cohen R, Schifitto G. Patterns of white matter injury in HIV infection after partial immune reconstitution: a DTI tract-based spatial statistics study. J Neuro-Oncol. 2013;19(1):10–23.
8. Wang B, Liu Z, Liu J, Tang Z, Li H, Tian J. Gray and white matter alterations in early HIV-infected patients: combined voxel-based morphometry and tract-based spatial statistics. J Magn Reson Imaging. 2016;43(6):1474–83.
9. Towgood KJ, Pitkanen M, Kulasegaram R, Fradera A, Kumar A, Soni S, Sibtain NA, Reed L, Bradbeer C, Barker GJ, et al. Mapping the brain in younger and older asymptomatic HIV-1 men: frontal volume changes in the absence of other cortical or diffusion tensor abnormalities. Cortex. 2012;48(2):230–41.
10. Tate DF, Sampat M, Harezlak J, Fiecas M, Hogan J, Dewey J, McCaffrey D, Branson D, Russell T, Conley J, et al. Regional areas and widths of the midsagittal corpus callosum among HIV-infected patients on stable antiretroviral therapies. J Neuro-Oncol. 2011;17(4):368–79.
11. Gongvatana A, Cohen RA, Correia S, Devlin KN, Miles J, Kang H, Ombao H, Navia B, Laidlaw DH, Tashima KT. Clinical contributors to cerebral white matter integrity in HIV-infected individuals. J Neuro-Oncol. 2011;17(5):477–86.
12. Muller-Oehring EM, Schulte T, Rosenbloom MJ, Pfefferbaum A, Sullivan EV. Callosal degradation in HIV-1 infection predicts hierarchical perception: a DTI study. Neuropsychologia. 2010;48(4):1133–43.
13. Smith SM, Jenkinson M, Johansen-Berg H, Rueckert D, Nichols TE, Mackay CE, Watkins KE, Ciccarelli O, Cader MZ, Matthews PM. Tract-based spatial statistics: Voxelwise analysis of multi-subject diffusion data. NeuroImage. 2006;31(4):1487–505.
14. Ackermann C, Andronikou S, Saleh MG, Laughton B, Alhamud AA, van der Kouwe A, Kidd M, Cotton MF, Meintjes EM. Early antiretroviral therapy in HIV-infected children is associated with diffuse white matter structural abnormality and Corpus callosum sparing. AJNR Am J Neuroradiol. 2016; 37(12):2363–9.
15. Nakamoto BK, Jahanshad N, McMurtray A, Kallianpur KJ, Chow DC, Valcour VG, Paul RH, Marotz L, Thompson PM, Shikuma CM. Cerebrovascular risk factors and brain microstructural abnormalities on diffusion tensor images in HIV-infected individuals. J Neuro-Oncol. 2012;18(4):303–12.
16. Song SK, Sun SW, Ramsbottom MJ, Chang C, Russell J, Cross AH. Dysmyelination revealed through MRI as increased radial diffusion of water. NeuroImage. 2002;17(3):1429–36.
17. Hoare J, Fouche JP, Phillips N, Joska JA, Donald KA, Thomas K, Stein DJ. Clinical associations of white matter damage in cART-treated HIV-positive children in South Africa. J Neuro-Oncol. 2015;21(2):120–8.
18. Zhuang Y, Qiu X, Wang L, Ma Q, Mapstone M, Luque A, Weber M, Tivarus M, Miller E, Arduino RC, et al. Combination antiretroviral therapy improves cognitive performance and functional connectivity in treatment- naïve HIV-infected individuals. J Neuro-Oncol. 2017;23(5):704–12.
19. Cysique LA, Soares JR, Geng G, Scarpetta M, Moffat K, Green M, Brew BJ, Henry RG, Rae C. White matter measures are near normal in controlled HIV infection except in those withcognitive impairment and longer HIV duration. J Neuro-Oncol. 2017;23(4):539–47.
20. Liu H, Xu E, Liu J, Xiong H. Oligodendrocyte injury and pathogenesis of HIV-1-associated neurocognitive disorders. Brain Sci. 2016;6(3):E23.
21. Xuan A, Wang GB, Shi DP, Xu JL, Li YL. Initial study of magnetic resonance diffusion tensor imaging in brain white matter of early aids patients. Chin Med J. 2013;126(14):2720–4.
22. Heaps-Woodruff JM, Wright PW, Ances BM, Clifford D, Paul RH. The impact of human immune deficiency virus and hepatitis C coinfection on white matter microstructural integrity. J Neuro-Oncol. 2016;22(3):389–99.
23. Wright PW, Vaida FF, Fernández RJ, Rutlin J, Price RW, Lee E, Peterson J, Fuchs D, Shimony JS, Robertson KR, et al. Cerebral white matter integrity during primary HIV infection. AIDS. 2015;29(4):433–42.
24. Cohen RA, Harezlak J, Schifitto G, Hana G, Clark U, Gongvatana A, Paul R, Taylor M, Thompson P, Alger J, et al. Effects of nadir CD4 count and duration of HIV infection on brain volumes in the HAART era. J Neuro-Oncol. 2010;16(1):25–32.
25. Seider TR, Gongvatana A, Woods AJ, Chen H, Porges EC, Cummings T, Correia S, Tashima K, Cohen RA. Age exacerbates HIV-associated white matter abnormalities. J Neuro-Oncol. 2016;22(2):201–12.
26. Gandhi NS, Skolasky RL, Peters KB, Moxley RT 4th, Creighton J, Roosa HV, Selnes OA, McArthur J, Sacktor N. A comparison of performance-based measures of function in HIV-associated neurocognitive disorders. J Neuro-Oncol. 2011;17(2):159–65.
27. Carey CL, Woods SP, Gonzalez R, Conover E, Marcotte TD, Grant I, Heaton RK, HNRC Group. Predictive validity of global deficit scores in detecting neuropsychological impairment in HIV infection. J Clin Exp Neuropsychol. 2004;26(3):307–19.
28. Jenkinson M, Beckmann CF, Behrens TE, Woolrich MW, Smith SM. FSL. NeuroImage. 2012;62(2):782–90.
29. Li R, Tang Z, Mi H, Zhao J, Yuan D, Li H. Diffusion tensor imaging study of early white matter integrity in HIV-infected patients: a tract-based spatial statistics analysis. Radiology of Infectious Diseases. 2015; 2(4):183–91.
30. Winkler AM, Ridgway GR, Webster MA, Smith SM, Nichols TE. Permutation inference for the general linear model. NeuroImage. 2014;92:381–97.
31. Smith SM, Nichols TE. Threshold-free cluster enhancement: addressing problems of smoothing, threshold dependence and localisation in cluster inference. NeuroImage. 2009;44(1):83–98.
32. Peluso MJ, Meyerhoff DJ, Price RW, Peterson J, Lee E, Young AC, Walter R, Fuchs D, Brew BJ, Cinque P, et al. Cerebrospinal fluid and neuroimaging biomarker abnormalities suggest early neurological injury in a subset of individuals during primary HIV infection. J Infect Dis. 2013;207(11):1703–12.
33. Ragin AB, Wu Y, Gao Y, Keating S, Du H, Sammet C, Kettering CS, Epstein LG. Brain alterations within the first 100 days of HIV infection. Ann Clin

Transl Neurol. 2015;2(1):12–21.

34. Valcour V, Chalermchai T, Sailasuta N, Marovich M, Lerdlum S, Suttichom D, Suwanwela NC, Jagodzinski L, Michael N, Spudich S, et al. Central viral invasion and inflammation during acute HIV infection. J Infect Dis. 2012; 206(2):275–82.

35. Shiramizu B, Gartner S, Williams A, Shikuma C, Ratto-Kim S, Watters M, Aguon J, Valcour V. Circulating proviral HIV DNA and HIV-associated dementia. AIDS. 2005;19(1):45–52.

36. Sun SW, Liang HF, Trinkaus K, Cross AH, Armstrong RC, Song SK. Noninvasive detection of cuprizone induced axonal damage and demyelination in the mouse corpus callosum. Magn Reson Med. 2006; 55(2):302–8.

37. MacDonald CL, Dikranian K, Bayly P, Holtzman D, Brody D. Diffusion tensor imaging reliably detects experimental traumatic axonal injury and indicates approximate time of injury. J Neurosci. 2007;27(44):11869–76.

38. Li J, Wu G, Wen Z, Zhang J, Lei H, Gui X, Lin F. White matter development is potentially influenced in adolescents with vertically transmitted HIV infections: a tract-based spatial statistics study. AJNR Am J Neuroradiol. 2015;36(11):2163–9.

39. Pfefferbaum A, Rosenbloom MJ, Rohlfing T, Kemper CA, Deresinski S, Sullivan EV. Frontostriatal fiber bundle compromise in HIV infection without dementia. AIDS. 2009;23(15):1977–85.

40. Corrêa DG, Zimmermann N, Doring TM, Wilner NV, Leite SC, Cabral RF, Fonseca RP, Bahia PR, Gasparetto EL. Diffusion tensor MR imaging of white matter integrity in HIV-positive patients with planning deficit. Neuroradiology. 2015;57(5):475–82.

41. O'Connor EE, Jaillard A, Renard F, Zeffiro TA. Reliability of white matter microstructural changes in HIV infection: meta-analysis and confirmation. AJNR Am J Neuroradiol. 2017;38(8):1510–9.

42. Ances BM, Roc AC, Korczykowski M, Wolf RL, Kolson DL. Combination antiretroviral therapy modulates the blood oxygen level-dependent aplitude in human immunodeficiency virus-seropositive patients. J Neuro-Oncol. 2008;14(5):418–24.

43. Sainz T, Serrano-Villar S, Diaz L, González Tomé MI, Gurbindo MD, de José MI, Mellado MJ, Ramos JT, Zamora J, Moreno S, et al. The CD4/CD8 ratio as a marker T-cell activation, senescence and activation/exhaustion in treated HIV-infected children and young adults. AIDS. 2013;27(9):1513–6.

44. Gongvatana A, Schweinsburg BC, Taylor MJ, Theilmann RJ, Letendre SL, Alhassoon OM, Jacobus J, Woods SP, Jernigan TL, Ellis RJ, et al. White matter tract injury and cognitive impairment in human immunodeficiency virusinfected individuals. J Neuro-Oncol. 2009;15(2):187–95.

45. Stubbe-Drger B, Deppe M, Mohammadi S, Keller SS, Kugel H, Gregor N, Evers S, Young P, Ringelstein EB, Arendt G, et al. Early microstructural white matter changes in patients with HIV: a diffusion tensor imaging study. BMC Neurol. 2012;12:23.

46. Nir TM, Jahanshad N, Busovaca E, Wendelken L, Nicolas K, Thompson PM, Valcour VG. Mapping white matter integrity in elderly people with HIV. Hum Brain Mapp. 2014;35(3):975–92.

47. Schmahmann JD, Smith EE, Eichler FS, Filley CM. Cerebral white matter: neuroanatomy, clinical neurology, and neurobehavioral correlates. Ann N Y Acad Sci. 2008;1142:266–309.

18

Dyke-Davidoff-Masson syndrome

Anna Misyail Abdul Rashid[1] and Mohamad Syafeeq Faeez Md Noh[2*] ⓘ

Abstract

Background: Dyke-Davidoff-Masson syndrome is a rare condition of unknown frequency resulting from brain injury due to a multitude of causes; especially in early life. Characteristics include cerebral hemiatrophy/hypoplasia, contralateral hemiparesis, seizures, and compensatory osseous hypertrophy.

Case presentation: We present a case of a 13-year-old girl who initially presented with headaches, followed by episodic complex-partial seizures; which was controlled via medication. She also had right sided hemiparesis. Computed tomography (CT) showed evidence of left parieto-temporal infarct with cerebral atrophy. Complementary magnetic resonance imaging (MRI) did not reveal additional information. Workup for young stroke was negative. Upon further evaluation by Neuroradiology, features suggesting Dyke-Davidoff-Masson syndrome were confirmed. Patient has been under Neurology follow up since.

Conclusions: Due to its rarity, Dyke-Davidoff-Masson syndrome may easily be missed by the majority of treating clinicians. Knowledge of its features on imaging enables timely and accurate diagnosis – allowing appropriate management.

Keywords: Dyke-Davidoff-Masson syndrome, Computed tomography (CT), Magnetic resonance imaging (MRI)

Background

Dyke-Davidoff-Masson syndrome (DDMS) is a rare neurological condition of unknown frequency, with available literature mostly from case reports/series [1–3]. Most affected patients are among the pediatric population. Due to its rarity, it may be misdiagnosed or under-reported by the majority of clinicians. We describe a patient who was initially thought to have young stroke of unknown etiology; eventually diagnosed having DDMS via imaging findings.

Case presentation

A 13-year-old girl presented to us for further management of episodic complex-partial seizures and right hemiparesis. She initially had episodes of headaches starting at the age of 7. Mother noticed that she had accompanying right sided weakness; which prompted medical attention. Initial evaluation revealed power of 4/5 on the right side, with reduced sensation and brisk reflexes. Minimal facial asymmetry was evident.

* Correspondence: msf.mdnoh@gmail.com
[2]Department of Imaging, Faculty of Medicine and Health Sciences, Universiti Putra Malaysia, Serdang, Malaysia
Full list of author information is available at the end of the article

A head CT was done, which revealed left parieto-temporal infarct, with cerebral atrophy. Complementary MRI was of no significant additional value. Workup for young stroke, which included protein S, protein C, anti-thrombin III, anti-phospholipid antibody, anti-cardiolipin antibody, and lupus anticoagulant were negative; she was subsequently put on routine follow up. One year after the initial presentation, her mother noticed new onset of brief moments of the child mumbling followed by blank stare and drowsiness, prior regaining consciousness. She was diagnosed as having complex-partial seizures, and initiated on syrup sodium valproate 200 mg bd. Upon further evaluation of the previous imaging studies, in addition to the left sided infarct, we noticed that the left cerebral hemisphere was universally atrophic with ventricular enlargement. There was also evidence of calvarial thickening on the ipsilateral side, and hyperpneumatization of the left frontal sinus (Fig. 1). A final diagnosis of DDMS was made. Patient has been on regular Neurology follow up since.

Discussion and conclusions

In 1933, Dyke, Davidoff, and Masson described 9 patients with clinical characteristics of hemiparesis, facial

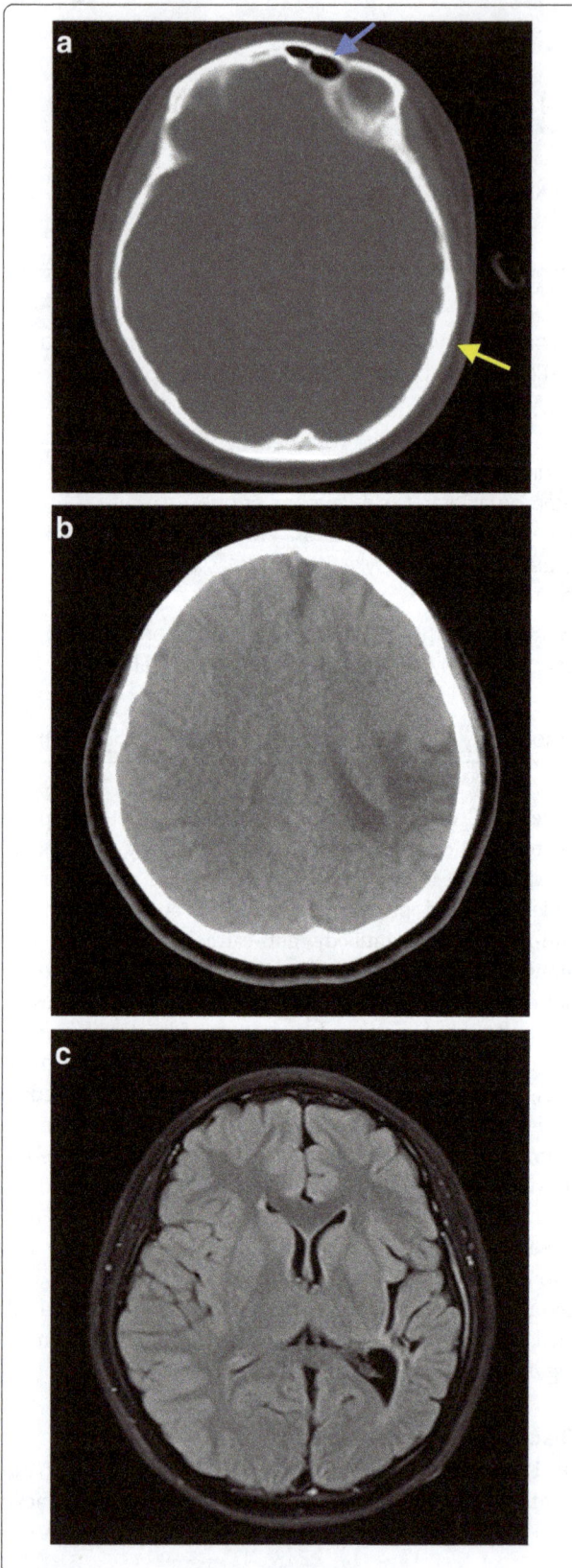

Fig. 1 CT (**a**, **b**) and MRI (**c**) images, in axial section showing. **a** CT image in bone window showing hyperpneumatization of the left frontal sinus (blue arrow) with compensatory calvarial thickening (yellow arrow). **b** CT image (non-contrasted) showing the left parieto-temporal infarct. **c** MRI T2 FLAIR image showing left cerebral hemiatrophy, with dilated left lateral ventricle. Focal encephalomalacia and gliotic changes are also noted

asymmetry, seizures, and mental retardation noted to have pneumatoencephalographic changes on skull radiograph [4]. CT and MRI features of this entity include cerebral hemiatrophy, ipsilateral ventriculomegaly, hyperpneumatization of the sinuses on the affected side, and compensatory calvarial thickening [1, 3, 5]. Affected patients are largely from the paediatric population; however, occurrence in adult patients have been reported [3]. Common causes include congenital anomalies, perinatal hypoxia, intracranial hemorrhage, and infections [1].

Clinically, patients may have seizures, mental retardation, contralateral hemiparesis, and facial asymmetry. Our patient initially had headaches, followed by episodic complex-partial seizures. Birth history did not reveal any hypoxic-ischemic events. There was also no history to suggest intra-uterine/perinatal infection. Only after head CT, an infarct was diagnosed; and patient was treated symptomatically. The MRI that followed did not add any additional information. To the unaccustomed, subtle findings on CT/MRI may easily be missed. We were able to accurately diagnose the imaging features after consulting with Neuroradiology. Understandably, the rarity of this condition makes accurate diagnosis a challenge – as evident in our experience.

Imaging via CT and MRI proves to be of significant value; enabling correct diagnosis and institution of appropriate management. These two imaging modalities are valuable in that they provide cross sectional images, with thin slices, and post processing capabilities. Pertinent imaging features for DDMS include cerebral hemiatrophy/hypoplasia, hyperpneumatization of the paranasal sinuses, and compensatory osseous hypertrophy. These radiological features will become more evident with time, as the patient gets older. There have been reports suggesting calvarial involvement, as in our experience, points to cerebral damage occurring during the intrauterine period or before the age of 3 [6–8]. Our patient, interestingly, did not have the clinical history or features to suggest an early life event which may lead to cerebral damage.

In essence, due to the rarity of this syndrome, it may be easily misdiagnosed by the untrained eye. CT and MRI are powerful imaging modalities to diagnose the pertinent imaging features associated with this syndrome. Knowledge of the clinical presentation, risk factors, and imaging features is therefore indispensable for appropriate patient management.

Abbreviations
CT: Computed tomography; DDMS: Dyke-Davidoff-Masson syndrome;
MRI: Magnetic resonance imaging

Authors' contributions
MSF drafted the manuscript and was responsible for overall content, images, and literature review. AM examined the patient and obtained the clinical history. Both authors read and approved the manuscript for publication.

Competing interests
The authors declare that they have no competing interests.

Author details
[1]Department of Medicine, Faculty of Medicine and Health Sciences, Universiti Putra Malaysia, Serdang, Malaysia. [2]Department of Imaging, Faculty of Medicine and Health Sciences, Universiti Putra Malaysia, Serdang, Malaysia.

References
1. Verma R, Sahu R. Dyke-Davidoff-Masson syndrome. BMJ Case Reports. 2012. https://doi.org/10.1136/bcr-2012-006729.
2. Piro E, Piccione M, Marrone G, Giuffre M, Corsello G. Dyke-Davidoff-Masson syndrome: case report of fetal unilateral ventriculomegaly and hypoplastic left middle cerebral artery. Ital J Pediatr. 2013;39:32.
3. Roy U, Panwar A, Mukherjee A, Biswas D. Adult presentation of dyke-Davidoff-Masson syndrome: a case report. Case Rep Neurol. 2016;8:20–6.
4. Dyke CG, Davidoff LM, Masson CB. Cerebral hemiatrophy and homolateral hypertrophy of the skull and sinuses. Surg Gynecol Obstet. 1933;57:588–600.
5. Gokce E, Beyhan M, Sade R. Radiological imaging findings of dyke-Davidoff-Masson syndrome. Acta Neurol Belg. 2017;117(4):885–93.
6. Arora R, Rani JY. Dyke-Davidoff-Masson syndrome: imaging features with illustration of two cases. Quant Imaging Med Surg. 2015;5(3):469–71.
7. Atalar MH, Icagasioglu D, Tas F. Cerebral hemiatrophy (dyke-Davidoff-Masson syndrome) in childhood: clinicoradiological analysis of 19 cases. Pediatr Int. 2007;49(1):70–5.
8. Uduma FU, Emejulu JK, Motah M, Okere PC, Ongolo PC, Muna W. Differential diagnoses of cerebral hemiatrophy in childhood: a review of literature with illustrative report of two cases. Glob J Health Sci. 2013;5(3):195–207.

19

Prucalopride inhibits the glioma cells proliferation and induces autophagy via AKT-mTOR pathway

Hong Qiao[1], Yong-Bo Wang[2], Yu-Mei Gao[2] and Li-Li Bi[3*]

Abstract

Backgrounds: Glioma is the most fatal primary brain glioma in central nervous system mainly attributed to its high invasion. Prucalopride, a Serotonin-4 (5-HT4) receptor agonist, has been reported to regulate neurodevelopment. This study aimed to investigate the influence of the Prucalopride on glioma cells and unveil underlying mechanism.

Methods: In this study, glioma cells proliferation was evaluated by Cell counting kit-8 (CCK8). Wound healing and transwell assay were used to test cellular migration and invasion. Flow cytometry was utilized to determine cellular apoptosis rate. Apoptosis related markers, autophagy markers, and protein kinase B (AKT)-mammalian target of rapamycin (mTOR) pathway key molecules were detected using western blot assay.

Results: As a result, the proliferation, migration and invasiveness of glioma cells were impaired by Prucalopride treatment, the apoptosis rate of glioma cells was enhanced by Prucalopride stimulation, accompanied by the increased pro-apoptosis proteins Bax and Cleaved caspase-3 and decreased anti-apoptosis protein Bcl-2. Prucalopride significantly promoted autophagy by increased expression level of Beclin 1 and LC3-II, while decreased expression level of p62. Prucalopride administration resulted in obvious inhibitions of key molecules of AKT-mTOR pathway, including phosphorylated- (p-) AKT, p-mTOR and phosphorylated-ribosomal p70S6 kinase (p-P70S6K).

Conclusions: Taking together, these results indicate that Prucalopride may be likely to play an anti-tumor role in glioma cells, which suggests potential implications for glioma promising therapy alternation in the further clinics.

Keywords: Prucalopride, Glioma, Proliferation, Autophagy, AKT-mTOR pathway

Background

Glioma is known as the most frequently malignant primary brain tumor in humans, with annual incidence about 5 out of 100,000 persons [1, 2]. In spite of current progressive therapeutics for glioma, patients eventually yield this disease, seen from the poor overall survival of about 12–15 months [3]. Vigorous proliferation and uncontrollable invasion have been the barriers for clearing out glioma, and therapeutic options for which are groping, but most of these are limited. Accordingly, more efficient treatment strategies directing toward glioma have remained urgent presently.

Previous studies have suggested that the Serotonin (5-Hydroxytryptamine, 5-HT)-4 (5-HT$_4$) receptor is richly distributed in the brain [4–6]. 5-HT$_4$ receptors are identified as neurogenerative and neuroprotective actions, which are vital to maintenance of a normal enteric nervous system [6–8]. It is well known that activity of 5-HT$_4$ receptors facilitates neurogenesis of injured enteric neuron and neural stem cells in the anastomotic ileum [9, 10]. Another study has documented that the 5-HT$_4$ receptor represses the formation of neurites in neurons and relates with regulation of neural development [11, 12]. Activation of 5-HT$_4$ receptors is demonstrated to improve memory performances [13]. Importantly, serotonin is reported to modulate some of cancer, namely placenta and choriocarcinoma cells [14], breast cancer cell [15], human prostate cancer tissue and cell [16]. Another report has demonstrated that a selective 5-HT$_4$ receptor

* Correspondence: bi4533@126.com
[3]Department of Medical Instruments, Second Affiliated Hospital of Mudanjiang Medical University, Mudanjiang, Heilongjiang 157009, People's Republic of China
Full list of author information is available at the end of the article

agonist, mosapride citrate inhibits the proliferative activity of human umbilical vein endothelial cells [17]. However, little is known about the effect of 5-HT4 receptor on glioma.

Prucalopride, a first-in-class dihydrobenzofuran-carboxamide derivative, is a highly selective, potent, and specific serotonin 5-HT$_4$ receptor agonist with enterokinetic properties [18]. It is initially applied to treat constipation and other gastrointestinal disorders [19]. It is reported to exert a neuroprotection role in human neuroblastoma [20]. Prucalopride has been documented to associate with cholinergic neurotransmission [21]. Prucalopride is found to play a positively promotive function in stimulating Dopamine release which relieves depression or anxiety disorder [22]. Johnson et al. determined that Prucalopride increased acetylcholine level in prefrontal cortex [23]. In all, above observations indicates that Prucalopride regulates neurodevelopment. Nonetheless, it remains unclear whether and how Prucalopride is involved in the regulation of cell proliferation, metastasis and apoptosis in glioma cells.

Hence, the present study aimed to investigate the functional actions of Prucalopride on the proliferation, migration and apoptosis of human glioma cells as well as explore the possible mechanism underlying the anti-tumor effects of Prucalopride on glioma cells. Herein, the results of this study suggested that Prucalopride inhibited glioma cells proliferation and migration as well as induced apoptosis and autophagy, which was probably modulated by suppression of protein kinase B (AKT)- mammalian target of rapamycin (mTOR) signaling. These findings obtained from our investigations implicate that Prucalopride may be a potential therapeutic drug for the treatment of glioma.

Methods

Cell culture

Glioma U251 cell line was obtained from the Shanghai Institute for Life Science, Chinese Academy of Sciences (Shanghai, China). Glioma U87 cell line and normal human astrocyte SVG p12 were purchased from American Type Culture Collection (Manassas, VA, USA). Cells were cultured in RPMI-1640 medium supplemented with 10% fetal bovine serum (FBS), 100 U/ml penicillin and 100 µg/ml streptomycin (Invitrogen, Thermo Scientific, Waltham, MA, USA) at 37 °C under a humidified atmosphere of 5% CO_2.

Cell counting kit-8 (CCK-8) assay

Growth of the cell lines was evaluated using a CCK-8 (Beyotime Institute of Biotechnology, Shanghai, China) assay according to the manufacturer's protocol. Cells (10^3 cells/well) were seeded into 96-well plates and cultured for 24 h. Then, cells were incubated with different concentrations of Prucalopride (0, 0.1, 1, 10, 20, 50, 100 µM) and cultured for an additionally 72 h. For

CCK-8 detection, 10 µl of CCK-8 solution was added into the wells and the cells were incubated at 37 °C for 1.5 h. The absorbance (optical density, OD) of cells was determined at 450 nm using a microplate reader (Bio-Rad, Hercules, CA, USA). The following experiment drug concentration (10 µM) was chosen from the series of the gradient concentration. Afterward, cells were incubated with Prucalopride (10 µM) and vehicle (DMSO, 0.1% in culture media) for 24, 48 and 72 h. Cells viabilities were measured by CCK-8 assay and OD values were measured as above described.

Migration and invasion assays

After Prucalopride treatments for 48 h, cell capabilities of invasion and migration were examined by 24-well transwell chamber with or without Matrigel matrix (BD Bioscience, San Jose, CA, USA) following the instructions of the manufacturer. To evaluate cell migration, U251 cells (1 × 10^5/ml) in 100 µl serum-free media were plated into top chamber of transwell migration chamber and 500 µl medium containing with 10% FBS was added into the lower chambers. Following incubation at 37 °C for 24 h, the filter was gently removed from the chamber and the remaining cells on the upper surface of the filter were wiped off with a cotton-tipped swab. The cells that had migrated on the lower surface of the filter were fixed with 4% paraformaldehyde for 10 min and stained with 0.5% crystal violet for 15 min. The number of migrated cells was counted from five random fields (× 200) under a microscope (Olympus, Tokyo, Japan). For invasion assay, transwell chamber was covered with Matrigel before a procedure similar to that for the migration assay was performed.

Flow cytometry evaluation of apoptosis

To examine apoptosis, cells were double-stained with an Annexin V-Fluorescein isothiocyanate (FITC)/propidium iodide (PI) Apoptosis Detection kit (Beyotime Institute of Biotechnology) according to the manufacturer's protocol. After Prucalopride treatments for 48 h, the cells were harvested, washed with cold phosphate-buffered saline (PBS), resuspended with binding buffer. Then cells were incubated with 5 µl Annexin-V-FITC reagent under room temperature for 5 min and were stained by PI reagent. The percentages of apoptosis cells were then analyzed by FACS Calibur flow cytofluorometry (BD Biosciences, San Jose, CA, USA) for the early apoptotic (Annexin V$^+$ and PI$^-$) and late apoptotic (Annexin V$^+$ and PI$^+$) cells. The apoptotic rate was determined using CellQuest software (BD Biosciences).

Western blot analysis

After Prucalopride treatments for 48 h, cells proteins were extracted with radioimmunoprecipitation assay

(RIPA) lysis buffer (Beyotime Institute of Biotechnology) and proteins concentrations were tested by a Bicinchoninic acid (BCA) protein assay (Beyotime Institute of Biotechnology). Following, equal amounts of protein were separated by 10% sodium dodecyl sulfate polyacrylamide gel electrophoresis (SDS-PAGE), and were transferred onto poly vinylidene difluoride (PVDF) membranes, then were blocked with 5% non-fat milk in Tris-buffered saline buffer with Tween-20. Afterwards, the PVDF membranes were incubated with primary antibody against LC3 (dilution 1:1, 000), Beclin-1 (dilution 1:1, 000), p62 (dilution 1:1, 000), AKT (dilution 1:1, 000), mTOR (dilution 1:1, 000), phosphorylated- (p-) AKT (dilution 1:1, 000), p-mTOR (dilution 1:1, 000) and phosphorylated-ribosomal p70S6 kinase (p-P70S6K) (dilution 1:1, 000) (Cell Signaling Technology, Inc., Danvers, MA, USA), GAPDH (Beyotime, dilution 1: 1000) and following with horseradish peroxidase-conjugated secondary antibodies (dilution 1:5, 000, Cell Signaling Technology, Inc.). Finally, proteins were visualized by enhanced chemiluminescence (ECL) kit (Millipore, Boston, MA, USA) and protein bands were measured with Image J software (National Institutes of Health (NIH), Stapleton, NY, USA).

Statistical analysis

All data were expressed as means ± standard deviation (SD). Differences between the control and experimental results were tested by Student's t-test (two-tailed) and one-way analysis of variance (ANOVA). A difference was considered statistically significant when the P value was deemed < 0.05 (*) or < 0.01 (**). All statistical analyses were carried out by SPSS version 22.0 (SPSS Inc., Chicago, IL, USA). All assays were performed three times.

Results

Prucalopride inhibited glioma cells growth

To investigate the effect of Prucalopride on the proliferation of glioma cells, CCK-8 was conducted. A dose response in proliferation was observed as a decrease in U251 cells from 0.1 to 100 μM of Prucalopride, while the viability of SVG p12 cells was inhibited by Prucalopride beyond 50 μM (Fig. 1a). Consequently, 10 μM of Prucalopride was selected to perform following experiments. The IC_{50} value was 9.942 ± 0.346 μM. In addition, U251 and U87 cells proliferation was assessed by measuring the OD values at increasing time-points. As shown in Fig. 1b, OD values of U251 and U87 cells were significantly reduced as compared to untreated cells in a temporal manner. These results suggested that Prucalopride impeded growth of glioma cells.

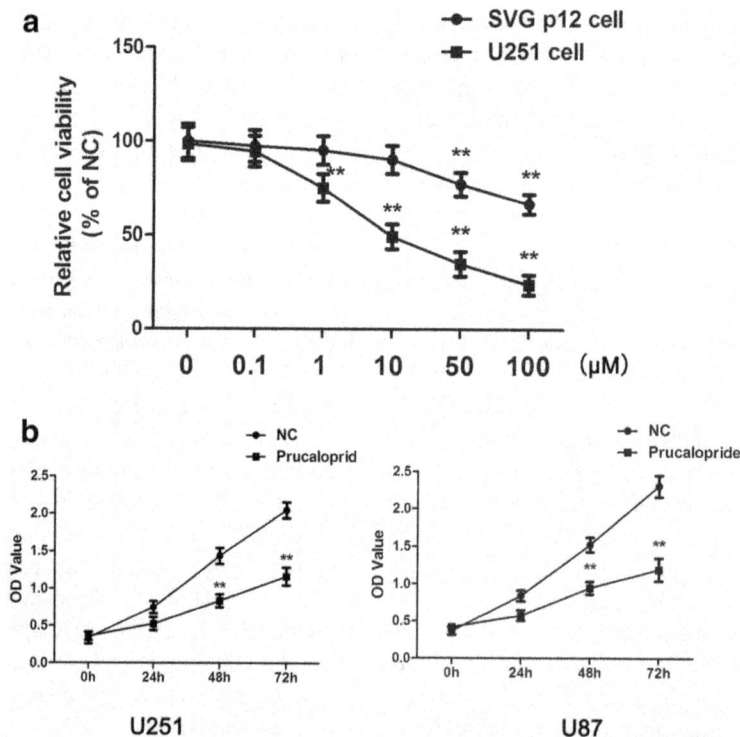

Fig. 1 The suppressive effect of Prucalopride on glioma cells proliferation. **a** The viabilities of U251 and SVG p21 cells treated by Prucalopride with 0, 0.1, 1. 10, 50, 100 μM. **$P < 0.01$ versus control group (0 μM Prucalopride group). **b** The OD values of U251 and U87 cells treated by Prucalopride with 10 μM (the following experiments were performed according to the concentration) after 0, 24, 48 and 72 h. The data are presented as the means ± SD, **$P < 0.01$ versus NC group. Each assay was conducted in triplicate

Prucalopride reduced glioma cells invasion and migration

To examine the function of Prucalopride on glioma cells invasion and migration, transwell migration and invasion assays were performed. As shown in Fig. 2, the number of migrated cells was markedly decreased in Prucalopride group (32 ± 2) compared with NC group (85 ± 4) ($P < 0.05$). Similarly, the number of invaded cells was significantly suppressed in Prucalopride group (18 ± 5), as compared with NC group (34 ± 2) ($P < 0.05$). These data showed that the capabilities of glioma cells migration and invasion were inhibited by Prucalopride.

Autophagy was induced by Prucaloprid

To explore whether Prucaloprid affected autophagy in glioma cells, the classical autophagic markers, including Beclin-1, LC3- I/II and p62 were analyzed by western blot. Consistent with our predictions, Beclin-1 was observed to be upregulated while LC3-I/II and p62 was downregulated evidently (Fig. 3, $P < 0.05$), indicating that Prucaloprid promoted autophagy in glioma cells.

Prucaloprid induced glioma cells apoptosis

To define the role of Prucalopride on glioma cells apoptosis, flow cytometry assay and western blot assay were carried out. As showed in Fig. 4a, the apoptosis rates of U251 and U87 cells in Prucalopride group was increased significantly in comparison with NC group ($P < 0.05$). Molecularly, we further examined the apoptosis related markers, namely Bcl-2, Bax and Cleaved caspase-3 using the western blot assay. The levels of anti-apoptosis protein Bcl-2 was obviously downregulated while pro-apoptosis proteins Bax and Cleaved caspase-3 were markedly upregulated in Prucalopride group compared with NC group (Fig. 4b, $P < 0.05$). Above of these results suggested that Prucalopride induced apoptosis of glioma cells.

AKT/mTOR activity was influenced by Prucaloprid

To gain insight into the molecular mechanism by which Prucalopride regulated glioma cell proliferation and migration, we thus tested the effect of Prucalopride on the activation of AKT/mTOR signaling pathway in U251

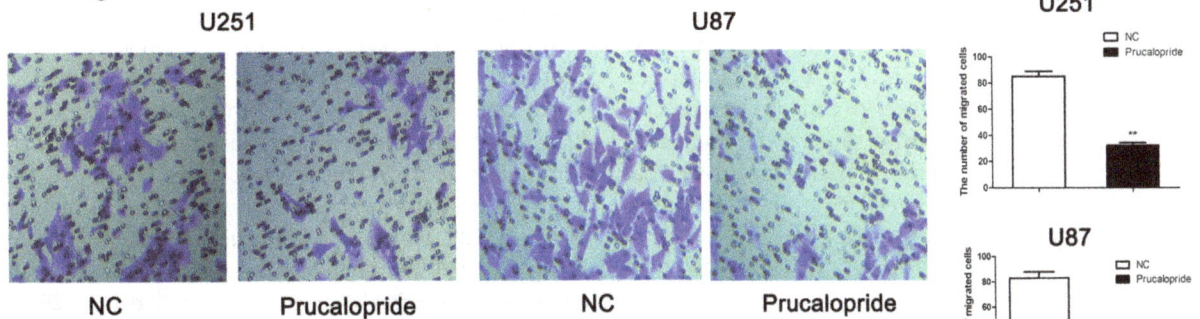

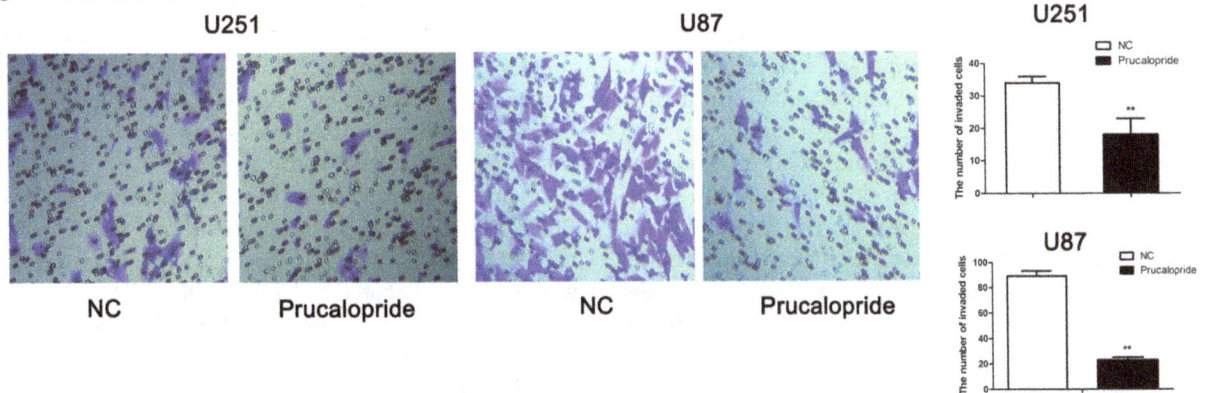

Fig. 2 The capabilities of glioma cells migration and invasion were inhibited by Prucalopride. **a** The number of migrated cells was counted under a microscope (×200) and quantitative analysis was shown in the right. **b** The number of invaded cells was counted under a microscope (×200) and quantitative analysis was shown in the right. The data are presented as the means ± SD, $^{**}P < 0.01$ versus NC group. Each assay was conducted in triplicate

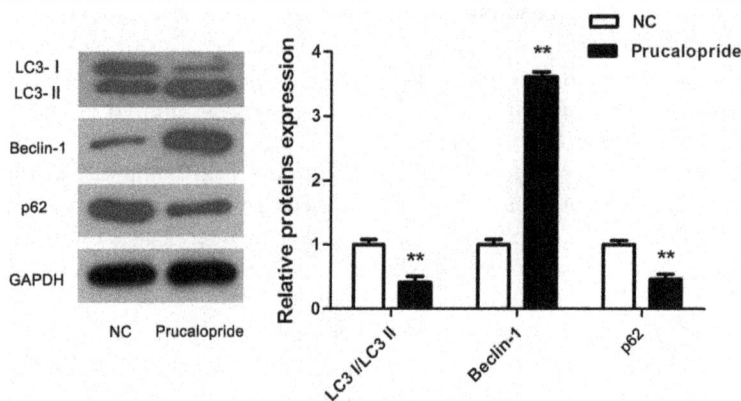

Fig. 3 Induced effect of Prucalopride on glioma cells autophagy. Classic markers of autophagy were tested using western blot assay. The data are presented as the means ± SD, $^{**}P < 0.01$ versus NC group. Each assay was conducted in triplicate

cells using western blot assay. To rule out the effect of Prucalopride dose on AKT/mTOR signaling pathway, 0.1 μM concentration was selected as the comparison of dose impact. As shown in Fig. 5, the levels of p-AKT and p-mTOR were decreased while total of AKT and mTOR were no detectable changes in 10 μM Prucalopride group on comparing the NC and 0.1 μM Prucalopride groups ($P < 0.05$, $P > 0.05$ respectively). Moreover, the p-P70S6K level was downregulated in Prucalopride group compared with NC and 0.1 μM Prucalopride groups ($P < 0.05$). Whereas levels of proteins in Prucalopride groups were no significant differences compared with those in NC group. These data suggested that AKT/mTOR signaling may involve in the anti-tumor effect of Prucalopride in glioma cells.

Discussion

In the current study, we demonstrated that Prucalopride played an inhibiting role in glioma cells proliferation, migration and invasion as well as a promoting effect in glioma cells apoptosis. In addition, autophagy was induced by Prucalopride treatment. Furthermore, the activity of AKT-mTOR signaling was suppressed by Prucalopride. Collectively, these data suggest Prucalopride might be a potential clinical application for glioma.

The regulation of tumor cell proliferation, migration, invasion and apoptosis by Prucalopride, a 5-HT$_4$ receptor agonist, has been investigated in this study. The OD values of glioma cells were decreased by administration of Prucalopride. The number of migrated and invaded glioma cells was reduced by Prucalopride treatment. Further, it was observed that apoptosis rate of glioma cells was increased after Prucalopride treatment, in support of this, the pro-apoptosis markers Cleaved caspase-3 and Bax were up-regulated while anti-apoptosis marker Bcl-2 was down-regulated by Prucalopride. A previous research by Takeshi et al.

demonstrated that another Selective 5-HT4 Receptor Agonist, mosapride citrate also exerted antiangiogenic and anti-proliferative effects of human umbilical vein endothelial cells [17]. Another study showed that 5-HT$_4$ receptor acted as a tumor suppressor role in ovarian carcinogenesis [24]. All in all, these evidence indicate that Prucalopride performs a potential anti-tumor role in glioma.

Autophagy is a highly conserved catabolic process that captures, degrades, and recycles damaged organelles, waste macro-molecules and other substances in cells [25, 26]. It is considered as a survival mechanism conventionally improves the survival of cells [27]. Autophagy can be activated in many types of cells, including gliomas [28]. However, paradoxically, it is increasingly being applied to facilitate cancer cell death, called autophagic or type II programmed cell death [29, 30]. To explore whether autophagy mediates anti-tumor action of Prucalopride in glioma, in this study, markers of autophagy were examined. The results showed that and Beclin-1 was increased while LC3-I/II and p62 were decreased by Prucalopride administration. Our investigations, in combination with previous studies, suggest that autophagy is induced by Prucalopride in glioma, implying a significant role of autophagy involved in tumor-inhibitory role by Prucalopride.

To gain some insight into the molecular mechanisms of Prucalopride-mediated anti-cancer action in glioma cells, the AKT-mTOR signaling pathway was assessed. It is well-established that the AKT-mTOR signaling pathway plays a crucial role in the regulation of cell proliferation and cell survival in wide array of tumor cells, usually linked with oncogenesis, including gliomas [31–33]. PI3K phosphorylation and its product phosphorylated- phosphatidylinositol 3,4,5-triphosphate (p-I3-P) with AKT binding site, thus AKT is phosphorylated. The p-AKT activated mTOR phosphorylation, which is followed by

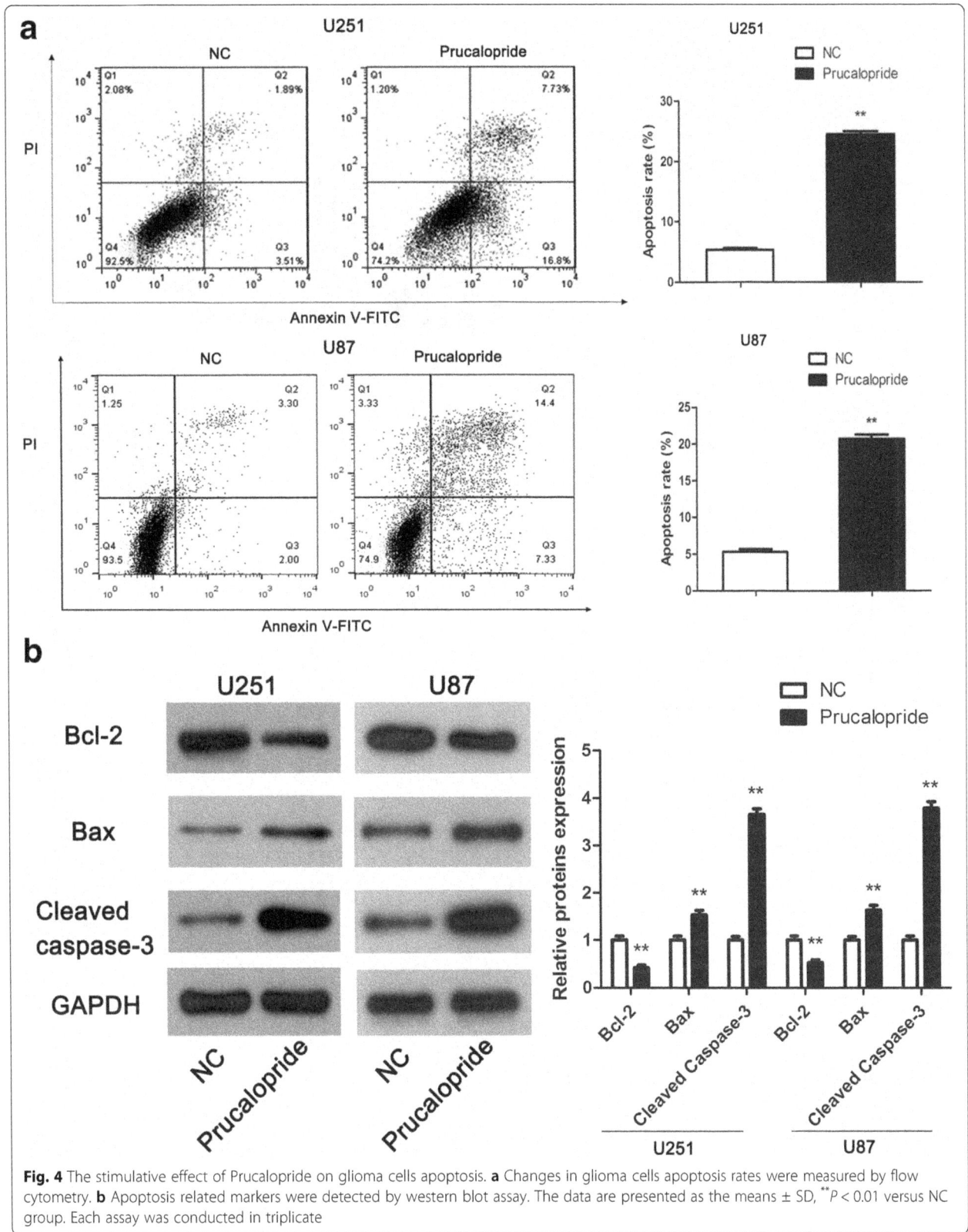

Fig. 4 The stimulative effect of Prucalopride on glioma cells apoptosis. **a** Changes in glioma cells apoptosis rates were measured by flow cytometry. **b** Apoptosis related markers were detected by western blot assay. The data are presented as the means ± SD, $^{**}P < 0.01$ versus NC group. Each assay was conducted in triplicate

the down-regulation of phosphorylated p70S6K, a major effector of mTOR in the downstream of the mTOR signaling pathway [34]. Down-regulation of phosphorylated p70S6K induces autophagy [35]. Thereby, the PI3K/AKT/mTOR/p-P70S6K has been known to be frequently implicated to modulate the initiation of autophagy [36–38]. It

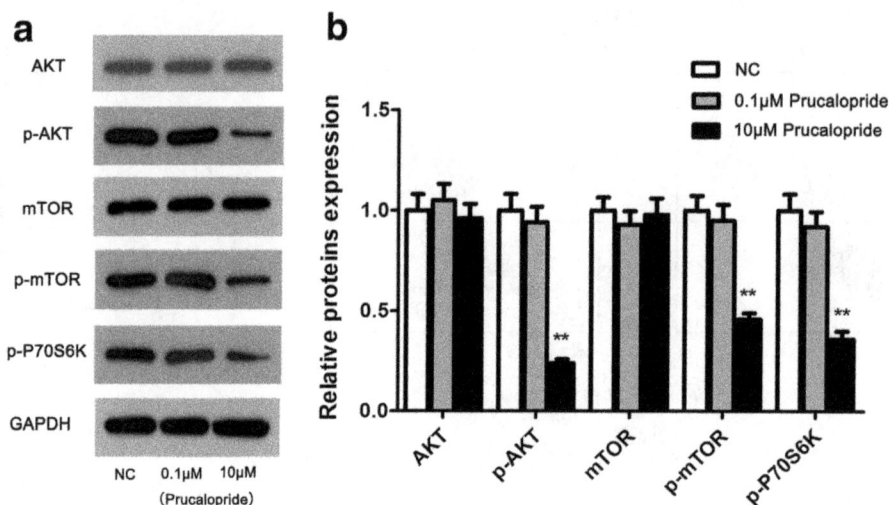

Fig. 5 Activity of AKT/mTOR signaling was suppressed by Prucalopride. **a** AKT/mTOR signaling key proteins were examined using western blot assay. **b** Densitometry analysis of proteins bands. The data are presented as the means ± SD, $^{**}P < 0.01$ versus NC group. Each assay was conducted in triplicate

was reported that autophagy mediated of suppressing glioma cells proliferation via involvement of this signaling [39]. Yu-Chen et al. revealed that autophagy formation was participated in the glioma cells growth inhibition through regulating this signaling [40]. Overall, above data demonstrated that the AKT-mTOR signaling was involved in the anti-tumor action of Prucalopride on glioma cells. In spite of this, limitations of the current work should be acknowledged that this study has examined merely U251 and U87 cells, further studies are needed to illuminate the molecular basis involved in this process through more cell lines and even animal model construction.

Conclusions

In conclusion, the findings of the present study suggested that Prucalopride exerted anti-proliferative, anti-migratory and anti-invasive effects in glioma cells, aside from this, it also developed an inductive action of autophagy occurrence on glioma cells. These effects were impelled by Prucalopride possibly via inhibiting AKT-mTOR signaling. This work indicates Prucalopride might function as a cancer suppressive agent for glioma, implying Prucalopride would be a promising candidate drug treatment for glioma in the further clinic.

Abbreviations
5-HT4: Serotonin-4; AKT: Protein kinase B; Annexin V-FITC/PI: Annexin V-Fluorescein isothiocyanate/propidium iodide; ANOVA: One-way analysis of variance; mTOR: Mammalian target of rapamycin; OD: Optical density; P70S6K: Ribosomal p70S6 kinase; SD: Standard deviation; SDS-PAGE: Sulfate polyacrylamide gel electrophoresis

Authors' contributions
LLB and HQ conceived and designed the study and wrote the article. HQ, YBW and YMG performed experiments and acquisition of data, analyzed the data and interpreted the data. All authors have read and approved the final manuscript.

Competing interests
The authors declare that they have no competing interests.

Author details
[1]Department of General Affairs Section, Second Affiliated Hospital of Mudanjiang Medical University, Mudanjiang, Heilongjiang 157009, People's Republic of China. [2]Department of Respiratory Medicine, Second Affiliated Hospital of Mudanjiang Medical University, Mudanjiang, Heilongjiang 157009, People's Republic of China. [3]Department of Medical Instruments, Second Affiliated Hospital of Mudanjiang Medical University, Mudanjiang, Heilongjiang 157009, People's Republic of China.

References
1. Wen PY, Kesari S. Malignant gliomas in adults. N Engl J Med. 2008;359(5): 492–507.
2. Omuro A, DeAngelis LM. Glioblastoma and other malignant gliomas: a clinical review. Jama. 2013;310(17):1842–50.
3. Clarke J, Penas C, Pastori C, Komotar RJ, Bregy A, Shah AH, Wahlestedt C, Ayad NG. Epigenetic pathways and glioblastoma treatment. Epigenetics. 2013;8(8):785–95.
4. Bockaert J, Claeysen S, Compan V, Dumuis A. 5-HT(4) receptors: history, molecular pharmacology and brain functions. Neuropharmacology. 2008; 55(6):922–31.
5. Licht CL, Marcussen AB, Wegener G, Overstreet DH, Aznar S, Knudsen GM. The brain 5-HT4 receptor binding is down-regulated in the flinders sensitive line depression model and in response to paroxetine administration. J Neurochem. 2009;109(5):1363–74.
6. Tesseur I, Pimenova AA, Lo AC, Ciesielska M, Lichtenthaler SF, De Maeyer JH, Schuurkes JA, D'Hooge R, De Strooper B. Chronic 5-HT4 receptor activation decreases Abeta production and deposition in hAPP/PS1 mice. Neurobiol Aging. 2013;34(7):1779–89.

7. Gershon MD. 5-HT4-mediated neuroprotection: a new therapeutic modality on the way? Am J Physiol Gastrointest Liver Physiol. 2016;310(10):G766–7.

8. Liu MT, Kuan YH, Wang J, Hen R, Gershon MD. 5-HT4 receptor-mediated neuroprotection and neurogenesis in the enteric nervous system of adult mice. J Neurosci. 2009;29(31):9683–99.

9. Takaki M, Goto K, Kawahara I, Nabekura J. Activation of 5-HT4 receptors facilitates neurogenesis of injured enteric neurons at an anastomosis in the lower gut. J Smooth Muscle Res. 2015;51:82–94.

10. Goto K, Kawahara I, Inada H, Misawa H, Kuniyasu H, Nabekura J, Takaki M. Activation of 5-HT4 receptors facilitates neurogenesis from transplanted neural stem cells in the anastomotic ileum. J Physiol Sci. 2016;66(1):67–76.

11. Kvachnina E, Liu G, Dityatev A, Renner U, Dumuis A, Richter DW, Dityateva G, Schachner M, Voyno-Yasenetskaya TA, Ponimaskin EG. 5-HT7 receptor is coupled to G alpha subunits of heterotrimeric G12-protein to regulate gene transcription and neuronal morphology. J Neurosci. 2005;25(34):7821–30.

12. Kozono N, Ohtani A, Shiga T. Roles of the serotonin 5-HT4 receptor in dendrite formation of the rat hippocampal neurons in vitro. Brain Res. 2017; 1655:114–21.

13. Quiedeville A, Boulouard M, Hamidouche K, Da Silva Costa-Aze V, Nee G, Rochais C, Dallemagne P, Fabis F, Freret T, Bouet V. Chronic activation of 5-HT4 receptors or blockade of 5-HT6 receptors improve memory performances. Behav Brain Res. 2015;293:10–7.

14. Sonier B, Lavigne C, Arseneault M, Ouellette R, Vaillancourt C. Expression of the 5-HT2A serotoninergic receptor in human placenta and choriocarcinoma cells: mitogenic implications of serotonin. Placenta. 2005; 26(5):484–90.

15. Sonier B, Arseneault M, Lavigne C, Ouellette RJ, Vaillancourt C. The 5-HT2A serotoninergic receptor is expressed in the MCF-7 human breast cancer cell line and reveals a mitogenic effect of serotonin. Biochem Biophys Res Commun. 2006;343(4):1053–9.

16. Dizeyi N, Bjartell A, Hedlund P, Tasken KA, Gadaleanu V, Abrahamsson PA. Expression of serotonin receptors 2B and 4 in human prostate cancer tissue and effects of their antagonists on prostate cancer cell lines. Eur Urol. 2005; 47(6):895–900.

17. Nishikawa T, Tsuno NH, Shuno Y, Sasaki K, Hongo K, Okaji Y, Sunami E, Kitayama J, Takahashi K, Nagawa H. Antiangiogenic effect of a selective 5-HT4 receptor agonist. J Surg Res. 2010;159(2):696–704.

18. Frampton JE. Prucalopride. Drugs. 2009;69(17):2463–76.

19. Quigley EM. Prucalopride: safety, efficacy and potential applications. Ther Adv Gastroenterol. 2012;5(1):23–30.

20. Bianco F, Bonora E, Natarajan D, Vargiolu M, Thapar N, Torresan F, Giancola F, Boschetti E, Volta U, Bazzoli F, et al. Prucalopride exerts neuroprotection in human enteric neurons. Am J Physiol Gastrointest Liver Physiol. 2016; 310(10):G768–75.

21. Priem E, Van Colen I, De Maeyer JH, Lefebvre RA. The facilitating effect of prucalopride on cholinergic neurotransmission in pig gastric circular muscle is regulated by phosphodiesterase 4. Neuropharmacology. 2012;62(5–6): 2126–35.

22. Navailles S, Di Giovanni G, De Deurwaerdere P. The 5-HT4 agonist prucalopride stimulates L-DOPA-induced dopamine release in restricted brain regions of the Hemiparkinsonian rat in vivo. CNS Neurosci Ther. 2015; 21(9):745–7.

23. Johnson DE, Drummond E, Grimwood S, Sawant-Basak A, Miller E, Tseng E, McDowell LL, Vanase-Frawley MA, Fisher KE, Rubitski DM, et al. The 5-hydroxytryptamine4 receptor agonists prucalopride and PRX-03140 increase acetylcholine and histamine levels in the rat prefrontal cortex and the power of stimulated hippocampal theta oscillations. J Pharmacol Exp Ther. 2012;341(3):681–91.

24. Henriksen R, Dizeyi N, Abrahamsson PA. Expression of serotonin receptors 5-HT1A, 5-HT1B, 5-HT2B and 5-HT4 in ovary and in ovarian tumours. Anticancer Res. 2012;32(4):1361–6.

25. Hoyer-Hansen M, Jaattela M. Autophagy: an emerging target for cancer therapy. Autophagy. 2008;4(5):574–80.

26. Levine B, Kroemer G. Autophagy in the pathogenesis of disease. Cell. 2008; 132(1):27–42.

27. Rabinowitz JD, White E. Autophagy and metabolism. Science (New York, NY). 2010;330(6009):1344–8.

28. Liu R, Li J, Zhang T, Zou L, Chen Y, Wang K, Lei Y, Yuan K, Li Y, Lan J, et al. Itraconazole suppresses the growth of glioblastoma through induction of autophagy: involvement of abnormal cholesterol trafficking. Autophagy. 2014;10(7):1241–55.

29. Ding L, Wang Q, Shen M, Sun Y, Zhang X, Huang C, Chen J, Li R, Duan Y. Thermoresponsive nanocomposite gel for local drug delivery to suppress the growth of glioma by inducing autophagy. Autophagy. 2017;13(7):1176–90.

30. Swart C, Du Toit A, Loos B. Autophagy and the invisible line between life and death. Eur J Cell Biol. 2016;95(12):598–610.

31. Borders EB, Bivona C, Medina PJ. Mammalian target of rapamycin: biological function and target for novel anticancer agents. Am J Health Syst Pharm. 2010;67(24):2095–106.

32. Yap TA, Garrett MD, Walton MI, Raynaud F, de Bono JS, Workman P. Targeting the PI3K-AKT-mTOR pathway: progress, pitfalls, and promises. Curr Opin Pharmacol. 2008;8(4):393–412.

33. Shen X, Kan S, Liu Z, Lu G, Zhang X, Chen Y, Bai Y. EVA1A inhibits GBM cell proliferation by inducing autophagy and apoptosis. Exp Cell Res. 2017; 352(1):130–8.

34. Heinonen H, Nieminen A, Saarela M, Kallioniemi A, Klefstrom J, Hautaniemi S, Monni O. Deciphering downstream gene targets of PI3K/mTOR/p70S6K pathway in breast cancer. BMC Genomics. 2008;9:348.

35. Shinojima N, Yokoyama T, Kondo Y, Kondo S. Roles of the Akt/mTOR/p70S6K and ERK1/2 signaling pathways in curcumin-induced autophagy. Autophagy. 2007;3(6):635–7.

36. Wu YT, Tan HL, Huang Q, Ong CN, Shen HM. Activation of the PI3K-Akt-mTOR signaling pathway promotes necrotic cell death via suppression of autophagy. Autophagy. 2009;5(6):824–34.

37. Vucicevic L, Misirkic M, Janjetovic K, Vilimanovich U, Sudar E, Isenovic E, Prica M, Harhaji-Trajkovic L, Kravic-Stevovic T, Bumbasirevic V, et al. Compound C induces protective autophagy in cancer cells through AMPK inhibition-independent blockade of Akt/mTOR pathway. Autophagy. 2011; 7(1):40–50.

38. Surviladze Z, Sterk RT, DeHaro SA, Ozbun MA. Cellular entry of human papillomavirus type 16 involves activation of the phosphatidylinositol 3-kinase/Akt/mTOR pathway and inhibition of autophagy. J Virol. 2013; 87(5):2508–17.

39. Luo M, Liu Q, He M, Yu Z, Pi R, Li M, Yang X, Wang S, Liu A. Gartanin induces cell cycle arrest and autophagy and suppresses migration involving PI3K/Akt/mTOR and MAPK signalling pathway in human glioma cells. J Cell Mol Med. 2017;21(1):46–57.

40. Cheng YC, Hueng DY, Huang HY, Chen JY, Chen Y. Magnolol and honokiol exert a synergistic anti-tumor effect through autophagy and apoptosis in human glioblastomas. Oncotarget. 2016;7(20):29116–30.

20

Prevalence and risk factors of deep venous thrombosis in patients with longitudinally extensive transverse myelitis

Tian Song[1,2], Xindi Li[1,2], Yonghong Liu[3] and Xinghu Zhang[1,2]*

Abstract

Objective: Deep venous thrombosis (DVT) is a severe complication in longitudinally extensive transverse myelitis (LETM) patients. It may interfere with LETM treatment and delay the recovery of the spinal dysfunction. However, there is less data about the prevalence and risk factors of DVT in patients with LETM. We analyzed data retrospectively to ascertain the prevalence of DVT and the clinical risk factors for DVT.

Methods: Clinical data on 255 LETM patients were collected from medical records. All patients were performed color Doppler ultrasound(US) to screen DVT in both lower extremities when admitted. Clinical characteristics of LETM patients with DVT were compared with those without DVT using corresponding statistical methods. Multivariate logistic regression was performed to identify risk factors related to DVT.

Results: DVT were found in 11.8% patients with LETM. Univariate analysis showed that age, muscle force and elevated baseline D-dimer were risk factors for DVT. After multivariate logistic regression, age, dyslipidemia, segments of lesions, and elevated baseline D-dimer remained significant independent risk factors.

Conclusions: DVT is common in patients with LETM and related to patient's age, dyslipidemia, segments of lesions, and elevated baseline D-dimer. Early recognition of DVT and thrombosis prophylaxis are appropriate in patients with LETM.

Keywords: Deep venous thrombosis, Longitudinally extensive transverse myelitis, Clinical risk factors, Thrombosis prophylaxis

Background

Longitudinally extensive transverse myelitis (LETM) is defined as myelitis with lesion extending at least 3 continuous vertebral segments in length [1]. A number of conditions can be associated with LETM, including neuromyelitis optica spectrum disorder (NMOSD), spinal infarction, spinal dural arteriovenous fistulas, compressive lesions, metabolic disorders, neoplasm, infection [2]. NMOSD is the most frequent cause of LETM [2], which primarily attacks the optic nerves and spinal cord [3]. LETM causes complete or partial neurologic impairment of motor, sensory and autonomic system [2]. These conditions are associated with increased morbidity and mortality, and a high economic burden [4]. Venous thromboembolism (VTE) is known as one of the common complications of LETM [5].

VTE includes deep venous thrombosis (DVT) and pulmonary embolism (PE). VTE affects 1/1000 patients, costs $13.5 billion annually to treat, and claims 100,000 lives annually in the US [6]. The risk of VTE in individuals with LETM may has been underestimated despite several plausible mechanisms. Autoimmune disorder associated with LETM may upregulate procoagulants,

---

* Correspondence: xhzhtiantan@hotmail.com
[1]Neuroinfection and Neuroimmunology Center, Department of Neurology, Beijing Tiantan Hospital, Capital Medical University, 6 TiantanXili, Dongcheng District, Beijing 100050, People's Republic of China
[2]China National Clinical Research Center for Neurological Diseases, Beijing Tiantan Hospital, Capital Medical University, 6 TiantanXili, Dongcheng District, Beijing 100050, People's Republic of China
Full list of author information is available at the end of the article

downregulate anticoagulants and suppress fibrinolysis [7].

But so far, little is known about the risk factors for DVT seen in LETM patients as it relates to other conditions, such as postoperation [8, 9], cancer [10, 11] and connective tissue diseases [12, 13]. Therefore, we evaluated the prevalence and risk factors of DVT and PE among patients with LETM in this study.

Methods

We retrospectively collected the medical records of LETM inpatients from July 2011 to August 2014. All patients were performed color Doppler US to screen DVT in both lower extremities when admitted, regardless of symptoms and signs of DVT. US examinations were operated and interpreted by ultrasonic specialists. The deep veins of lower extremities and pelvis were screened at approximately 2-cm intervals in the transverse sections from the inguinal ligament to the ankle. A diagnosis of DVT was confirmed with the presence of visible embolus, dilated incompressible vessel, or abnormal flow pattern [14]. Similarly, D-dimer was tested in all patients when admitted, regardless of symptoms and signs of DVT. When patients complained dyspnea, tachypnea, or chest pain which could not be explained by other reasons, we tested PE using Computed Tomography Pulmonary Angiography (CTPA). Once VTE was detected, anticoagulant was administered.

Continuous variables were described by means±SDs, and categorical variables were described as percentages. Characteristics of patients with DVT were compared with those without DVT using corresponding statistical methods. Mann–Whitney U-test was performed for numerical variables (eg, patient's age, inpatient days, inpatient costs, etiology of LETM, length of lesion). Fisher exact probability test was applied for the association of DVT and qualitative variables (eg, sex, combined diseases, location of lesions, contrast-enhanced or not, elevated baseline D-dimer). Ridit analysis was performed for ordinal variables, such as muscle strength of lower limbs. Logistic regression analysis was performed to identify patient characteristics related to DVT. Statistical significance was defined as $P < 0.05$. All statistical analysis was performed by IBM SPSS statistical software version 21.0 (IBM, Armonk, NY, USA).

The study protocol was approved by the ethics committee of Beijing Tiantan Hospital. Informed consent was signed by all patients or their legal representatives.

Results

There were 255 LETM patients enrolled in this study in total. The diagnostic criteria for NMOSD were met in 116 patients (45.5%). In other 139 patients, an alternative specific diagnosis was made: infectious, 57; clinically isolated syndrome (CIS), 47; vascular myelopathy, 9; neoplastic, 5; compressive, 3; nutritional, 3; neurosarcoidosis, 2; and idiopathic, 13. 68 NMOSD cases were at first attack, and 48 cases were recurrent. These patients (186 women, 69 men) ranged in age from 15 to 77 years (mean 41.3 years). DVT was identified in 30 patients, corresponding to 11.8% of LETM cases, and 4 cases were symptomatic DVT. Symptomatic PE was confirmed in 1 patient by CTPA.

Patients with DVT were at older age, had poorer muscle force of lower limbs and higher baseline D-dimer when compared to those without DVT (Table 1, $P < 0.001$). The associations of lipid disorder, smoking and lesion length with DVT were nearly significant ($P = 0.06$) in univariate analysis. The duration of hospitalization was obviously longer in patients with DVT than that without DVT (31.87 versus 18.95 days, $P < 0.001$). The hospital charges were higher in patients with DVT than patients absence of DVT (38,178 versus 17,153 CNY, $P < 0.001$). There were no differences in sex, comorbidity, etiology, location and enhancement of lesions, and coagulogram abnormal.

Multivariate logistic regression analysis presented that elderly patients showed higher likelihood of DVT with an OR of 1.10(95% CI 1.03–1.18). In addition, lipid disorder (OR0.07, 95%CI 0.01–0.51), lesion segments (OR1.53, 95%CI 1.14–2.05), elevated baseline D-dimer (OR18.40, 95%CI 3.32–101.89) were independent risk factors ($P < 0.05$) for occurrence of DVT (Table 2).

Discussion

This is a retrospective and observational study to identify the prevalence and risk factors of DVT in LETM patients. DVT prevalence among LETM inpatients in our study was 11.8%, obviously higher than that in non-surgical inpatients [11, 15], outpatients [16] and community population [17]. However, previous studies regarding to surgical and spinal cord lesion cases showed inconsistent DVT prevalence, ranging from 1.2% [18] to 27.6% [19]. This inconsistence can be explained by difference in population/race, sample size, DVT definition (symptomatic or asymptomatic).

Another primary aim of this study was to analyzed individual-level risk factors of DVT. Our data showed that age, dyslipidemia, lesion segments and elevated baseline D-dimer remained independent risk factors after adjustment for covariates. There are numerous published reports concerning the risk factors for DVT development in various diseases. A study about patients after spine surgery reported that risk factors for DVT included age and preoperative walking disability [20]. Immobility as a risk factor of DVT was also mentioned in neurosurgical patients, including cranial and spinal procedures [9]. However, there were different opinions. A Korean-based study reported that age and

Table 1 Characteristics of LETM patients with and without DVT

Variable	Total (N = 255)	With DVT (N = 30)	Without DVT (N = 225)	P value
Age (years), mean ± SD	41.3 ± 13.93	53.73 ± 11.94	39.65 ± 13.34	< 0.001
Sex, n(%)				
Men	69	7(23.33%)	62(27.56%)	0.62
Women	186	23(76.67%)	163(72.44%)	
Inpatient stays (days), mean ± SD	20.47 ± 9.90	31.87 ± 17.68	18.95 ± 7.14	< 0.001
Inpatient costs (CNY), mean ± SD	19,627.22±14,019.56	38,178.44 ± 30,309.69	17,153.73 ± 7190.18	< 0.001
Comorbidity, n(%)				
Hematological abnormality (anemia, leukopenia)	13(5.10%)	1(3.33%)	12(5.33%)	0.64
Connective tissue diseases	39(15.29%)	5(16.67%)	34(15.11%)	0.82
Thyroid dysfunction	22(8.63%)	3(10.00%)	19(8.44%)	0.78
Diabetes mellitus type 2	12(4.71%)	3(10.00%)	9(4.00%)	0.14
Hypertension	27(10.59%)	5(16.67%)	22(9.78%)	0.25
Dyslipidemia	80(31.37%)	5(16.67%)	75(33.33%)	0.06
Smoking	42(16.47%)	9(30%)	33(14.67%)	0.06
Etiology, n(%)				
NMOSD	116(45.49%)	13(43.33%)	103(45.78%)	0.85
First attack	68(26.67%)	6(20%)	62(27.56%)	0.38
Relapses	48(18.82%)	7(23.33%)	41(18.22%)	
Infection	57(22.35%)	9(30%)	48(21.33%)	0.35
CIS	47(18.43%)	4(13.33%)	43(19.11%)	0.62
Vascular myelopathy	9(3.53%)	1(3.33%)	8(3.56%)	0.71
Neoplastic	5(1.96%)	1(3.33%)	4(1.78%)	0.47
Compressive	3(1.18%)	0	3(1.33%)	1.00
Nutritional	3(1.18%)	0	3(1.33%)	1.00
Neurosarcoidosis	2(0.78%)	0	2(0.89%)	1.00
Idiopathic	13(5.10%)	2(6.67%)	11(4.89%)	0.66
Muscle strength of left leg, n (%)				
Grade 0	19(7.45%)	8(26.67%)	11(4.89%)	< 0.001
Grade 1	7(2.75%)	2(6.67%)	5(2.22%)	
Grade 2	14(5.49%)	5(16.67%)	9(4.00%)	
Grade 3	25(9.80%)	4(13.33%)	21(9.33%)	
Grade 4	73(28.63%)	5(16.67%)	68(30.22%)	
Grade 5	117(45.88%)	6(20.00%)	111(49.33%)	
Muscle strength of right leg, n (%)				
Grade 0	19(7.45%)	8(26.67%)	11(4.89%)	< 0.001
Grade 1	10(3.92%)	4(13.33%)	6(2.67%)	
Grade 2	11(4.31%)	4(13.33%)	7(3.11%)	
Grade 3	21(8.24%)	4(13.33%)	17(7.56%)	
Grade 4	68(26.67%)	8(26.67%)	60(26.67%)	
Grade 5	126(49.41%)	2(6.67%)	124(55.11%)	
Location of lesions, n (%)				
Cervical	204(80.00%)	25(83.33%)	179(79.56%)	0.63
Thoracic	133(52.16%)	17(56.67%)	116(51.56%)	0.60

Table 1 Characteristics of LETM patients with and without DVT *(Continued)*

Variable	Total (N = 255)	With DVT (N = 30)	Without DVT (N = 225)	P value
Lumbar	8(3.14%)	1(3.33%)	7(3.11%)	1.00
Segments of lesions, mean ± SD	5.20 ± 3.56	6.77 ± 4.98	5 ± 3.30	0.06
Enhancement of lesions, n (%)				
Yes	115(45.10%)	13(43.33%)	102(45.33%)	0.60
No	108(42.35%)	11(36.67%)	97(43.11%)	
Unknown	32(12.55%)	6(20.00%)	26(11.56%)	
Internals between LETM symptoms onset and US screening(days), mean ± SD	18.45 ± 7.40	21.40 ± 10.26	18.07 ± 6.87	0.025
Coagulogram abnormal, n (%)	108(42.35%)	14(46.67%)	94(41.78%)	0.61
Baseline D-dimer elevated, n (%)	24(9.41%)	17(56.67%)	7(3.11%)	<0.001

completeness of motor paralysis were not significantly associated with occurrence of DVT after spinal cord injury [21]. In our study, immobility appeared to be a risk factor in univariate analysis, but it was no longer independent risk factor after multivariate analysis. D-dimer values, in particular age-adjusted D-dimer cut-off values, have been confirmed to be associated with DVT [22, 23]. Our finding is in accordance with above researches. A review showed lipoprotein (a) was slightly but significantly associated with an increased risk of VTE (OR: 1.56, 95% CI: 1.36, 1.79), which included 10 studies, 13,541 patients [24]. Our study analyzed dyslipidemia as a whole including hyper/hypo-triglyceridemia and hyper/hypo- hypercholesteremia, instead of lipoprotein (a) individually. Much of the differences between studies may be due to small patient populations and different methods for assessment of DVT [25]. We have not searched literature focused on risk factors of DVT in LETM patients. Therefore,larger prospective studies will be needed to illuminate the risk factors for DVT and intrinsic mechanism.

The plausible mechanisms to explain the high prevalence of DVT in LETM patients remain unclear. Three main promoters to venous thrombosis included: venous stasis, hypercoagulable blood state and vascular endothelial injury (Virchow's triad) [26]. Immobility caused by

Table 2 Multivariate logistic regression analysis of significant risk factors for DVT in LETM patients

	P	OR(95% CI)
Age	0.004	1.104(1.032–1.181)
Dyslipidemia	0.009	0.07(0.01–0.51)
Segments of lesions	0.005	1.529(1.140–2.050)
Baseline D-dimer elevated	< 0.001	18.395(3.321–101.891)

spinal cord dysfunction can lead to venous stasis in LETM cases. There is some evidence that steroid use can increase procoagulant factors [27]. Most NMOSD and CIS patients in our study received high dose steroid pulse therapy. In addition, hospitalization also is a known risk factor for VTE [28]. Above elements may contribute to the high prevalence of DVT in LETM inpatients.

Several limitations to our analysis are worth noting. First limitation is lack of prospective control, which is inherent to observational studies. Second, the interval was not standardized between LETM symptom onset and US screening. The intervals in patients with DVT were significantly longer (P < 0.05, Table 1). The prevalence in our study might be underestimated because US screening was performed beyond the acute phase in some cases. Third, certain confounders were unavailable in our databases, such as body mass index(BMI) [29] and glucocorticoid usage [30], which are known as risk factors for DVT. Despite these limitations, our data is convincing for the large sample size and routine US screening for DVT.

Conclusion

In conclusion, this retrospective study demonstrated that patients with LETM had an increased risk for developing DVT. Therefore, it is important to identify the high-risk patients and initiate thrombosis prophylaxis promptly.

Abbreviations
BMI: body mass index; CIS: Clinical isolated syndrome; CNS: Central nervous system; CTPA: Computed Tomography Pulmonary Angiography; DVT: Deep venous thrombosis; LETM: Longitudinally extensive transverse myelitis; NMOSD: Neuromyelitis optica spectrum disorders; PE: Pulmonary embolism; US: Ultrasound; VTE: Venous thromboembolism

Acknowledgements
The authors thank the participants and all who were involved in this study.

Funding
This work was supported by Youth Research Fund of Beijing Tiantan Hospital (201403011).

Authors' contributions
ST contributed to study design, data analysis, manuscript writing and revising. LXD contributed to patient's clinical information collection and follow-up. LYH contributed to patient's clinical information collection and follow-up. ZXH contributed to study design and manuscript revising. All authors read and approved the final manuscript.

Competing interests
The authors declare that they have no competing interests.

Author details
[1]Neuroinfection and Neuroimmunology Center, Department of Neurology, Beijing Tiantan Hospital, Capital Medical University, 6 TiantanXili, Dongcheng District, Beijing 100050, People's Republic of China. [2]China National Clinical Research Center for Neurological Diseases, Beijing Tiantan Hospital, Capital Medical University, 6 TiantanXili, Dongcheng District, Beijing 100050, People's Republic of China. [3]Department of Neurology, Beijing Rehabilitation Hospital, Capital Medical University,Xixiazhuang, Shijingshan District, Beijing 100050, People's Republic of China.

References
1. Weinshenker BG, Wingerchuk DM, Vukusic S, Linbo L, Pittock SJ, Lucchinetti CF, et al. Neuromyelitis optica IgG predicts relapse after longitudinally extensive transverse myelitis. Ann Neurol. 2006;59:566–9.
2. Tobin WO, Weinshenker BG, Lucchinetti CF. Longitudinally extensive transverse myelitis. Curr Opin Neurol. 2014;27:279–89.
3. Wingerchuk DM, Banwell B, Bennett JL, Cabre P, Carroll W, Chitnis T, et al. International consensus diagnostic criteria for neuromyelitis optica spectrum disorders. Neurology. 2015;85:177–89.
4. ZhangBao J, Zhou L, Li X, Cai T, Lu J, Lu C, et al. The clinical characteristics of AQP4 antibody positive NMO/SD in a large cohort of Chinese Han patients. J Neuroimmunol. 2017;302:49–55.
5. Cushman M. Epidemiology and risk factors for venous thrombosis. Semin Hematol. 2007;44:62–9.
6. Behravesh S, Hoang P, Nanda A, Wallace A, Sheth RA, Deipolyi AR, et al. Pathogenesis of thromboembolism and endovascular management. Thrombosis. 2017;2017, 3039713.
7. Xu J, Lupu F, Esmon CT. Inflammation, innate immunity and blood coagulation. Hamostaseologie. 2010;30:5–6, 8-9.
8. Sebastian AS, Currier BL, Kakar S, Nguyen EC, Wagie AE, Habermann ES, et al. Risk factors for venous thromboembolism following thoracolumbar surgery: analysis of 43,777 patients from the American College of Surgeons National Surgical Quality Improvement Program 2005 to 2012. Global Spine J. 2016;6:738–43.
9. Rolston JD, Han SJ, Bloch O, Parsa AT. What clinical factors predict the incidence of deep venous thrombosis and pulmonary embolism in neurosurgical patients? J Neurosurg. 2014;121:908–18.
10. Faiz AS, Khan I, Beckman MG, Bockenstedt P, Heit JA, Kulkarni R, et al. Characteristics and risk factors of Cancer associated venous thromboembolism. Thromb Res. 2015;136:535–41.
11. Mellema WW, van der Hoek D, Postmus PE, Smit EF. Retrospective evaluation of thromboembolic events in patients with non-small cell lung cancer treated with platinum-based chemotherapy. Lung Cancer. 2014;86:73–7.
12. Lee JJ, Pope JE. A meta-analysis of the risk of venous thromboembolism in inflammatory rheumatic diseases. Arthritis Res Ther. 2014;16:435.
13. Kim SC, Schneeweiss S, Liu J, Solomon DH. Risk of venous thromboembolism in patients with rheumatoid arthritis. Arthritis Care Res (Hoboken). 2013;65:1600–7.
14. Liu LP, Zheng HG, Wang DZ, Wang YL, Hussain M, Sun HX, et al. Risk assessment of deep-vein thrombosis after acute stroke: a prospective study using clinical factors. CNS Neurosci Ther. 2014;20:403–10.
15. Lawall H, Hoffmanns W, Hoffmanns P, Rapp U, Ames M, Pira A, et al. Prevalence of deep vein thrombosis (DVT) in non-surgical patients at hospital admission. Thromb Haemost. 2007;98:765–70.
16. Shulman RM, Buchan C, Bleakney RR, White LM. Low prevalence of unexpected popliteal DVT detected on routine MRI assessment of the knee. Clin Imaging. 2016;40:79–85.
17. Ho WK, Hankey GJ, Eikelboom JW. The incidence of venous thromboembolism: a prospective, community-based study in Perth. Western Australia Med J Aust. 2008;189:144–7.
18. Maiser S, Adil MM, Roohani P, Tariq N. Patients with transverse myelitis who developed venous thromboembolism while hospitalized have increased rate for inpatient mortality. J Neuroimmunol. 2013;261:120–2.
19. Do JG, Kim DH, Sung DH. Incidence of deep vein thrombosis after spinal cord injury in Korean patients at acute rehabilitation unit. J Korean Med Sci. 2013;28:1382–7.
20. Tominaga H, Setoguchi T, Tanabe F, Kawamura I, Tsuneyoshi Y, Kawabata N, et al. Risk factors for venous thromboembolism after spine surgery. Medicine. 2015;94:e466.
21. Do JG, Kim DH, Sung DH. Incidence of deep vein thrombosis after spinal cord injury in Korean patients at acute rehabilitation unit. J Korean Med Sci. 2013;28:1382.
22. Haase C, Joergensen M, Ellervik C, Joergensen MK, Bathum L. Age- and sex-dependent reference intervals for D-dimer: evidence for a marked increase by age. Thromb Res. 2013;132:676–80.
23. Broen K, Scholtes B, Vossen R. Predicting the need for further thrombosis diagnostics in suspected DVT is increased by using age adjusted D-dimer values. Thromb Res. 2016;145:107–8.
24. Dentali F, Gessi V, Marcucci R, Gianni M, Grandi AM, Franchini M. Lipoprotein(a) as a risk factor for venous thromboembolism: a systematic review and meta-analysis of the literature. Semin Thromb Hemost. 2017.
25. Guyatt GH, Eikelboom JW, Gould MK, Garcia DA, Crowther M, Murad MH, et al. (2012) Approach to outcome measurement in the prevention of thrombosis in surgical and medical patients: antithrombotic therapy and prevention of thrombosis, 9th ed: American College of Chest Physicians Evidence-Based Clinical Practice Guidelines. Chest 141: e185S-e194S.
26. Kumar DR, Hanlin E, Glurich I, Mazza JJ, Yale SH. Virchow's contribution to the understanding of thrombosis and cellular biology. Clin Med Res. 2010;8:168–72.
27. Girolami A, de Marinis GB, Bonamigo E, Treleani M, Vettore S. Arterial and venous thromboses in patients with idiopathic (immunological) thrombocytopenia: a possible contributing role of cortisone-induced hypercoagulable state. Clin Appl Thromb Hemost. 2013;19:613–8.
28. Heit JA, Melton LR, Lohse CM, Petterson TM, Silverstein MD, Mohr DN, et al. Incidence of venous thromboembolism in hospitalized patients vs community residents. Mayo Clin Proc. 2001;76:1102–10.
29. Holst AG, Jensen G, Prescott E. Risk factors for venous thromboembolism: results from the Copenhagen City heart study. Circulation. 2010;121:1896–903.
30. Johannesdottir SA, Horvath-Puho E, Dekkers OM, Cannegieter SC, Jorgensen JO, Ehrenstein V, et al. Use of glucocorticoids and risk of venous thromboembolism: a nationwide population-based case-control study. JAMA Intern Med. 2013;173:743–52.

21

Diagnostic and prognostic value of the optic nerve sheath diameter with respect to the intracranial pressure and neurological outcome of patients following hemicraniectomy

Yuzhi Gao, Qiang Li, Chunshuang Wu, Shaoyun Liu and Mao Zhang[*]

Abstract

Background: In cases showing cerebrospinal fluid (CSF) redistribution as a compensatory mechanism in acute intracranial hypertension, the optic nerve sheath diameter (ONSD) can be used to estimate intracranial pressure (ICP). However, it remains unclear whether the ONSD can be applied in patients with skull defects after a craniectomy, because the primary injury or surgical craniectomy may alter the dynamics of the CSF circulation or structure of the optical nerve sheath. This study explored the value of the ONSD in patients after a hemicraniectomy.

Methods: This prospective observational study enrolled patients after a hemicraniectomy. All patients underwent invasive ICP monitoring and ocular ultrasound within 6 h postoperatively. We followed the patients for 6 months and evaluated them using the Glasgow Outcome Score (GOS), classifying the outcome as favorable (GOS 4–5) or unfavorable (GOS 1–3). We evaluated the ONSD in both according to the ICP and neurological outcome.

Results: Of the 33 enrolled patients, 20 (60.6%) had an unfavorable outcome at 6 months. Disagreement was seen in the ONSD measurements between the eyes [craniectomy side (ONSDips) and opposite side (ONSDcon)]. The intraclass correlation coefficient between ONSDips and ONSDcon was 0.745 ($p < 0.001$). ONSD had no significant correlation with ICP in Spearman correlation analysis (ONSDips $r = 0.205$, $p = 0.252$; ONSDcon $r = 0.164$, $p = 0.362$). Receiver operator characteristic (ROC) curve analysis revealed that the GCS, Helsinki computed tomography (CT) score, pupil reaction, and ONSDcon measured after the craniectomy were significantly associated with a poor outcome. ONSDcon > 5.5 mm predicted a poor outcome, with an area under the ROC curve of 0.717 (95% confidence interval, 0.534–0.860, $p = 0.02$), 70% sensitivity, and 69.2% specificity.

Conclusions: After hemicraniectomy, the ONSD measured on ultrasound was unreliable for evaluating ICP, but showed potential prognostic value for a poor neurological outcome.

Keywords: Optical nerve sheath diameter, Intracranial pressure, Hemicraniectomy, Neurological outcome

* Correspondence: z2jzk@zju.edu.cn
Department of Emergency Medicine, Second Affiliated Hospital, Zhejiang University School of Medicine, No. 88, Jiefang Road, Hangzhou City 310009, Zhejiang Province, China

Background

The optic nerve sheath diameter (ONSD) is often taken as a proxy of intracranial hypertension in brain injury patients [1–3]. The space surrounding the optic nerve is a continuation of the intracranial subarachnoid space. With the compensatory redistribution of cerebrospinal fluid (CSF) seen in cases of intracranial hypertension, the raised intracranial pressure (ICP) instantaneously distends the ONSD [4]. In traumatic brain injury (TBI) and post-cardiac arrest patients, the ONSD calculated based on ultrasound or computed tomography (CT) image is correlated with the invasive ICP [5, 6]. An increase in ONSD from the baseline CT was associated with an unfavorable neurological outcome [7–9]. Although measurement of ONSD by portable ultrasound is feasible and convenient, there are still obstacles to its widespread clinical application [5, 10]. Moreover, some studies found no correlation between ONSD and ICP [11, 12]. Primary brain injury or decompression craniectomy (DC) may alter CSF hydrodynamics or destroy the optic nerve sheath [13, 14]. Therefore, it remains unclear whether ONSD can be applied in patients with skull defects after DC. This study explored the value of the ONSD calculated based on ultrasound images in patients with skull defects following hemicraniectomy.

Methods

Setting and participants

This observational study was conducted in a 16-bed intensive care unit (ICU) affiliated with an academic hospital in eastern China. The research protocol was approved by the second Hospital affiliated Zhejiang University Institutional Review Board prior to the start of recruitment and data collection. Almost all of the enrolled neurocritical patients had no ability to express themselves at early stage. So after admitted to our unit, the doctor had a talk with the patients' immediate family members (spouse, children, parents, et ac) and then they signed an informed consent about patient-related medical treatment. We screened all patients who underwent invasive ICP monitoring after a hemicraniectomy. Exclusion criteria were age < 18 years, ONSD measurement unavailable within 6 h postoperatively, ocular trauma or pre-existing ocular disease, and unsuitable optic nerve sheath images.

Study protocol

To avoid operator differences, one experienced doctor (WC) performed the ocular ultrasound for every eligible patient and then numbered and stored the ONSD images. Blinded to the ONSD measurements, another doctor (LQ) was in charge of collecting the relevant data from the ocular ultrasound examinations. Before collecting the data, we ensured that the ICP monitors had been zeroed. We followed the patients for 6 months after the injury and evaluated them using the Glasgow Outcome Score (GOS). We classified the patient outcomes as unfavorable (GOS 1, dead; GOS 2, vegetative state; GOS 3, severe disability) and favorable (GOS 4, moderate disability; GOS 5, return to normal life). Two experienced doctors (LS and GY) rechecked the ONSD images and recorded the data. Instead of averaging the values for the two eyes, we classified the ONSD measurements from both eyes into ipsilateral ONSD (craniectomy side, ONSDips) and contralateral ONSD (the side opposite the craniectomy, ONSDcon) according to the side of the craniectomy. Then, we analyzed the ONSD measurements according to the ICP and outcome.

ONSD measurement

A portable ultrasound machine (M9, Mindray, Shenzhen, China) with a linear array probe (13–6 MHz) was used. As described by Blehar et al. [15], we determined ONSD in the visual axis by placing the probe over the closed eyelid. The probe was moved slightly until the optic nerve appeared as a linear hypoechoic object with defined margins behind the globe. After freezing the screen image, we determined ONSD manually 3 mm behind the globe with mechanical calipers (Fig. 1).

Management of neurocritical patients

All postoperative neurocritical patients received standard intensive care according to the guidelines for management of TBI or intracranial hemorrhage. Ventilation was used to maintain normal oxygenation (PaO_2 80–120 mmHg, $PaCO_2$ 35–45 mmHg). Midazolam, fentanyl, or sufentanil was infused continuously for sedation and analgesia. Hyperosmolar therapy with 20% mannitol or 3% hypertonic saline was applied when the ICP exceeded 20 mmHg. The cerebral perfusion pressure was maintained at 60~70 mmHg with fluids and norepinephrine as needed. Hypothermia treatment, neuromuscular blocking drugs, and barbiturates were used if indicated clinically.

Statistics analysis

Variables with normal distributions are expressed as means ± SD, and those with non-normal distributions as medians with interquartile range (IQR). Categorical variables are expressed as n (%). We used Student's t-test or the Kolmogorov–Smirnov test to compare baseline characteristics between patients with favorable and unfavorable outcomes. We constructed

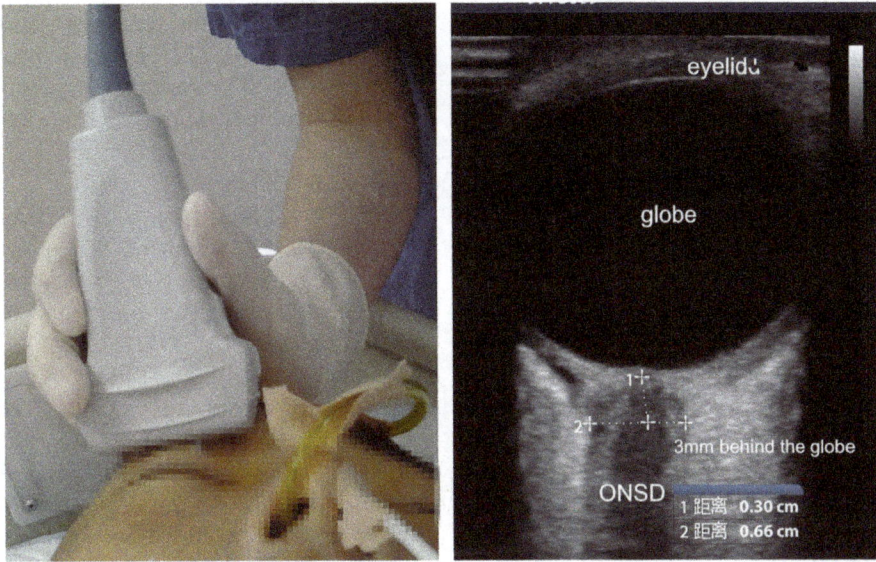

Fig. 1 Illustration of ONSD performance and B-mode image of ONSD measurement. A linear high frequency probe placed on the closed eye in transverse visual axis plane, and then adjusted the depth and angle of ultrasound to show the image of ONSD clearly, measure the width of ONSD at 3 mm behind the globe. ONSD optical nerve sheath diameter

Bland–Altman plots and used intraclass correlation coefficient (ICC) analysis to determine the agreement between ONSDips and ONSDcon. Spearman rank correlation was used to evaluate the association of both ONSD measurements with ICP. Receiver operator characteristic (ROC) curves were used to analyze predictors of an unfavorable outcome at 6 months (GOS 1–3). The cutoff values of predictors of a poor outcome (GOS 1–3) were determined using ROC curves. Then, we calculated the sensitivity, specificity, positive predictive value (PPV), and negative predictive value (NPV) for each cutoff. Statistical analyses were performed using MedCalc for Windows software (ver. 11.4; MedCalc Software). P-values < 0.05 were considered to be statistically significant.

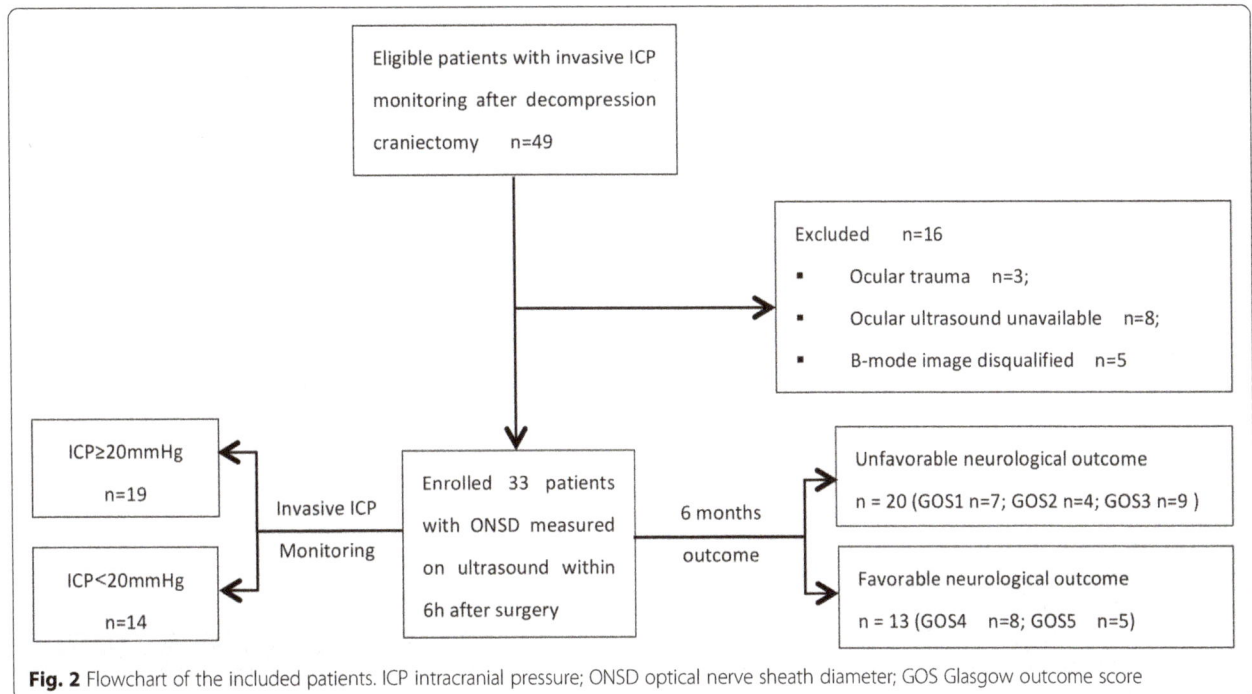

Fig. 2 Flowchart of the included patients. ICP intracranial pressure; ONSD optical nerve sheath diameter; GOS Glasgow outcome score

Results

Baseline characteristics

During the study period, there were 49 potentially eligible patients, 16 of whom were excluded because ocular ultrasound was unavailable ($n = 8$), they had ocular trauma ($n = 3$), or the ONSD image was inadequate ($n = 5$). Figure 2 shows a flowchart of the included patients. Of the 33 enrolled patients, 31 (93.9%) had TBI. The outcome at 6 months was favorable (GOS 4–5) in 13 patients (39.4%). Table 1 summarizes the baseline characteristics according to the 6-month neurological outcome. Univariate analysis revealed that the baseline Helsinki CT score, GCS, pupil light reflex before surgery, and ONSDcon after craniectomy were associated with an unfavorable neurological outcome. We found no significant differences in sex, age, reason for surgery, ICP, or ICU stay duration between the patients with unfavorable and favorable outcomes.

In total, 33 paired ONSD measurements of both eyes were obtained from the patients within 6 h after hemicraniectomy. Bland–Altman analysis yielded a mean difference in the bilateral ONSD measurements of 0.07

mm. The limits of agreement were – 0.91 and 1.05 mm, and 9.1% (3/33) of the plots were outside the limits of agreement (Fig. 3). The interclass correlation coefficient of the two ONSD measurements was 0.745 (95% confidence interval [CI]: 0.574–0.867, $p < 0.001$).

ONSD vs. ICP

The ICP had a non-normal distribution, with a median (IQR) of 22 (9–27) mmHg. We applied nonparametric Spearman rank correlation to analyze the relationship between ONSD and ICP, and found no significant correlation (ipsilateral $r = 0.205$, $p = 0.252$; contralateral $r = 0.164$, $p = 0.362$) (Fig. 4). ROC curves for ICP ≥ 20 mmHg were drawn for the ONSD measurements of both eyes. The ONSD of both eyes did not predict a raised ICP (ipsilateral: area under the curve [AUC] = 0.686, 95% CI: 0.502–0.836, $p = 0.05$; contralateral: AUC = 0.677, 95% CI: 0.492–0.828, $p = 0.66$).

ONSD vs. outcome

ROC curve analysis revealed that the cut-off value of ONSDcon for predicting an unfavorable outcome was

Table 1 Baseline characteristics

		Neurological outcome (6 months)		
	All	Unfavorable GOS 1–3	Favorable GOS4–5	p-value
Number of patients	33	20 (60.6%)	13 (39.4%)	–
Age, y	46.6 ± 14.9	47.9 ± 15.0	46.5 ± 14.1	0.552
Sex (male), n (%)	25 (75.8%)	15 (45.5%)	10 (30.3%)	0.619
Causes of surgery, n (%)				0.474
Traumatic brain injury	31 (93.9%)	14 (42.4%)	17 (51.5%)	–
Hemorrhage stroke	2 (6.1%)	2 (6.1%)	0	–
Initial Glasgow coma score (GCS)				0.008
3–8	22 (66.7%)	17 (51.5%)	5 (15.2%)	–
≥ 9	11 (33.3%)	3 (9.1%)	8 (24.2%)	–
Initial Pupil light reflex (n %)				0.039
Both react	20 (60.6%)	9 (27.3%)	11 (33.3%)	
1 reacts	3 (9.1%)	2 (6.1%)	1 (3.0%)	
None reacts	10 (30.3%)	9 (27.3%)	1 (3.0%)	
Helsinki CT score	6 ± 3	7 ± 2	4 ± 3	0.013
ICU duration (day)	8 (6–12)	9 (8–13)	7 (3–12)	0.079
Hospital discharge (day)	19 ± 9	17 ± 8	22 ± 10	0.134
Data during ocular ultrasound performed within 6 h after craniectomy				
ICP (mmHg)	22 (9–27)	26 (24–32)	14 (9–16)	0.668
MAP (mmHg)	89 (81–97)	89 (82–97)	86 (80–96)	0.337
CPP (mmHg)	68 ± 18	69 ± 20	67 ± 16	0.812
Ipsilateral ONSD (mm)	5.9 ± 0.7	6.0 ± 0.7	5.8 ± 0.5	0.164
Contralateral ONSD (mm)	5.8 ± 0.7	6.1 ± 0.7	5.5 ± 0.7	0.018

CT computerized tomography, *ICU* intensive care unit, *ICP* intracranial pressure, *MAP* mean arterial pressure, *CPP* cerebral perfusion pressure, *ONSD* optic nerve sheath diameter, *GOS* glasgow outcome score, GOS 1 dead, GOS 2 vegetative state, GOS 3 severe disability, GOS 4 moderate disability, GOS 5 back to normal life with or without mild disability

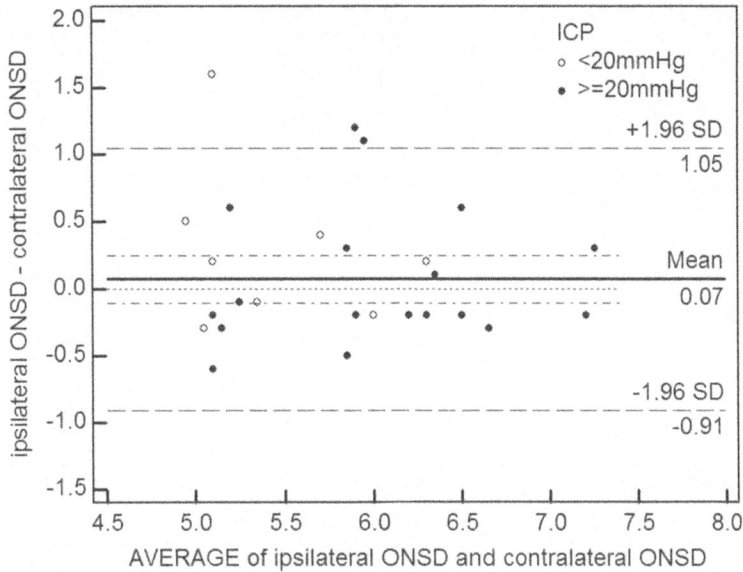

Fig. 3 Bilateral ONSD measurements agreement and difference. Bland-Altman plots display the agreement of ipsilateral ONSD and contralateral ONSD measured 3 mm behind the globe by ocular ultrasound. Continuous lines depict the mean of differences; dashed lines denote limits of agreement (mean ± 1.96 times of standard deviation)

5.5 mm (AUC = 0.717; 95% CI: 0.534–0.860, $p = 0.02$). The sensitivity and specificity of this cut-off value were 70 and 69.2%, respectively. The PPV of a poor outcome was 100% when ONSD > 6.6 mm. The cutoff value of the Helsinki CT score for predicting a poor outcome was 5 (AUC = 0.831, 95% CI: 0.660–0.938, $p < 0.001$), and the sensitivity and specificity were 85 and 69.2%, respectively (see Table 2). On ROC curve analysis, there was no significant difference between the ONSDcon and Helsinki CT score in terms of predicting a poor outcome ($p = 0.301$).

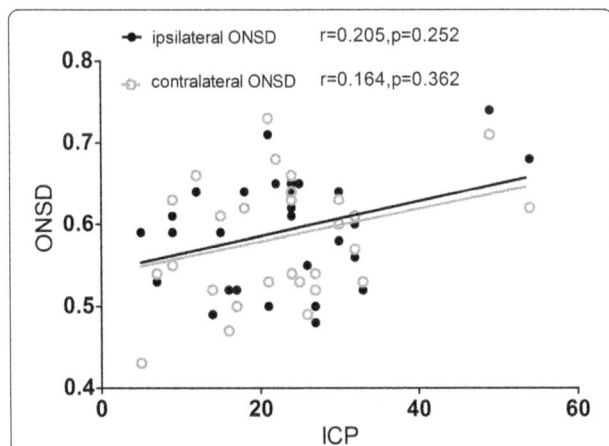

Fig. 4 Scatter diagrams of bilateral ONSDs and ICP. There was no significant correlation between bilateral ONSDs and ICP respectively ($p > 0.05$). ONSD optical nerve sheath diameter; ICP intracranial pressure

Discussion

Our data revealed that ONSD was not reliable for non-invasive evaluation of ICP in patients after a hemicraniectomy. First, the ONSD calculated based on postoperative ultrasound images had no correlation with ICP. Second, the diagnostic value of ONSD with respect to a raised ICP (≥ 20 mmHg) was variable in patients after craniectomy. A few studies have reported a weak correlation between ONSD and ICP [11, 12]. Several factors might explain our results; first, the effect of DC complications, such as subdural hygroma and post-traumatic hydrocephalus, on CSF hydrodynamics has been neglected [13]. Surgical craniectomy could reduce the secretion of CSF, affect its outflow, or cause a redistribution of CSF; these altered CSF hydrodynamics might prevent the ONSD from shrinking after the intracranial hypertension relieved by DC [14]. Damage to the optic nerve sheath might also delay or prevent the reversal of ONSD distension [11]. In addition, the standard range of ONSD is inconsistent among studies where a study including a large sample of healthy Chinese adults gave a reference range of ONSD of 4.7–5.4 mm [16].

In TBI and post-cardiac arrest patients, drugs and hypothermia therapy often influence the early prognosis. A few studies have explored the prognostic value of ONSD, calculated based on the initial CT, with respect to the outcome in TBI and post-cardiac arrest patients [7, 8, 17]. In our post-hemicraniectomy patients, increased ONSD was associated with unfavorable outcomes (GOS 1–3). The ONSD reflects the severity of the primary brain injury induced by the initial increase

Table 2 Parameters in prediction of six months unfavorable outcome (GOS 1–3)

	Cutoff	AUC	95% CI	Sens/Spec(%)	PPV/NPV(%)	p-value
Unfavorable outcome (GOS 1–3)						
Ipsilateral ONSD (mm)	6.2	0.642	0.457–0.801	45/84.6	81.8/50	0.15
	6.5			15/100	100/43.3	
Contralateral ONSD (mm)	5.5	0.717	0.534–0.860	70/69.2	73.7/57.1	0.02
	6.6			20/100	100/44.8	
ICP (mmHg)	17	0.638	0.453–0.798	70/53.9	70/53.8	0.17
	33			10/100	100/41.9	
Helsinki CT score	5	0.831	0.660–0.938	85/69.2	81/75	< 0.001
	7			45/100	100/54.2	

ONSD optic nerve sheath diameter, ICP intracranial pressure, GOS glasgow outcome score, AUC area under curve, 95% CI 95% confidence intervals, Sens sensitivity, Spec specificity, PPV positive prediction value, NPV negative prediction value

in the ICP, where primary brain injury plays an important role in the neurological prognosis [18]. Although the ONSD was not correlated with the ICP, ONSDcon was significantly greater in patients with unfavorable outcomes (6.1 ± 0.7 vs. 5.5 ± 0.7 mm, $p = 0.018$). The ROC curve analysis indicated that ONSDcon has potential value for predicting an unfavorable outcome. The cutoff value of ONSDcon was 5.5 mm (AUC = 0.717, $p = 0.02$), with a PPV of 100% when ONSDcon > 6.6 mm. As Rajajee et al. surmised, the relationship between ICP and ONSD is contingent on a close temporal association [11]. In our study, primary brain injury and craniectomy itself altered the dynamics of the CSF circulation and structure of the optical nerve sheath, which may have delayed the reversal of ONSD distension after DC. Increased ONSD measured after a craniectomy with a normal or low ICP indicates either severe primary injury or altered CSF hydrodynamics. Such post-craniectomy patients tend to have a poor prognosis.

The bilateral difference in ONSD measurements was another unexpected finding. We classified the ONSD measurements into ONSDips and ONSDcon according to the side of the craniectomy, rather than the right and left side. The patients who underwent hemicraniectomy had non-diffuse primary brain injuries, where higher pressure and greater ONSD might occur on the side with more severe injury [12]. Therefore, we analyzed ONSDips and ONSDcon separately, rather than using the average, including only the larger value in the analyses, as done in previous studies.

Some errors may have influenced our results, for example in terms of the reliability of the ONSD measurements [5, 10]. The ONSD can be measured in the transverse or sagittal plane. Blehar et al. showed that different ONSD measurement methods yielded different values, where more shadowing artifacts arising from the optic disc were observed in the visual axis plane [15]. Therefore, in our study, a single experienced physician performed the ocular ultrasound and used the visual axis

transverse plane for the ONSD measurements. We also rechecked the ultrasound images to ensure that unsuitable images were excluded, to avoid measurement errors.

Conclusions

ONSD was not a reliable index in the noninvasive evaluation of ICP in patients after hemicraniectomy. Due to the influence of the primary brain injury or the craniectomy itself, damage to the optic nerve sheath delayed the reversal of ONSD distention, while the altered CSF hydrodynamics prevented CSF redistribution as a compensatory mechanism in acute intracranial hypertension. Ultrasound measurement of ONSD has potential prognostic value for a poor outcome in patients after hemicraniectomy. An increased ONSD induced by initial intracranial hypertension before DC can reflect the severity of the primary brain injury, which plays an important role in the neurological prognosis.

Abbreviations
CSF: Cerebral spinal fluid; DC: Decompression craniectomy; GOS: Glasgow outcome score; ICP: Intracranial pressure; NPV: Negative prediction value; ONSD: Optical nerve sheath diameter; PPV: Positive prediction value; TBI: Traumatic brain injury

Acknowledgments
Not applicable.

Funding
Not applicable.

Authors' contributions
The corresponding author (ZM) was in charge of study design. The first author (GY) was responsible for manuscript writing and cooperated with the rest three authors (WC, LS and LQ) in clinical research work. LQ was in charge of data collection and data analysis. WC was the ocular ultrasound operator during the study. Apart from assisting data collection, LS was also responsible for the relevant literature review. All authors have read and approved the publication of this manuscript.

Competing interests
The authors declare that they have no competing interests.

References
1. Rajajee V, Vanaman M, Fletcher JJ, Jacobs TL. Optic nerve ultrasound for the detection of raised intracranial pressure. Neurocrit Care. 2011;15(3):506–15.
2. Geeraerts T, Launey Y, Martin L, Pottecher J, Vigué B, Duranteau J, Benhamou D. Ultrasonography of the optic nerve sheath may be useful for detecting raised intracranial pressure after severe brain injury. Intens Care Med. 2007;33(10):1704–11.
3. Geeraerts T, Merceron S, Benhamou D, Vigué B, Duranteau J. Non-invasive assessment of intracranial pressure using ocular sonography in neurocritical care patients. Intens Care Med. 2008;34(11):2062–7.
4. Robba C, Bacigaluppi S, Cardim D, Donnelly J, Bertuccio A, Czosnyka M. Non-invasive assessment of intracranial pressure. Acta Neurol Scand. 2016;134(1):4–21.
5. Dubourg J, Javouhey E, Geeraerts T, Messerer M, Kassai B. Ultrasonography of optic nerve sheath diameter for detection of raised intracranial pressure: a systematic review and meta-analysis. Intens Care Med. 2011;37(7):1059–68.
6. Ohle R, McIsaac SM, Woo MY, Perry JJ. Sonography of the optic nerve sheath diameter for detection of raised intracranial pressure compared to computed tomography: a systematic review and meta-analysis. J Ultrasound Med. 2015;34(7):1285–94.
7. Chelly J, Deye N, Guichard JP, Vodovar D, Vong L, Jochmans S, Thieulot-Rolin N, Sy O, Serbource-Goguel J, Vinsonneau C, et al. The optic nerve sheath diameter as a useful tool for early prediction of outcome after cardiac arrest: a prospective pilot study. RESUSCITATION. 2016;103:7–13.
8. Sekhon MS, McBeth P, Zou J, Qiao L, Kolmodin L, Henderson WR, Reynolds S, Griesdale DEG. Association between optic nerve sheath diameter and mortality in patients with severe traumatic brain injury. Neurocrit Care. 2014; 21(2):245–52.
9. Hwan Kim Y, Ho Lee J, Kun Hong C, Won Cho K, Hoon Yeo J, Ju Kang M, Weon Kim Y, Yul Lee K, Joo Kim J, Youn Hwang S. Feasibility of optic nerve sheath diameter measured on initial brain computed tomography as an early neurologic outcome predictor after cardiac arrest. Acad Emerg Med. 2014;21(10):1121–8.
10. MORETTI R, PIZZI B. Ultrasonography of the optic nerve in neurocritically ill patients. ACTA ANAESTH SCAND. 2011;55(6):644–52.
11. Rajajee V, Fletcher JJ, Rochlen LR, Jacobs TL. Comparison of accuracy of optic nerve ultrasound for the detection of intracranial hypertension in the setting of acutely fluctuating vs stable intracranial pressure: post-hoc analysis of data from a prospective, blinded single center study. Crit Care. 2012;16(3):R79.
12. Strumwasser A, Kwan RO, Yeung L, Miraflor E, Ereso A, Castro-Moure F, Patel A, Sadjadi J, Victorino GP. Sonographic optic nerve sheath diameter as an estimate of intracranial pressure in adult trauma. J Surg Res. 2011;170(2):265–71.
13. Czosnyka M, Copeman J, Czosnyka Z, McConnell R, Dickinson C, Pickard JD. Post-traumatic hydrocephalus: influence of craniectomy on the CSF circulation. J Neurol Neurosurg Psychiatry. 2000;68(2):246–8.
14. Shapiro K, Fried A, Takei F, Kohn I. Effect of the skull and dura on neural axis pressure-volume relationships and CSF hydrodynamics. J Neurosurg. 1985;63(1):76.
15. Blehar DJ, Gaspari RJ, Montoya A, Calderon R. Correlation of visual axis and coronal axis measurements of the optic nerve sheath diameter. J Ultrasound Med. 2008;27(3):407–11.
16. Chen H, Ding GS, Zhao YC, Yu RG, Zhou JX. Ultrasound measurement of optic nerve diameter and optic nerve sheath diameter in healthy Chinese adults. BMC Neurol. 2015;15(1):106.
17. Chae MK, Ko E, Lee JH, Lee TR, Yoon H, Hwang SY, Cha WC, Shin TG, Sim MS, Jo IJ, et al. Better prognostic value with combined optic nerve sheath diameter and grey-to-white matter ratio on initial brain computed tomography in post-cardiac arrest patients. RESUSCITATION. 2016;104:40–5.
18. Soldatos T, Karakitsos D, Chatzimichail K, Papathanasiou M, Gouliamos A, Karabinis A. Optic nerve sonography in the diagnostic evaluation of adult brain injury. Crit Care. 2008;12(3):R67.

22

Relationship between *ABCB1* 3435TT genotype and antiepileptic drugs resistance in Epilepsy

Malek Chouchi[1,2*†], Wajih Kaabachi[3†], Hedia Klaa[2], Kalthoum Tizaoui[3], Ilhem Ben-Youssef Turki[2] and Lamia Hila[4]

Abstract

Background: Antiepileptic drugs (AEDs) are effective medications available for epilepsy. However, many patients do not respond to this treatment and become resistant. Genetic polymorphisms may be involved in the variation of AEDs response. Therefore, we conducted an updated systematic review and a meta-analysis to investigate the contribution of the genetic profile on epilepsy drug resistance.

Methods: We proceeded to the selection of eligible studies related to the associations of polymorphisms with resistance to AEDs therapy in epilepsy, published from January 1980 until November 2016, using Pubmed and Cochrane Library databases. The association analysis was based on pooled odds ratios (ORs) and 95% confidence intervals (CIs).

Results: From 640 articles, we retained 13 articles to evaluate the relationship between ATP-binding cassette sub-family C member 1 (*ABCB1*) C3435T polymorphism and AEDs responsiveness in a total of 454 epileptic AEDs-resistant cases and 282 AEDs-responsive cases. We found a significant association with an OR of 1.877, 95% CI 1.213–2.905. Subanalysis by genotype model showed a more significant association between the recessive model of *ABCB1* C3435T polymorphism (TT vs. CC) and the risk of AEDs resistance with an OR of 2.375, 95% CI 1.775–3.178 than in the dominant one (CC vs. TT) with an OR of 1.686, 95% CI 0.877–3.242.

Conclusion: Our results indicate that *ABCB1* C3435T polymorphism, especially TT genotype, plays an important role in refractory epilepsy. As genetic screening of this genotype may be useful to predict AEDs response before starting the treatment, further investigations should validate the association.

Keywords: Epilepsy, Antiepileptic drugs, Resistance, *ABCB1* C3435T polymorphism, Meta-analysis

Background

Epilepsy is a chronic neurological worldwide disorder [1]. Most cases of epileptic patients respond to antiepileptic drugs (AEDs). However, about one-third of epileptic patients develop recurrent seizures, despite the efficacy of treatment at the optimal dose regimen. They are then, considered resistant to antiepileptic treatment [2]. The international league against epilepsy (ILAE) redefined refractory epilepsy in 2010 as the persistence of seizures after two adequate trials of appropriate and tolerated AEDs [3].

The exact mechanism of refractory epilepsy is not well understood. Two main hypotheses are potentially involved in the biological mechanism of AEDs resistance: transporter and target hypotheses. The transporter hypothesis supports the overexpression of drug efflux transporters at the blood–brain barrier (BBB) reducing AEDs access to the brain. The target hypothesis contends that the changes in drug intracellular target sites

---

* Correspondence: chch.m@hotmail.fr

†Equal contributors

[1]Department of Genetic, Tunis El Manar University, Faculty of Medicine of Tunis, 15 Jebel Lakhdhar street, La Rabta, 1007 Tunis, Tunisia

[2]Department of Child Neurology, National Institute Mongi Ben Hmida of Neurology, UR12SP24 Abnormal Movements of Neurologic Diseases, Jebel Lakhdhar street, La Rabta, 1007 Tunis, Tunisia

Full list of author information is available at the end of the article

(receptors) result in decreased sensitivity of AEDs [4, 5]. Therefore, the two mechanisms prevent pharmacological effects of antiepileptic at cerebral sites initiating seizures. It seems that genetic polymorphisms of drug transporter and target genes have a potential impact on the resistance to treatment: they may be responsible for the mechanisms of intractable epilepsy [5–7] by changing the function of genes products [8–10] and leading to the AEDs failure [4, 11–14]. Moreover, other authors have suggested that they may involve the prognosis of newly treated epilepsy [15]. Since drug-resistant epilepsy represents a major problem in the control of seizures, the researchers focused on the genetic profile to try to better understand the pharmacoresistance for a more effective treatment.

Since drug resistance often occurs in patients with multiple AEDs, the multidrug transporter hypothesis is considered better than the target hypothesis to explain the phenomenon of AEDs resistant epilepsy. However, the two hypotheses may complement each other. Given that drug transport mechanisms are the candidate mechanisms underlying AEDs resistance [16], many studies took significantly into consideration the association between efflux transporters overexpression inducing recurrent seizures.

Bioavailability and response to medication in epilepsy are mainly influenced by atp-binding cassette (ABC) transporter superfamily. The atp-binding cassette subfamily b member 1 (ABCB1) and the atp-binding cassette sub-family c member 2 (ABCC2) also known as multidrug resistance protein 1 (MDR1) and multidrug resistance protein 2 (MDR2), located at the membrane of BBB endothelial cells, are members of the ABC superfamily. They are the most studied candidate genes in pharmacoresistant epilepsy [5]. P-glycoprotein (P-gp) was the first human ABC protein that has been discovered [17]. ABCB1 gene encodes it and it affects a wide range of drugs distribution in target compartments [18–20]. The C3435T polymorphism is the most investigated polymorphism in the ABCB1 gene (single nucleotide polymorphism (SNP) in exon 26) and it has received the most attention. It has been associated with the variations in the expression levels of P-gp [21]. Previous studies focusing on the association between ABCB1 C3435T polymorphism and drug-resistant epilepsy showed discordant findings. Several studies have supported the hypothesis of this association (alleles, genotypes or haplotypes) to AEDs resistance [22–37]. However, a number of studies conducted on epileptic patients from different regions and ethnicities failed to confirm this result [38–42]. Subsequently, the opposed findings stimulated some previous meta-analyses of which the majority indicated that no association existed [43–49]. Besides, G1249A polymorphism is one of the common polymorphisms in the ABCC2 gene (SNP in exon 10). The overexpression of the ABCC2 transporter protein reduces AEDs

levels in brain tissues, which is a risk factor for pharmacoresistant epilepsy. A genotypic association between this polymorphism and responsiveness to AEDs has been suggested in Asian populations [50, 51]. However, other studies published contradictory results and they did not find any association [42, 52–56]. Furthermore, only two meta-analyses investigated its role in drug-resistant epilepsy and found that ABCC2 G1249A polymorphism was significantly associated with the decreased risk of AED resistance [57, 58].

Among their pharmacological effects, some AEDs may block voltage-dependent sodium channels [59, 60], which stimulate the researchers to investigate the potential link between drug-resistant epilepsy and polymorphisms in channels genes like SCN1A gene. This gene is the most studied drug target gene in epilepsy and it exhibits an intronic polymorphism IVS5-91G > A, one of the most common polymorphisms (SNP at intron splice donor site of exon 5). It alters the proportion of human brain NaV1.1-5N (exon 5N) and NaV1.1-5A (exon 5A) proteins, but the functional impact of the splicing on NaV1.1 is unknown. The correlation between SCN1A IVS5-91G > A polymorphism and maximum doses of Oxcarbazepine (OXC) may have a potential effect on resistant to epilepsy. The same study found the same correlation for ABCC2 G1249A polymorphism [61]. An additional study reported a genotypic association of SCN1A IVS5-91G > A polymorphism with the response to Carbamazepine (CBZ)/OXC [51, 62], and another one showed its role on pharmacoresponse to CBZ via an effect on GABAergic cortical interneurons [63]. However, other studies [64–66] and only one meta-analysis [67] were unable to replicate this association.

Overall, even the most considered polymorphisms that may explain mechanisms of pharmacoresistant epilepsy, showed contradictory and inclusive results. Therefore, we assembled pharmacogenetics (PGt) and pharmacogenomics (PGx) studies reporting associations between AEDs resistant epilepsy and eventual polymorphisms. Then, we performed an updated meta-analysis to clarify their role in response to AEDs.

Methods

We defined search strategy, study selection criteria, data elements and methods for study quality assessment.

Data sources and literature searches

We conducted a literature search using Pubmed and Cochrane Library with English-language restriction from January 1980 to November 2016. The key words used in the search strategy were: "anti-epileptic drug(s)", "antiepileptic drug(s)", "anti epileptic drug(s)" and "epilepsy" and "efficacy", "intractable", "refractory", "resistance", "resistant", "response to treatment", "pharmacoresistance", "pharmacoresistant" and "genetic factor(s)", "genotype(s)", "pharmacogenetic(s)", "pharmacogenomic(s)", "polymorphism(s)", "variant(s)", "variation(s)", "SNP(s)". We did not search of additional publications. The reported results followed the preferred reporting items for systematic reviews and meta-analyses guidelines (PRISMA).

Eligibility and inclusion criteria

For eligibility, we retained full-text publications showing a relationship between genetic polymorphisms and responsiveness of AEDs in epilepsy (monotherapy or polytherapy).

The included studies met the following criteria: 1) Original research articles reported a genotypic evaluation of polymorphisms and resistant epilepsy to antiepileptic treatment. 2) Studies compared AEDs-resistant cases with AEDs-responsive cases. 3) Studies showed sufficient individual genotype frequencies for specific genotype model. 4) At least three studies on the same polymorphism were available in order to avoid the non-pertinence of the results and the high risk of bias.

Data extraction

Two independent authors performed the data eligibility, they extracted the following information from each included study: first author, publication year, ethnicity of the study population, the number of cases and controls, genotype model for each polymorphism, age, gender, aetiology, type of epilepsy, and AEDs administered.

Data synthesis and analysis

We calculated the association between polymorphisms and AEDs resistant epilepsy using individual and overall odds ratios (OR) with corresponding 95% confidence intervals (CIs) by Forest Plot (Comprehensive Meta-Analysis Version 3, USA). The P-value determined the significance of the combined ORs. If the P-value (P) < 0.05, we considered the pooled ORs statistically significant [68]. The Z-value showed uniformisation of values and their position in the full distribution of values in the program. The I^2 statistic test assessed statistical heterogeneity among included studies; if I^2 < 50%, fixed-effects model pooled study data and if $I^2 \geq 50\%$, random-effects model pooled it [69]. Additionally, we performed subgroup analysis using genotype model to quantify the reported association between polymorphisms and AEDs resistant epilepsy in each reported genotypic model. To identify publication bias between the included studies, we applied Funnel plot and Egger's regression tests. The graph of Funnel plot reflected publication bias. Egger's test assessed and confirmed funnel plot's results: P < 0.05 determined the existence of bias [70].

Results

Evidence base

We identified a total of 640 potentially relevant articles. We excluded a total of 591 publications from the further analysis: abstract, articles showing absence of associations between polymorphisms and AEDs resistant epilepsy for insufficient data, case reports, duplicated articles, letter to the editors, meta-analysis, not epileptic studies, not human reports, researches about other treatments than AEDs, review articles and studies not related to associations between polymorphisms and AEDs resistant epilepsy (Fig. 1).

Among the 49 reports that met eligibility requirements], 39 reviewed an association between polymorphisms and epilepsy drug resistance [22–37, 50, 51, 62, 71–90]. We identified the majority of polymorphisms in AEDs transporter genes: ABCB1 and ABCC2. We also found other polymorphisms in AEDs target genes: gamma-aminobutyric acid-a receptor alpha1-subunit (GABRA1), gamma-aminobutyric acid-a receptor alpha2-subunit (GABRA2), gamma-aminobutyric acid-a receptor alpha3-subunit (GABRA3), sodium channel nav1.1 (SCN1A), sodium channel nav1.2 (SCN2A), in other potential genes as apolipoprotein e (ApoE), cytochrome p450 1a1 (CYP1A1), cytochrome p450 family member 2c9 (CYP2C9), gamma-aminobutyric acid transporter 3 (GAT3), glutathione s-transferases mu 1 (GSTM1) and solute ligand carrier family 6 member a4 (SLC6A4). We summarized the characteristics of polymorphisms implicated in AEDs resistance in different ethnic groups (Table 1). We excluded 10 full-text studies for insufficient data (Fig. 1). Only 13 met the inclusion criteria and constituted the data set for this analysis [22–29, 31, 33–36] (Table 2).

Data analysis

We carried out a meta-analysis to evaluate the relationship between ABCB1 C3435T polymorphism and AEDs resistance among AEDs-resistant patients vs. AEDs-responsive patients. The included studies were heterogeneous for the study characteristics. The analysis of data showed that 454 of 1653 AEDs-resistant patients (27.465%) and 282 of 1732 AEDs-responsive patients (16.282%) were included in the statistical analysis [22–29, 31, 33–36]. The frequency of AEDs-resistant cases was higher than AEDs-responsive patients. We divided the age of cases and controls into three subgroups: >20 years, 20–40 years, and <40 years. We divided the gender of cases and controls into two subgroups: males >50% and males <50%. A total of eight included studies were conducted in Asia [22, 23, 27–29, 34–36], three studies in Europe [25, 26, 31], one study in Egypt [24] and one another in Australia [33]. We classified the cases by epilepsy syndrome (idiopathic, cryptogenic or symptomatic epilepsy) [22, 23, 28, 31, 34, 36] or by

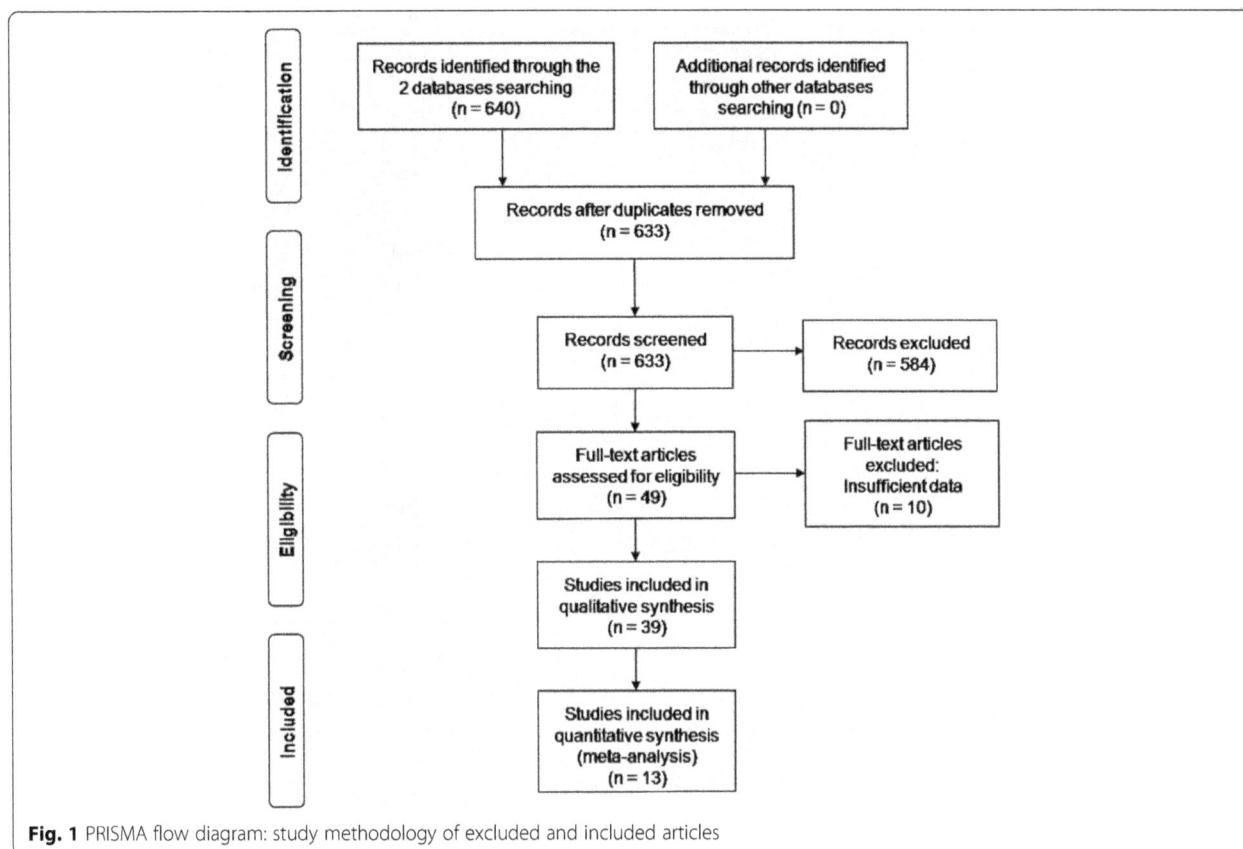

Fig. 1 PRISMA flow diagram: study methodology of excluded and included articles

seizure types (generalized or partial seizures) [22–24, 28, 29, 31, 33, 35, 36]. However, the classifications of cases by epilepsy syndrome were not mentioned in seven studies [24–27, 29, 33, 35] and the classifications of cases by seizure types were not mentioned in three studies [26, 27, 34]. Two studies were stratified by epilepsy syndrome [28, 31] and three studies were stratified by seizure types [29, 33, 35]. Cases were treated with AEDs polytherapy in seven studies [23, 26–29, 35, 36]. Only one study reported association between *ABCB1* C3435T polymorphism and cases with Phenytoin (PHT) therapy, the administration of PHT as monotherapy or polytherapy was not mentioned [24]. However, AEDs were not specified in five studies [22, 25, 27, 31, 33]. We summarized the characteristics of the available included studies in Table 2.

Association of *ABCB1* C3435T polymorphism with the susceptibility to AEDs resistance

The heterogeneity among the included studies was high ($I^2 = 82.961\%$, $P < 10^{-3}$) and we used a random-effects model [22–29, 31, 33–36]. The summary OR was 1.877, 95% CI 1.213–2.905, $P = 0.005$ showing that *ABCB1* C3435T was significantly associated with AEDs resistance (Fig. 2).

For the robustness of our findings, we used subanalysis by dominant (CC vs. TT) and recessive (TT vs. CC) genotype models. The heterogeneity among the nine included studies was high ($I^2 = 87.843\%$, $P < 10^{-3}$) in the dominant model [22–29, 31]. The summary OR was 1.686, 95% CI 0.877–3.242, $P = 0.117$ under a random-effects model (Fig. 3). The analysis of the recessive model revealed that the heterogeneity was absent ($I^2 = 0.000\%$, $P = 0.727$) among the four included studies [33–36]. The summary OR was 2.375, 95% CI 1.775–3178, $P < 10^{-3}$ under a fixed-effects model (Fig. 4). Therefore, the results of our present meta-analysis indicates that the association of *ABCB1* C3435T polymorphism with the risk of AEDs resistance, exists and it is more significant in *ABCB1* 3435TT genotype than in 3435CC genotype.

Analysis of publication bias

For the association between *ABCB1* C3435T polymorphism, *ABCB1* 3435CC, and 3435TT genotype models with AEDs resistance, Funnel Plot showed asymmetrical appearances (Figs. 5, 6 and 7) and Egger's regression test showed that $P = 0.413$, $P = 0.492$, and $P = 0.085$, respectively, were more than 0.05. The two tests demonstrated a significant publication bias.

Discussion

Epilepsy is a serious health problem affecting about 65 million people worldwide and manifesting many

Table 1 Characteristics of reviewed studies reporting associations between polymorphisms and AEDs resistance epilepsy

Gene	Polymorphism	Genotype model	Ethnicity	Reference
ABCB1	c.1199G > A (rs2229109)	GA vs. GG	Mexican	Escalante-Santiago et al. 2014 [71]
	c.1236T > C (rs1128503)	CC + CT vs. TT	Iranian	Maleki et al. 2010 [72]
	c.2677G > T/A (rs2032582)	AT + AG vs. GG + GT + TT	Mexican	Escalante-Santiago et al. 2014 [71]
		TT vs. GG + GT	European	Sánchez et al. 2010 [31]
			Malaysian	Subenthiran et al. 2013 [37]
		TT vs. GG		Subenthiran et al. 2013 [73]
			Japanese	Seo et al. 2006 [36]
	c.3435C > T (rs1045642)	CC vs. TT	Chinese	Hung et al. 2005 [22]
				Hung et al. 2007 [23]
			Egyptian	Ebid et al. 2007 [24]
			European	Sánchez et al. 2010 [31]
				Siddiqui et al. 2003 [25]
				Stasiołek et al. 2016 [26]
			Indian	Taur et al. 2014 [27]
			Iranian	Sayyah et al. 2011 [28]
			Thai	Keangpraphun et al. 2015 [29]
		CC vs. CT + TT	European	Basic et al. 2008 [30]
				Sánchez et al. 2010 [31]
		CC + CT vs. TT		Soranzo et al. 2004 [32]
		CT vs. CC + TT	Iranian	Sayyah et al. 2011 [28]
		TT vs. CC	Australian	Tan et al. 2004 [33]
			Chinese	Kwan et al. 2007 [34]
			Indian	Shaheen et al. 2014 [35]
			Japanese	Seo et al. 2006 [36]
		TT vs. CT + CC	Malaysian	Subenthiran et al. 2013 [37]
ABCC2	c.-24C > T (rs717620)	CT + TT vs. CC	Chinese	Qu et al. 2012 [74]
	c.-1019A > G (rs2804402)	AA vs. AG + GG	Indian	Grover et al. 2012 [75]
	c.-1549G > A (rs1885301)	GG vs. GA + AA		
	c.1249G > A (rs2273697)	AA vs. GG	Malaysian	Sha'ari et al. 2014 [50]
			Japanese	
		GA vs. GG	Chinese	
		GA + AA vs. GG		
		GA vs. GG + AA		Ma et al. 2014 [51]
	c.3972C > T (rs3740066)	CT vs. CC CC + TT vs. CC	Malaysian Chinese	Sha'ari et al. 2014 [50]
		CT + TT vs. CC		Qu et al. 2012 [74]
		TT vs. CC + CT	Mexican	Escalante-Santiago et al. 2014 [71]
ApoE	c.388T > C (rs429358), c.526C > T (rs7412)	e3/4 vs. e3/3 + e2/3	European	Sporiš et al. 2005 [76]
	c.388T > C (rs429358)	e4 vs. e2 + e3	Chinese	Gong et al. 2016 [77]

Table 1 Characteristics of reviewed studies reporting associations between polymorphisms and AEDs resistance epilepsy *(Continued)*

CYP1A1	IVS1 + 606C > A (rs2606345)	CC + CA vs. AA CC vs. CA + AA	Indian	Grover et al. 2010 [78]
CYP2C9	c.1075A > C (rs1057910)	CYP2C9*3/*3 vs. CYP2C9*1/*1+ CYP2C9*1/*3	European	Seven et al. 2014 [79]
GABRA1	IVS11 + 15A > G (rs2279020)	GG vs. AA + AG	Indian	Kumari et al. 2010 [80]
				Kumari et al. 2011 [81]
	c.74 + 448C > T (rs6883877)	CC vs. TC + TT	Thai	Hung et al. 2013 [82]
GABRA2	g.46240004A > G (rs511310)	GG vs. AA + AG		
GABRA3	c.-27 + 37622A > G (rs4828696)	TT vs. CC + CT		
GAT3	c.1572C > T (rs2272400)	CT + TT vs. CC	Korean	Kim et al. 2011 [83]
GSTM1	GSTM1*0	GSTM1- vs. GSTM1+	Chinese	Liu et al. 2002 [84]
SCN1A	c.3184A > G (rs2298771)	AA vs. AG + GG		Wang et al. 2014 [85]
		AG + GG vs. AA		Zhou et al. 2012 [86]
		AG vs. AA + GG	Egyptian	Abo El Fotoh et al. 2016 [87]
	IVS5-91G > A (rs3812718)	AA vs. AG + GG	Japanese	Ma et al. 2014 [51]
				Abe et al. 2008 [62]
SCN2A	IVS7-32A > G (rs2304016)	AA vs. AG + GG	Chinese	Kwan et al. 2008 [88]
SLC6A4	5-HTTLPR	L/L vs. S/L + S/S	European	Hecimovic et al. 2010 [89]
	STin2 VNTR	12/12 vs. 10/10	Argentinean	Kauffman et al. 2009 [90]
		12/12 vs. 10/12 + 10/10	European	Hecimovic et al. 2010 [89]

Abbreviation: ABCB1 atp-binding cassette sub-family b member 1, *ABCC2* atp-binding cassette subfamily c member 2, *ApoE* apolipoprotein e, *CYP1A1* cytochrome p450 1a1, *CYP2C9* cytochrome p450 family member 2c9, *GABRA1* gamma-aminobutyric acid-a receptor alpha1-subunit, *GABRA2* gamma-aminobutyric acid-a receptor alpha2-subunit, *GABRA3* gamma-aminobutyric acid-a receptor alpha3-subunit, *GAT3* gamma-aminobutyric acid transporter 3, *GSTM1* glutathione s-transferases mu 1, *SCN1A* sodium channel nav1.1, *SCN2A* sodium channel nav1.2, *SLC6A4* solute ligand carrier family 6 member a4

syndromes and types of seizures [60]. Since uncontrollable seizures increase morbidity and mortality, drug-resistant epilepsy is one of the major problems that physicians encounter. Recurrent seizures can devastate patients and their families. Therefore, drug-resistant epilepsy still remains one of the main challenges for epileptologists.

Since that genetic polymorphisms may play a role in response to AEDs [10], we conducted an updated systematic review in order to summarize the impact of polymorphisms in *ABCB1, ABCC2, ApoE, CYP1A1, CYP2C9, GABRA1, GABRA2, GABRA3, GAT3, GSTM1, SCN1A, SCN2A,* and *SLC6A4* genes on AEDs resistant epilepsy. Our meta-analysis concerned only the association between *ABCB1* C3435T polymorphism and drug-resistant epilepsy, which revealed a significant risk to pharmacoresistance (OR = 1.877, 95% CI 1.213–2.905, P = 0.005) (Fig. 2). Some studies confirmed our results [22–37]. Nevertheless, many other reports failed to prove an association between *ABCB1* C3435T polymorphism and refractory epilepsy [38–42, 91–96].

The first publication showed that drug-resistant patients compared to drug-responsive patients, were more likely to have the CC genotype than the TT genotype (P = 0.006) [25]. Zimprich et al. confirmed the result [97]. Moreover, many studies indicated that the CC genotype were more prevalent in drug-resistant epilepsy [12, 16–23]. However, three Asian studies [34–36] and one Australian study [33] showed the opposite association of TT genotype high frequency. In addition, our meta-analysis showed that patients resistant to AEDs were more likely to have *ABCB1* 3435TT genotype (OR = 2.375, 95% CI 1.775–3.178, $P < 10^{-3}$) than 3435CC genotype (OR = 1.686, 95% CI 0.877–3.242, P = 0.117) (Figs. 3 and 4).

Due to these controversial results, meta-analyses were made in order to clarify the association between *ABCB1* C3435T polymorphism and drug-resistant epilepsy. The majority suggest that the *ABCB1* C3435T polymorphism may not be involved in the response to AEDs [58–62]. The study of Bournissen et al. showed no association of *ABCB1* C3435T polymorphism with risk of drug resistance in overall and in the subgroup analysis by ethnicity (Asian and Caucasian populations) (n = 3371 subjects) [43]. The first study of Haerian et al. demonstrated the lack of allelic association with the risk of drug resistance under fixed and random effects models (n = 6755

Table 2 Summary of studies included into meta-analysis

Polymorphism	Genotype Model	Ethnicity	Total No.		Male %/Female %	Mean Age (years)	Aetiology of epilepsy	Type of epilepsy	AEDs	Reference
ABCB1 c.3435C>T	CC vs. TT	Chinese	Cases	331	56.193/43.807	39.1±11 [a] 38.5±13.4 [b]	Cryptogenic Cryptogenic, idiopathic	Generalized, partial	-	Hung et al., 2005 [22]
			Controls	-	-	-			-	Hung et al., 2007 [23]
			Cases	331	-	40.11±11 [a] 39.5±13.4 [b]	Cryptogenic Cryptogenic, idiopathic	Generalized, partial	CBZ, CNZ, GBP, LTG, OXC, PB, PHT, TPM, VGB, VPA	
			Controls	287	-	41±10.9			-	
		Egyptian	Cases	100	56/44	35.9±8.42	-	Generalized, partial	PHT [a]	Ebid et al., 2007 [24]
			Controls	50	64/36	38.6±10.32	-		-	
		European	Cases	289	49.827/50.173	27.0±18.5 [a] 26.0±19.8 [b]	Various [d]	Generalized, partial	-	Sánchez et al., 2010 [31]
			Controls	-	-	-			-	
			Cases	315	-	-	-	Generalized, partial	-	Siddiqui et al., 2003 [25]
			Controls	200	-	-			-	
			Cases	173	50.289/49.711	8.5±4.84 [a] 8.2±4.019 [b]	-	-	CBZ, GBP, LEV, LTG, OXC, TPM	Stasiolek et al., 2016 [26]
			Controls	98	53.061/46.939	8.3±4.64	-	-	-	
		Indian	Cases	115	73.215/26.786	34.69±10.06 [a] 38.02±11.46 [b]	-	-	CBZ, PB, PHT	Taur et al., 2014 [27]
			Controls	-	-	-			-	
		Iranian	Cases	332	52.711/47.289	28.8±11 [a] 27±13 [b]	Various [d]	Generalized, partial	CBZ, CNZ, LEV, LTG, OXC, PB, PHT, PRI, TPM, VPA	Sayyah et al., 2011 [28]
			Controls	-	-	-			-	
		Thai	Cases	110	52.727/47.273	41.96±12.19 [a] 46.65±12.65 [b]	-	Generalized, partial	CBZ, PB, PHT, VPA	Keangpraphun et al., 2015 [29]
			Controls	-	-	-			-	
ABCB1 c.3435C>T	TT vs. CC	Australian	Cases	609	-	-	-	Generalized, partial	-	Tan et al., 2004 [33]
			Controls	-	-	-			-	
		Chinese	Cases	746	-	-	Various [d]	-	-	Kwan et al., 2007 [34]
			Controls	-	-	-			-	
		Indian	Cases	220	65.455/34.545	8.1±2.47 [e]	Various [d]	-	CBZ, CLB, LEV, OXC, PHT, VPA	Shaheen et al., 2013 [35]

Table 2 Summary of studies included into meta-analysis (Continued)

Population	Group	N	Genotype	Age	Epilepsy classification	Epilepsy etiology	AEDs	Reference
	Controls	220	65.455/34.545	38.3±12.2 [f]	Generalized, partial	–	–	–
Japanese	Cases	210	56.667/43.333	10.5±4.5 [e] 37±10 [f]	Generalized, partial	Various [d]	AZA, CBZ, CLB, CNZ, DZP, ESM, Ethotoin, NTZ, PB, PHT, VPA, ZNS	Seo et al., 2006 [36]
				18.0±9.6 [a] 16.5±9.5 [b]				
	Controls	–	–	–	–	–	–	–

Abbreviation: AEDs anti-epileptic drugs, ABCB1 atp-binding cassette sub-family b member 1, AZA acetazolamide, CBZ carbamazepine, CLB clobazam, CNZ clonazepam, DZP diazepam, ESM ethosuximide, GBP gabapentin, LEV levetiracetam, LTG lamotrigine, NTZ nitrozepam, OXC oxcarbazepine, PB phenobarbital, PHT phenytoin, PRI primidone, TPM topiramate, VGB vigabatrin, VPA valproate, ZNS zonisamide, – = no data, [a] AEDs-resistant cases, [b] AEDs-responsive cases, [c] Administration of PHT as monotherapy or polytherapy was not mentioned, [d] Idiopathic, cryptogenic, symptomatic, [e] <15 years, [f] >15 years

Meta Analysis

Study name	Statistics for each study					Odds ratio and 95% CI
	Odds ratio	Lower limit	Upper limit	Z-Value	P-Value	
Hung et al. [16]	4.772	2.789	8.166	5.701	0.000	
Hung et al. [17]	0.415	0.247	0.696	-3.330	0.001	
Ebid et al. [18]	8.000	2.756	23.218	3.825	0.000	
Sánchez et al. [12]	1.889	1.086	3.284	2.254	0.024	
Siddiqui et al. [19]	2.044	1.132	3.691	2.371	0.018	
Stasiołek et al. [20]	2.526	1.291	4.944	2.705	0.007	
Taur et al. [21]	0.208	0.066	0.655	-2.683	0.007	
Sayyah et al. [22]	2.020	0.915	4.460	1.740	0.082	
Keangpraphun et al. [23]	1.483	0.672	3.271	0.976	0.329	
Tan et al. [26]	2.094	1.183	3.706	2.537	0.011	
Kwan et al. [27]	2.514	1.436	4.399	3.228	0.001	
Shaheen et al. [28]	2.928	1.711	5.009	3.921	0.000	
Seo et al. [15]	1.848	0.922	3.705	1.730	0.084	
Overall	**1.877**	**1.213**	**2.905**	**2.826**	**0.005**	
(I^2 = 82.961%, P = 0.000)						

Cases   Controls

Meta Analysis

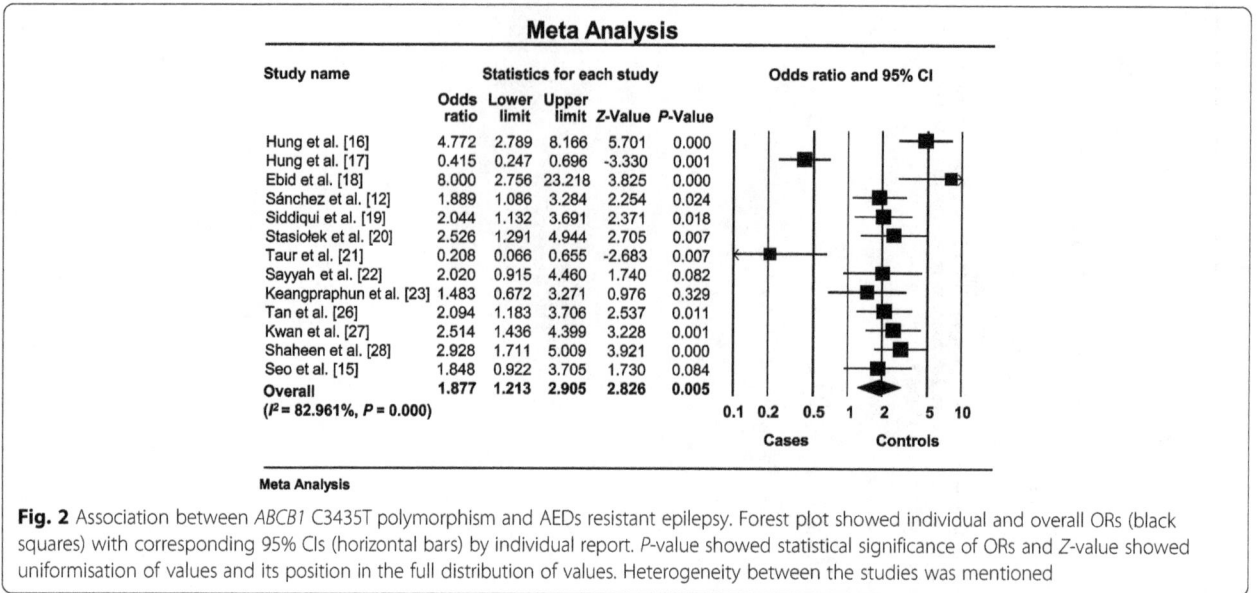

Fig. 2 Association between *ABCB1* C3435T polymorphism and AEDs resistant epilepsy. Forest plot showed individual and overall ORs (black squares) with corresponding 95% CIs (horizontal bars) by individual report. *P*-value showed statistical significance of ORs and *Z*-value showed uniformisation of values and its position in the full distribution of values. Heterogeneity between the studies was mentioned

subjects) [44] and the second study of Haerian et al. showed no significant association of *ABCB1* alleles, genotypes, and haplotypes with recurrent seizures (*n* = 7067 patients) [45]. In the two studies, subanalysis of studies by ethnicity (Asian and Caucasian populations) yielded similar findings. Nurmohamed et al. failed to find a statistical significance between genotypes of *ABCB1* C3435T polymorphism in cases and controls (*n* = 3996 subjects) [46]. No allelic neither genotypic association of *ABCB1* C3435T polymorphism with childhood risk of drug resistance was found in overall and in the subgroup analysis by ethnicity (Asian and Caucasian populations) (*n* = 1249 subjects) in the study of Sun et al. [47]. Recently, two meta-analyses have indicated that CC genotype was associated with recurrent seizures in Caucasians. However, none of the genetic comparisons

exhibited a significant association in Asians [63, 64]. In our knowledge, no another meta-analysis showed the same result as ours. Overall, meta-analyses stratified by genotype genetic models in the overall studies, indicate that the polymorphism may not play a major role in drug resistance to AEDs [46] and similar results are found in the subgroup analysis for the Asian and the Caucasian populations [43–45, 47]. However, other meta-analyses show a significant association in a specific ethnic subgroup [63, 64]. These discrepant results are mainly due to the small sample size, which is a common problem in association studies leading to underpowered genotypic results. Worldwide collaboration between different centers is then necessary to increase the sample size. In addition, ethnicity is another factor that may affect the results. An allele may become more common in ethnic subgroup but

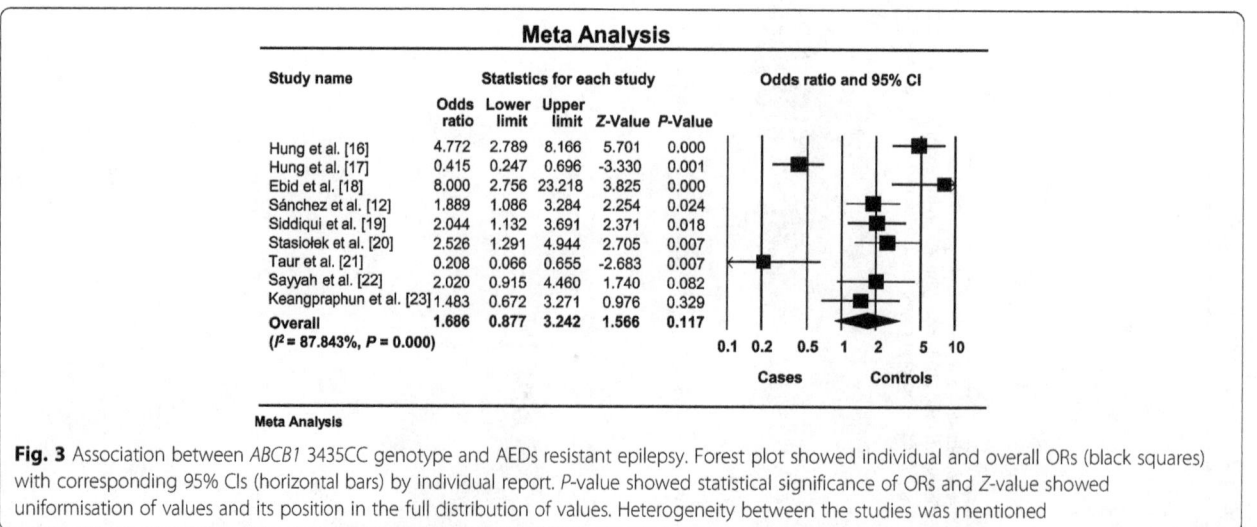

Meta Analysis

Study name	Statistics for each study					Odds ratio and 95% CI
	Odds ratio	Lower limit	Upper limit	Z-Value	P-Value	
Hung et al. [16]	4.772	2.789	8.166	5.701	0.000	
Hung et al. [17]	0.415	0.247	0.696	-3.330	0.001	
Ebid et al. [18]	8.000	2.756	23.218	3.825	0.000	
Sánchez et al. [12]	1.889	1.086	3.284	2.254	0.024	
Siddiqui et al. [19]	2.044	1.132	3.691	2.371	0.018	
Stasiołek et al. [20]	2.526	1.291	4.944	2.705	0.007	
Taur et al. [21]	0.208	0.066	0.655	-2.683	0.007	
Sayyah et al. [22]	2.020	0.915	4.460	1.740	0.082	
Keangpraphun et al. [23]	1.483	0.672	3.271	0.976	0.329	
Overall	**1.686**	**0.877**	**3.242**	**1.566**	**0.117**	
(I^2 = 87.843%, P = 0.000)						

Cases   Controls

Meta Analysis

Fig. 3 Association between *ABCB1* 3435CC genotype and AEDs resistant epilepsy. Forest plot showed individual and overall ORs (black squares) with corresponding 95% CIs (horizontal bars) by individual report. *P*-value showed statistical significance of ORs and *Z*-value showed uniformisation of values and its position in the full distribution of values. Heterogeneity between the studies was mentioned

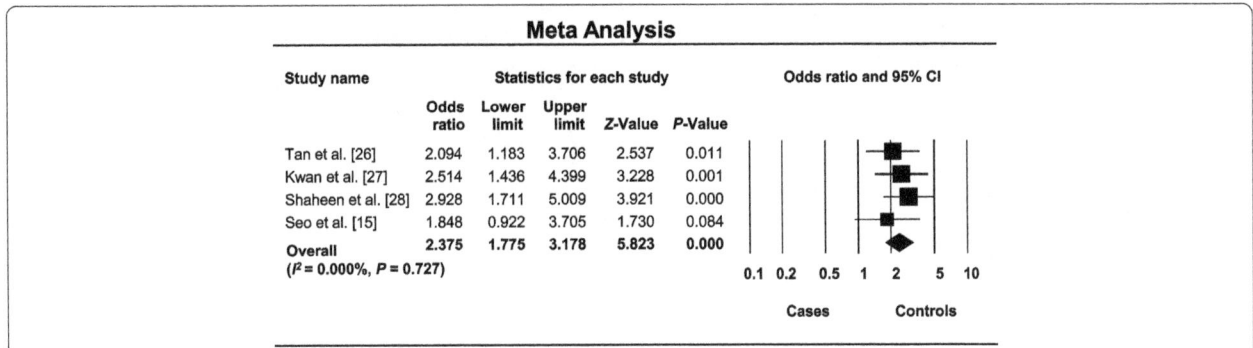

Fig. 4 Association between *ABCB1* 3435TT genotype and AEDs resistant epilepsy. Forest plot showed individual and overall ORs (black squares) with corresponding 95% CIs (horizontal bars) by individual report. *P*-value showed statistical significance of ORs and *Z*-value showed uniformisation of values and its position in the full distribution of values. Heterogeneity between the studies was mentioned

not in another, which may affect the response to AEDs [45]. However, four meta-analyses show no evidence that the *ABCB1* C3435T polymorphism is associated with the risk of resistance to AEDs in Asians and Caucasians [43–45, 47]. Therefore, meta-analysis startified by ethnicity are needed to increase in order to confirm the ethnic-dependence of AEDs resistant epilepsy.

AEDs transporters have contribute in pharmacoresistant epilepsy. In fact, the most studied AEDs transporter proteins like membrane proteins, are ABC transporter superfamily members. They are ATP-dependent drug efflux pumps for specific AED and are mainly encoded by *ABCB1* gene. ABCB1 protein or P-gp was transporte AED in the BBB [72]. P-gp activity can be affected by *ABCB1* polymorphisms reducing plasmatic levels of AEDs and minimizing antiepileptic treatment efficiency in epileptic patients [98, 99]. If genetic background affects the expression of P-gp, then penetration of AEDs in the brain might depend on the patient's genotype [16, 18].

Homozygous TT genotype is associated with decreased P-gp expression [4, 100].

Compared to literature search supporting conflicting results, our results show a higher contribution of *ABCB1* 3435TT genotype on response to AEDs. Our findings may contribute to exhibit the implication of genetic markers in refractory epilepsy before starting the treatment. In order to have a better AEDs therapeutic response, the identification of new potential genetic markers become necessary against pharmcoresistance in epilepsy. This will lead to a better understanding of drug resistance mechanisms in epilepsy. Furthermore, it will be extremely important for individual AEDs selection, early surgery feasibility and development of new efficacious treatments.

Limitations

Our analysis is consistent to our strategy search, inclusion criteria and statistical parameters. However, it may be limited due to several factors: 1) Few number of

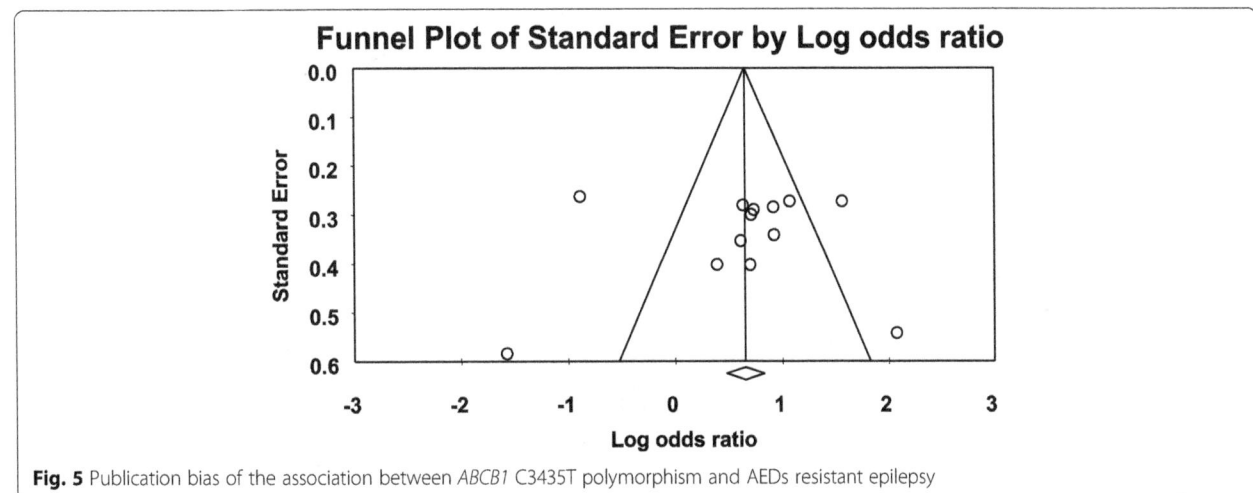

Fig. 5 Publication bias of the association between *ABCB1* C3435T polymorphism and AEDs resistant epilepsy

Funnel Plot of Standard Error by Log odds ratio

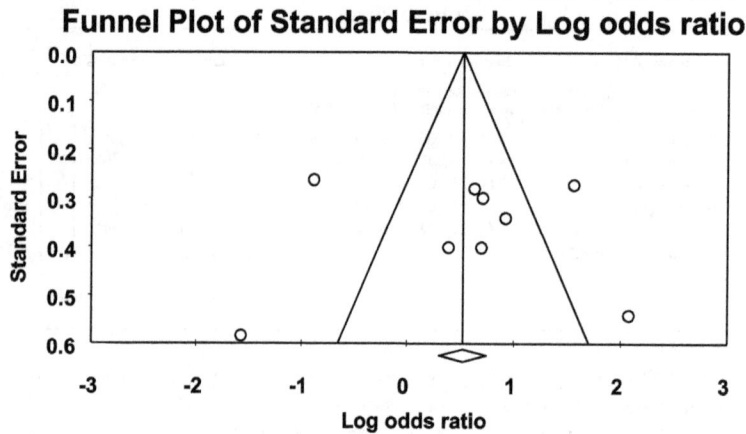

Fig. 6 Publication bias of the association between *ABCB1* 3435CC genotype model and AEDs resistant epilepsy

included studies is insufficient to carry out a subgroup analysis by ethnicity. In addition, the ethnicities in the included studies are heterogeneous. PGt and PGx studies of AEDs resistance should be performed by ethnicity. 2) Publication bias and heterogeneity might have an impact on the meta-analysis results. 3) Most of the included studies match different types of epilepsy with different AEDs. The affinity of each AED for ABC transporters is variable. In fact, Valproic acid (VPA) is a widely used AED and it is not transported by P-gp [101]. Thereby, the association between *ABCB1* C3435T polymorphism and drug resistance epilepsy could be affected. Correlation between PGt and PGx results with specific AED should be required. 4) Different inclusion criteria are used to classify AEDs-resistant patients in the included studies, subsequently, the interpretation of the meta-analysis results become very complex. In fact, AEDs-resistant patients were defined as patients who had at least one seizure per month or 10 seizures over the previous year, despite two or more AEDs at

therapeutic dosages and/or serum drug concentrations in three studies [22, 28, 34]. In other reports, drug resistance was defined as the occurrence of at least four seizures over the year despite more than three appropriate and tolerated AEDs for the epilepsy syndrome [25, 31, 33]. In some studies, it was defined as the failure of two appropriate and tolerated AEDs trials [27, 29], with a poor clinical outcome and recurrent seizures [35], or the occurrence of any types of seizures for a minimum of one year at the same dose of AEDs [36], or any seizures during the past three months [24] and more than 10 seizures over the year [23].

Conclusions
Various studies have yielded contradictory findings regarding the relationship between *ABCB1* C3435T polymorphism and AEDs resistance in epilepsy. In the current meta-analysis, we demonstrate the existence of a statistical significant association between *ABCB1* 3435TT genotype

Funnel Plot of Standard Error by Log odds ratio

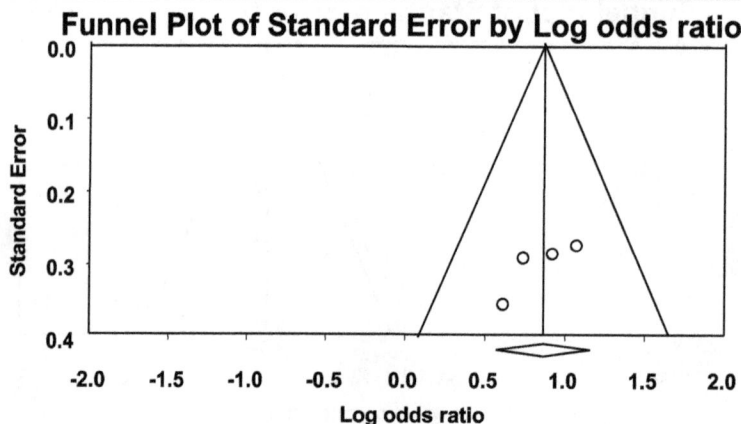

Fig. 7 Publication bias of the association between *ABCB1* 3435TT genotype model and AEDs resistant epilepsy

and refractory epilepsy. Therefore, the screening of *ABCB1* gene for this polymorphism in the future might be useful to decide the best treatment option for each patient and to predict the treatment outcome for new epileptic patients. However, considering the few number of included studies and the significant publication bias found in this meta-analysis, further investigations should be helpful to validate the use of this polymorphism in treatment decisions.

Abbreviations

ABC: atp-binding cassette; *ABCB1*: atp-binding cassette sub-family b member 1; *ABCC2*: atp-binding cassette sub-family c member 2; AEDs: Antiepileptic drugs; *ApoE*: Apolipoprotein e; BBB: Blood–brain barrier; CBZ: Carbamazepine; CIs: Confidence intervals; *CYP1A1*: Cytochrome p450 1a1; *CYP2C9*: Cytochrome p450 family member 2c9; *GABRA1*: Gamma-aminobutyric acid-a receptor alpha1-subunit; *GABRA2*: Gamma-aminobutyric acid-a receptor alpha2-subunit; *GABRA3*: Gamma-aminobutyric acid-a receptor alpha3-subunit; *GAT3*: Gamma-aminobutyric acid transporter 3; *GSTM1*: Glutathione s-transferases mu 1; ILAE: International league against epilepsy; *MDR*1: Multidrug resistance protein 1; *MDR2*: Multidrug resistance protein 2; ORs: Odds ratios; OXC: Oxcarbazepine; *P*: P-value; P-gp: P-glycoprotein; PGt: Pharmacogenetics; PGx: Pharmacogenomics; PHT: Phenytoin; PRISMA: Preferred reporting items for systematic reviews and meta-analyses guidelines; *SCN1A*: Sodium channel nav1.1; *SCN2A*: Sodium channel nav1.2; *SLC6A4*: Solute ligand carrier family 6 member a4; SNP: Single nucleotide polymorphism; VPA: Valproic acid

Acknowledgements
Not applicable.

Funding
Not applicable.

Authors' contributions
M.C. and W.K. contributed equally to this work: designed the study, collected the data, conducted the analyses and wrote the manuscript. K.T. helped to perform the outcome analyses. H.K., I.B.Y.T. and L.H. revised the manuscript. All authors read and approved the final document.

Competing interests
The authors declare that they have no competing interests.

Author details
[1]Department of Genetic, Tunis El Manar University, Faculty of Medicine of Tunis, 15 Jebel Lakhdhar street, La Rabta, 1007 Tunis, Tunisia. [2]Department of Child Neurology, National Institute Mongi Ben Hmida of Neurology, UR12SP24 Abnormal Movements of Neurologic Diseases, Jebel Lakhdhar street, La Rabta, 1007 Tunis, Tunisia. [3]Division of Histology and Immunology Division, Department of Basic Sciences, Faculty of Medicine of Tunis, 15 Jebel Lakhdhar street, La Rabta, 1007 Tunis, Tunisia. [4]Department of Genetic, Faculty of Medicine of Tunis, 15 Jebel Lakhdhar street, La Rabta, 1007 Tunis, Tunisia.

References
1. Depont C. The potential of pharmacogenetics in the treatment of epilepsy. Eur J Pedaetric Neurol. 2006;10(2):57–65.
2. Moshé SL, Perucca E, Ryvlin P, Tomson T. Epilepsy: new advances. Lancet. 2015;385(9971):884–98.
3. Kwan P, Arzimanoglou A, Berg AT, Brodie MJ, Hauser WA, Mathern G, et al. Definition of drug resistant epilepsy: consensus proposal by the ad hoc Task Force of the ILAE Commission on Therapeutic Strategies. Epilepsia. 2010; 51(6):1069–77.
4. Lazarowski A, Czornyj L, Lubienieki F, Girardi E, Vazquez S, D'Giano C. ABC transporters during epilepsy and mechanisms underlying multidrug resistance in refractory epilepsy. Epilepsia. 2007;48 (Suppl 5):140–9.
5. Tishler DM, Weinberg KI, Hinton DR, Barbaro N, Annett GM, Raffel C. MDR1 gene expression in brain of patients with medically intractable epilepsy. Epilepsia. 1995;36(1):1–6.
6. Loscher W, Klotz U, Zimprich F, et al. The clinical impact of pharmacogenetics on the treatment of epilepsy. Epilepsia. 2009;50(1):1–23.
7. Cascorbi I. ABC transporters in drug-refractory epilepsy: limited clinical significance of pharmacogenetics? Clin Pharmacol Ther. 2010;87(1):15.
8. Rau T, Erney B, Gores R, Eschenhagen T, Beck J, Langer T. High-dose methotrexate in pediatric acute lymphoblastic leukemia: impact of ABCC2 polymorphisms on plasma concentrations. Clin Pharmacol Ther. 2006;80(5): 468–76.
9. de Jong FA, Scott-Horton TJ, Kroetz DL, McLeod HL, Friberg LE, Mathijssen RH, et al. Irinotecan-induced diarrhea: functional significance of the polymorphic ABCC2 transporter protein. Clin Pharmacol Ther. 2007;81:42–9.
10. Haenisch S, Zimmermann U, Dazert E, Wruck CJ, Dazert P, Siegmund W, et al. Influence of polymorphisms of ABCB1 and ABCC2 on mRNA and protein expression in normal and cancerous kidney cortex. Pharmacogenomics J. 2007;7(1):56–65.
11. Sisodiya SM, Martinian L, Scheffer GL, van der Valk P, Cross JH, Scheper RJ, et al. Major vault protein, a marker of drug resistance, is upregulated in refractory epilepsy. Epilepsia. 2003;44(11):1388–96.
12. Schmidt D, Loscher W. Drug resistance in epilepsy: putative neurobiologic and clinical mechanisms. Epilepsia. 2005;46(6):858–77.
13. Kubota H, Ishihara H, Langmann T, Schmitz G, Stieger B, Wieser HG, et al. Distribution and functional activity of P-glycoprotein and multidrug resistanceassociated proteins in human brain microvascular endothelial cells in hippocampal sclerosis. Epilepsy Res. 2006;68(3): 213–28.
14. Remy S, Beck H. Molecular and cellular mechanisms of pharmacoresistance in epilepsy. Brain. 2006;129(Pt 1):18–35.
15. Speed D, Hoggart C, Petrovski S, Tachmazidou I, Coffey A, Jorgensen A, et al. A genome-wide association study and biological pathway analysis of epilepsy prognosis in a prospective cohort of newly treated epilepsy. Hum Mol Genet. 2013;23(1):247–58.
16. Kwan P, Brodie MJ. Potential role of drug transporters in the pathogenesis of medically intractable epilepsy. Epilepsia. 2005;46(2):224–35.
17. Potschka H, Fedrowitz M, Löscher W. P-glycoprotein and multidrug resistance-associated protein are involved in the regulation of extracellular levels of the major antiepileptic drug carbamazepine in the brain. Neuroreport. 2001;12(16):3557–60.
18. Loscher W, Potschka H. Blood-brain barrier active efflux transporters: ATP-binding cassette gene family. NeuroRx. 2005;2(1):86–98.
19. Fromm MF. Importance of P-glycoprotein at blood-tissue barriers. Trends Pharmacol Sci. 2004;25(8):423–9.
20. Sarkadi B, Homolya L, Szakács G, Váradi A. Human multidrug resistance ABCB and ABCG transporters: participation in a chemoimmunity defense system. Physiol Rev. 2006;86(4):1179–236.
21. Tate SK, Sisodiya SM. Multidrug resistance in epilepsy: a pharmacogenomic update (review). Exp Opin Pharmacother. 2007;8(10):1441–9.
22. Hung CC, Tai JJ, Lin CJ, Lee MJ, Liou HH. Complex haplotypic effects of the ABCB1 gene on epilepsy treatment response. Pharmacogenomics. 2005;6(4): 411–7.
23. Hung CC, Jen Tai J, Kao PJ, Lin MS, Liou HH. Association of polymorphisms in NR1I2 and ABCB1 genes with epilepsy treatment responses. Pharmacogenomics. 2007;8(9):1151–8.
24. Ebid AH, Ahmed MM, Mohammed SA. Therapeutic drug monitoring and clinical outcomes in epileptic Egyptian patients: a gene polymorphism perspective study. Ther Drug Monit. 2007;29(3):305–12.
25. Siddiqui A, Kerb R, Weale ME, Brinkmann U, Smith A, Goldstein DB, et al. Association of multidrug resistance in epilepsy with a polymorphism in the drug-transporter gene ABCB1. N Engl J Med. 2003;348(15):1442–8.
26. Stasiołek M, Romanowicz H, Połatyńska K, Chamielec M, Skalski D, Makowska M, et al. Association between C3435T polymorphism of MDR1 gene and the

incidence of drug-resistant epilepsy in the population of Polish children. Behav Brain Funct. 2016;12(1):21.

27. Taur SR, Kulkarni NB, Gandhe PP, Thelma BK, Ravat SH, Gogtay NJ, et al. Association of polymorphism of CYP2C9, CYP2C19, and ABCB1, and activity of P-glycoprotein with response to anti-epileptic drugs. J Postgrad Med. 2014;60(3):265–9.

28. Sayyah M, Kamgarpour F, Maleki M, Karimipoor M, Gharagozli K, Shamshiri AR. Association analysis of intractable epilepsy with C3435T and G2677T/A ABCB1 gene polymorphisms in Iranian patients. Epileptic Disord. 2011;13(2):155–65.

29. Keangpraphun T, Towanabut S, Chinvarun Y, Kijsanayotin P. Association of ABCB1 C3435T polymorphism with phenobarbital resistance in Thai patients with epilepsy. J Clin Pharm Ther. 2015;40(3):315–9.

30. Basic S, Hajnsek S, Bozina N, Filipcic I, Sporis D, Mislov D, et al. The influence of C3435T polymorphism of ABCB1 gene on penetration of Phenobarbital across the blood-brain barrier in patients with generalized epilepsy. Seizure. 2008;17(6):524–30.

31. Sánchez MB, Herranz JL, Leno C, Arteaga R, Oterino A, Valdizán EM, et al. Genetic factors associated with drug-resistance of epilepsy: relevance of stratification by patient age and aetiology of epilepsy. Seizure. 2010;19(2):93–101.

32. Soranzo N, Cavalleri GL, Weale ME, Wood NW, Depondt C, Marguerie R, et al. Identifying candidate causal variants responsible for altered activity of the ABCB1 multidrug resistance gene. Genome Res. 2004;14(7):1333–44.

33. Tan NC, Heron SE, Scheffer IE, Pelekanos JT, McMahon JM, Vears DF, et al. Failure to confirm association of a polymorphism in ABCB1 with multidrug-resistant epilepsy. Neurology. 2004;63(6):1090–2.

34. Kwan P, Baum L, Wong V, Ng PW, Lui CH, Sin NC, et al. Association between ABCB1 C3435T polymorphism and drug-resistant epilepsy in Han Chinese. Epilepsy Behav. 2007;11(1):112–7.

35. Shaheen U, Prasad DK, Sharma V, Suryaprabha T, Ahuja YR, Jyothy A, et al. Significance of MDR1 gene polymorphism C3435T in predicting drug response in epilepsy. Epilepsy Res. 2014;108(2):251–6.

36. Seo T, Ishitsu T, Ueda N, Nakada N, Yurube K, Ueda K, et al. ABCB1 polymorphisms influence the response to antiepileptic drugs in Japanese epilepsy patients. Pharmacogenomics. 2006;7(4):551–61.

37. Subenthiran S, Abdullah NR, Joseph JP, Muniandy PK, Mok BT, Kee CC, et al. Linkage disequilibrium between polymorphisms of ABCB1 and ABCC2 to predict the treatment outcome of Malaysians with complex partial seizures on treatment with carbamazepine mono-therapy at the Kuala Lumpur Hospital. PLoS One. 2013;8(5), e64827.

38. Chen L, Liu CQ, Hu Y, Xiao ZT, Chen Y, Liao JX. Association of a polymorphism in MDR1 C3435T with response to antiepileptic drug treatment in ethic Han Chinese children with epilepsy. Zhongguo Dang Dai Er Ke Za Zhi. 2007;9(1):11–4.

39. Grover S, Bala K, Sharma S, Gourie-Devi M, Baghel R, Kaur H, et al. Absence of a general association between ABCB1 genetic variants and response to antiepileptic drugs in epilepsy patients. Biochimie. 2010;92(9):1207–12.

40. Ozgon GO, Bebek N, Gul G, Cine N. Association of MDR1 (C3435T) polymorphism and resistance to carbamazepine in epileptic patients from Turkey. Eur Neurol. 2009;59(1-2):67–70.

41. Sills GJ, Mohanraj R, Butler E, McCrindle S, Collier L, Wilson EA, et al. Lack of association between the C3435T polymorphism in the human multidrug resistance (MDR1) gene and response to antiepileptic drug treatment. Epilepsia. 2005;46(5):643–7.

42. Ufer M, Mosyagin I, Muhle H, Jacobsen T, Haenisch S, Hasler R, et al. Nonresponse to antiepileptic pharmacotherapy is associated with the ABCC2-24C > T polymorphism in young and adult patients with epilepsy. Pharmacogenet Genomics. 2009;19(5):353–62.

43. Bournissen FG, Moretti ME, Juurlink DN, Koren G, Walker M, Finkelstein Y. Polymorphism of the MDR1/ABCB1 C3435T drug-transporter and resistance to anticonvulsant drugs: a meta-analysis. Epilepsia. 2009;50(4):898–903.

44. Haerian BS, Roslan H, Raymond AA, Tan CT, Lim KS, Zulkifli SZ, et al. ABCB1 C3435T polymorphism and the risk of resistance to antiepileptic drugs in epilepsy: a systematic review and meta-analysis. Seizure. 2010;19(6):339–46.

45. Haerian BS, Lim KS, Tan CT, Raymond AA, Mohamed Z. Association of ABCB1 gene polymorphisms and their haplotypes with response to antiepileptic drugs: a systematic review and meta-analysis. Pharmacogenomics. 2011;12(5):713–25.

46. Nurmohamed L, Garcia-Bournissen F, Buono RJ, Shannon MW, Finkelstein Y. Predisposition to epilepsy–does the ABCB1 gene play a role? Epilepsia. 2010;51(9):1882–5.

47. Sun G, Sun X, Guan L. Association of MDR1 gene C3435T polymorphism with childhood intractable epilepsy: a meta-analysis. J Neural Transm (Vienna). 2014;121(7):717–24.

48. Li SX, Liu YY, Wang QB. ABCB1 gene C3435T polymorphism and drug resistance in epilepsy: evidence based on 8,604 subjects. Med Sci Monit. 2015;21:861–8.

49. Lv WP, Han RF, Shu ZR. Associations between the C3435T polymorphism of the ABCB1 gene and drug resistance in epilepsy: a meta-analysis. Int J Clin Exp Med. 2014;7(11):3924–32.

50. Sha'ari HM, Haerian BS, Baum L, Saruwatari J, Tan HJ, Rafia MH, et al. ABCC2 rs2273697 and rs3740066 polymorphisms and resistance to antiepileptic drugs in Asia Pacific epilepsy cohorts. Pharmacogenomics. 2014;15(4):459–66.

51. Ma CL, Wu XY, Zheng J, Wu ZY, Hong Z, Zhong MK. Association of SCN1A, SCN2A and ABCC2 gene polymorphisms with the response to antiepileptic drugs in Chinese Han patients with epilepsy. Pharmacogenomics. 2014; 15(10):1323–36.

52. Ufer M, von Stulpnagel C, Muhle H, Haenisch S, Remmler C, Majed A, et al. Impact of ABCC2 genotype on antiepileptic drug response in Caucasian patients with childhood epilepsy. Pharmacogenet Genomics. 2011;21:624–30.

53. Seo T, Ishitsu T, Oniki K, Abe T, Shuto T, Nakagawa K. ABCC2 haplotype is not associated with drug-resistant epilepsy. J Pharm Pharmacol. 2008;60(5):631–5.

54. Kim DW, Lee SK, Chu K, Jang IJ, Yu KS, Cho JY, et al. Lack of association between ABCB1, ABCG2, and ABCC2 genetic polymorphisms and multidrug resistance in partial epilepsy. Epilepsy Res. 2009;84(1):86–90.

55. Kwan P, Wong V, Ng PW, Lui CH, Sin NC, Wong KS, et al. Gene-wide tagging study of the association between ABCC2, ABCC5 and ABCG2 genetic polymorphisms and multidrug resistance in epilepsy. Pharmacogenomics. 2011;12(3):319–25.

56. Hilger E, Reinthaler EM, Stogmann E, Hotzy C, Pataraia E, Baumgartner C, et al. Lack of association between ABCC2 gene variants and treatment response in epilepsy. Pharmacogenomics. 2012;13(2):185–90.

57. Chen P, Yan Q, Xu H, Lu A, Zhao P. The effects of ABCC2 G1249A polymorphism on the risk of resistance to antiepileptic drugs: a meta-analysis of the literature. Genet Test Mol Biomarkers. 2014;18(2):106–11.

58. Wang Y, Tang L, Pan J, Li J, Zhang Q, Chen B. The recessive model of MRP2 G1249A polymorphism decrease the risk of drug-resistant in Asian Epilepsy: a systematic review and meta-analysis. Epilepsy Res. 2015;112:56–63.

59. Pi Piana C, Antunes Nde J, Della PO. Implications of pharmacogenetics for the therapeutic use of antiepileptic drugs. Expert Opin Drug Metab Toxicol. 2014;10(3):341–58.

60. Franco V, Perucca E. The pharmacogenomics of epilepsy. Expert Rev Neurother. 2015;15(10):1161–70.

61. Ma CL, Wu XY, Jiao Z, Hong Z, Wu ZY, Zhong MK, et al. SCN1A, ABCC2 and UGT2B7 gene polymorphisms in association with individualized oxcarbazepine therapy. Pharmacogenomics. 2015;16(4):347–60.

62. Abe T, Seo T, Ishitsu T, Nakagawa T, Hori M, Nakagawa K. Association between SCN1A polymorphism and carbamazepine-resistant epilepsy. Br J Clin Pharmacol. 2008;66(2):304–7.

63. Menzler K, Hermsen A, Balkenhol K, Duddek C, Bugiel H, Bauer S, et al. A common SCN1A splice-site polymorphism modifies the effect of carbamazepine on cortical excitability--a pharmacogenetic transcranial magnetic stimulation study. Epilepsia. 2014;55(2):362–9.

64. Zimprich F, Stogmann E, Bonelli S, Baumgartner C, Mueller JC, Meitinger T, et al. A functional polymorphism in the SCN1A gene is not associated with carbamazepine dosages in Austrian patients with epilepsy. Epilepsia. 2008; 49(6):1108–9.

65. Manna I, Gambardella A, Bianchi A, Striano P, Tozzi R, Aguglia U, et al. A functional polymorphism in the SCN1A gene does not influence antiepileptic drug responsiveness in Italian patients with focal epilepsy. Epilepsia. 2011;52(5):e40–4.

66. Yip TS, O'Doherty C, Tan NC, Dibbens LM, Suppiah V, et al. SCN1A variations and response to multiple antiepileptic drugs. Pharmacogenomics J. 2014; 14(4):385–9.

67. Haerian BS, Baum L, Kwan P, Tan HJ, Raymond AA, Mohamed Z, et al. SCN1A, SCN2A and SCN3A gene polymorphisms and responsiveness to

antiepileptic drugs: a multicenter cohort study and meta-analysis. Pharmacogenomics. 2013;14(10):1153–66.

68. Cochran WG. The combination of estimates from different experiments. Biometrics. 1954;10:101–29.

69. Higgins JP, Thompson SG, Deeks JJ, Altman DG. Measuring inconsistency in meta-analyses. BMJ. 2003;327(7414):557–60.

70. Begg CB, Berlin JA. Publication bias and dissemination of clinical research. J Natl Cancer Inst. 1989;81(2):107–15.

71. Escalante-Santiago D, Feria-Romero IA, Ribas-Aparicio RM, Rayo-Mares D, Fagiolino P, Vázquez M, et al. MDR-1 and MRP2 Gene Polymorphisms in Mexican Epileptic Pediatric Patients with Complex Partial Seizures. Front Neurol. 2014;5:184.

72. Maleki M, Sayyah M, Kamgarpour F, Karimipoor M, Arab A, Rajabi A, Gharagozli K, et al. Association between ABCB1-T1236C polymorphism and drug-resistant epilepsy in Iranian female patients. Iran Biomed J. 2010;14(3): 89–96.

73. Subenthiran S, Abdullah NR, Muniandy PK, Joseph JP, Cheong KC, Ismail Z, et al. G2677T polymorphism can predict treatment outcome of Malaysians with complex partial seizures being treated with Carbamazepine. Genet Mol Res. 2013;12(4):5937–44.

74. Qu J, Zhou BT, Yin JY, Xu XJ, Zhao YC, Lei GH, et al. ABCC2 polymorphisms and haplotype are associated with drug resistance in Chinese epileptic patients. CNS Neurosci Ther. 2012;18(8):647–51.

75. Grover S, Gourie-Devi M, Bala K, Sharma S, Kukreti R. Genetic association analysis of transporters identifies ABCC2 loci for seizure control in women with epilepsy on first-line antiepileptic drugs. Pharmacogenet Genomics. 2012;22(6):447–65.

76. Sporis D, Sertic J, Henigsberg N, Mahovic D, Bogdanovic N, Babic T. Association of refractory complex partial seizures with a polymorphism of ApoE genotype. J Cell Mol Med. 2005;9(3):698–703.

77. Gong JE, Qu J, Long HY, Long LL, Qu Q, Li XM, et al. Common variants of APOE are associated with anti-epileptic drugs resistance in Han Chinese patients. Int J Neurosci. 2016;2:1–6.

78. Grover S, Talwar P, Gourie-Devi M, Gupta M, Bala K, Sharma S, et al. Genetic polymorphisms in sex hormone metabolizing genes and drug response in women with epilepsy. Pharmacogenomics. 2010;11(11):1525–34.

79. Seven M, Batar B, Unal S, Yesil G, Yuksel A, Guven M. The effect of genetic polymorphisms of cytochrome P450 CYP2C9, CYP2C19, and CYP2D6 on drug-resistant epilepsy in Turkish children. Mol Diagn Ther. 2014;18(2):229–36.

80. Kumari R, Lakhan R, Kalita J, Misra UK, Mittal B. Association of alpha subunit of GABAA receptor subtype gene polymorphisms with epilepsy susceptibility and drug resistance in north Indian population. Seizure. 2010; 19(4):237–41.

81. Kumari R, Lakhan R, Garg RK, Kalita J, Misra UK, Mittal B. Pharmacogenomic association study on the role of drug metabolizing, drug transporters and drug target gene polymorphisms in drug-resistant epilepsy in a north Indian population. Indian J Hum Genet. 2011;17(Suppl1):S32–40.

82. Hung CC, Chen PL, Huang WM, Tai IJ, Hsieh TJ, Ding ST, et al. Gene-wide tagging study of the effects of common genetic polymorphisms in the α subunits of the GABA(A) receptor on epilepsy treatment response. Pharmacogenomics. 2013;14(15):1849–56.

83. Kim DU, Kim MK, Cho YW, Kim YS, Kim WJ, Lee MG, et al. Association of a synonymous GAT3 polymorphism with antiepileptic drug pharmacoresistance. J Hum Genet. 2011;56(9):640–6.

84. Liu CS, Tsai CS. Enhanced lipid peroxidation in epileptics with null genotype of glutathione S-transferase M1 and intractable seizure. Jpn J Pharmacol. 2002;90(3):291–4.

85. Wang P, Zhou Q, Sheng Y, Tang B, Liu Z, Zhou B. Association between two functional SNPs of SCN1A gene and efficacy of carbamazepine monotherapy for focal seizures in Chinese Han epileptic patients. Zhong Nan Da Xue Xue Bao Yi Xue Ban. 2014;39(5):433–41.

86. Zhou BT, Zhou QH, Yin JY, Li GL, Qu J, Xu XJ, et al. Effects of SCN1A and GABA receptor genetic polymorphisms on carbamazepine tolerability and efficacy in Chinese patients with partial seizures: 2-year longitudinal clinical follow-up. CNS Neurosci Ther. 2012;18(7):566–72.

87. Abo El Fotoh WM, Abd El Naby SA, Habib MS, ALrefai AA, Kasemy ZA. The potential implication of SCN1A and CYP3A5 genetic variants on antiepileptic drug resistance among Egyptian epileptic children. Seizure. 2016;41:75–80.

88. Kwan P, Poon WS, Ng HK, Kang DE, Wong V, Ng PW, et al. Multidrug resistance in epilepsy and polymorphisms in the voltage-gated sodium channel genes SCN1A, SCN2A, and SCN3A: correlation among phenotype, genotype, and mRNA expression. Pharmacogenet Genomics. 2008;18(11): 989–98.

89. Hecimovic H, Stefulj J, Cicin-Sain L, Demarin V, Jernej B. Association of serotonin transporter promoter (5-HTTLPR) and intron 2 (VNTR-2) polymorphisms with treatment response in temporal lobe epilepsy. Epilepsy Res. 2010;91(1):35–8.

90. Kauffman MA, Consalvo D, Gonzalez-Morón D, Aguirre F, D'Alessio L, Kochen S. Serotonin transporter gene variation and refractory mesial temporal epilepsy with hippocampal sclerosis. Epilepsy Res. 2009;85(2-3): 231–4.

91. Lakhan R, Misra UK, Kalita J, Pradhan S, Gogtay NJ, Singh MK, et al. No association of ABCB1 polymorphisms with drug-refractory epilepsy in a north Indian population. Epilepsy Behav. 2009;14(1):78–82.

92. Kim DW, Kim M, Lee SK, Kang R, Lee SY. Lack of association between C3435T nucleotide MDR1 genetic polymorphism and multidrug-resistant epilepsy. Seizure. 2006;15(5):344–7.

93. Leschziner GD, Andrew T, Leach JP, Chadwick D, Coffey AJ, Balding DJ, et al. Common ABCB1 polymorphisms are not associated with multidrug resistance in epilepsy using a gene-wide tagging approach. Pharmacogenet Genomics. 2007;17(3):217–20.

94. Shahwan A, Murphy K, Doherty C, Cavalleri GL, Muckian C, Dicker P, et al. The controversial association of ABCB1 polymorphisms in refractory epilepsy: an analysis of multiple SNPs in an Irish population. Epilepsy Res. 2007;73(2):192–8.

95. Vahab SA, Sen S, Ravindran N, Mony S, Mathew A, Vijayan N, et al. Analysis of genotype and haplotype effects of ABCB1 (MDR1) polymorphisms in the risk of medically refractory epilepsy in an Indian population. Drug Metab Pharmacokinet. 2009;24(3):255–60.

96. Zhou L, Cao Y, Long H, Long L, Xu L, Liu Z, et al. ABCB1, ABCC2, SCN1A, SCN2A, GABRA1 gene polymorphisms and drug resistant epilepsy in the Chinese Han population. Pharmazie. 2015;70(6):416–20.

97. Zimprich F, Sunder-Plassmann R, Stogmann E, Gleiss A, Dal-Bianco A, Zimprich A, et al. Association of an ABCB1 gene haplotype with pharmacoresistance in temporal lobe epilepsy. Neurology. 2004;63(6):1087–9.

98. Liang LP, Ho YS, Patel M. Mitochondrial superoxide production in kainate-induced hippocampal damage. Neuroscience. 2000;101(3):563–70.

99. Lason W, Chlebicka M, Rejdak K. Research advances in basic mechanisms of seizures and antiepileptic drug action. Pharmacol Rep. 2013;65(4):787–801.

100. Hoffmeyer S, Burk O, von Richter O, Arnold HP, Brockmöller J, Johne A, et al. Functional polymorphisms of the human multidrug-resistance gene: multiple sequence variations and correlation of one allele with P-glycoprotein expression and activity in vivo. Proc Natl Acad Sci U S A. 2000; 97(7):3473–8.

101. Baltes S, Fedrowitz M, Tortós CL, Potschka H, Löscher W. Valproic acid is not a substrate for P-glycoprotein or multidrug resistance proteins 1 and 2 in a number of in vitro and in vivo transport assays. J Pharmacol Exp Ther. 2007; 320(1):331–43.

23

Content validity and clinical meaningfulness of the HFMSE in spinal muscular atrophy

Maria C. Pera[1], Giorgia Coratti[1], Nicola Forcina[1], Elena S. Mazzone[1], Mariacristina Scoto[2], Jacqueline Montes[3], Amy Pasternak[4], Anna Mayhew[5], Sonia Messina[6], Maria Sframeli[6], Marion Main[2], Robert Muni Lofra[5], Tina Duong[7], Danielle Ramsey[2], Sally Dunaway[3], Rachel Salazar[3], Lavinia Fanelli[1], Matthew Civitello[8], Roberto de Sanctis[1], Laura Antonaci[1], Leonardo Lapenta[1], Simona Lucibello[1], Marika Pane[1], John Day[7], Basil T. Darras[4], Darryl C. De Vivo[3], Francesco Muntoni[2], Richard Finkel[8] and Eugenio Mercuri[1]* (ID)

Abstract

Background: Reports on the clinical meaningfulness of outcome measures in spinal muscular atrophy (SMA) are rare. In this two-part study, our aim was to explore patients' and caregivers' views on the clinical relevance of the Hammersmith Functional Motor Scale Expanded- (HFMSE).

Methods: First, we used focus groups including SMA patients and caregivers to explore their views on the clinical relevance of the individual activities included in the HFMSE. Then we asked caregivers to comment on the clinical relevance of possible changes of HFMSE scores over time. As functional data of individual patients were available, some of the questions were tailored according to their functional level on the HFMSE.

Results: Part 1: Sixty-three individuals participated in the focus groups. This included 30 caregivers, 25 patients and 8 professionals who facilitated the discussion.
The caregivers provided a comparison to activities of daily living for each of the HFMSE items.
Part 2: One hundred and forty-nine caregivers agreed to complete the questionnaire: in response to a general question, 72% of the caregivers would consider taking part in a clinical trial if the treatment was expected to slow down deterioration, 88% if it would stop deterioration and 97% if the treatment was expected to produce an improvement.
Caregivers were informed of the first three items that their child could not achieve on the HFMSE. In response 75% indicated a willingness to take part in a clinical trial if they could achieve at least one of these abilities, 89% if they could achieve two, and 100% if they could achieve more than 2.

Conclusions: Our findings support the use of the HFMSE as a key outcome measure in SMA clinical trials because the individual items and the detected changes have clear content validity and clinical meaningfulness for patients and their caregivers.

Keywords: Spinal muscular atrophy, Quality of life, Carers, Clinical trials

* Correspondence: eumercuri@gmail.com
[1]Pediatric Neurology, Catholic University, Largo Gemelli 8, 00168 Rome, Italy
Full list of author information is available at the end of the article

Background

Several efforts have been made recently to identify disease specific outcome measures for spinal muscular atrophy (SMA) patients. The Hammersmith Functional Motor Scale Expanded (HFMSE), a motor function scale specifically designed for SMA, is widely used in patients. [1–3] The activities included in the original Hammersmith scale and in the expanded version were chosen by clinicians because of their functional relevance after careful observation and evaluation of many SMA patients [1–3].

The potential for therapeutic benefit from interventions in SMA has highlighted the need to obtain reliable documented evidence of patient input to support the clinical meaningfulness of the measures used in natural history studies and in clinical trials [4–7].

The activities included in the HFMSE have been found to be extremely useful in clinical practice as an assessment and rehabilitation tool, and in natural history studies and clinical trials to establish disease progression [8–15]. However, no systematic study has been performed to determine if the individual activities included in the scale are also relevant for patients and their caregivers.

This approach, to include the patient perspective, has been strongly encouraged by the United States Food and Drug Administration (FDA) [16]. This regulatory agency has indeed suggested that patient reported scales should be used to determine the relevance of the observed functional changes [17].

One of the challenges is that SMA is clinically very heterogeneous; and, even when restricted to the type 2 and 3 phenotypes whose functional domains are covered by the HFMSE, the clinical severity still ranges from non-ambulant sitting patients with only a few points on the scale to ambulant patients who may be able to complete nearly all of the 33 items on the scale [8, 9].

Another significant challenge is the variability of SMA types 2 and 3 disease progression, as reported by recent natural history studies, and the various factors, such as age or functional level, that influence different trajectories [10].

Because of these and other challenges, it is may be difficult to determine a clinically meaningful change for patients at different ages and at different functional levels. Moreover, it is not clear if similar quantitative improvements in the scale, two points for example, have the same clinical meaning regardless of where the patients score on the HFMSE scale.

This paper describes a two part study reporting: (1) patients' and caregivers' view on the clinical relevance of the HFMSE, and (2) the possible changes of HFMSE scores over time. More specifically, in the first part we aimed to explore caregivers' and patients' views on the clinical meaningfulness of each individual HFMSE item, asking them to describe the implications between the activity being explored in the individual items and the consequences as it relates to activities of daily living. In the second part we collected caregivers' views on the relevance of possible changes on the HFMSE scale. The novelty of our approach was that, rather than just asking general open questions, we tailored them according to each participant's specific functional level based on their HFMSE score.

Methods

Part 1: Content validity of the HFMSE

The first part was based on patients' and caregivers' focus groups as we explored content validity of individual HFMSE items. This qualitative study was conducted in Italy between June and October 2015 as part of a collaborative project with the two main Italian SMA advocacy groups (Famiglie SMA and Asamsi). The study was approved by the Ethical Committees of all the participating centers (Catholic University, Rome; University of Messina, Messina; UCL Institute of Child Health & Great Ormond Street Hospital, London; Columbia University Medical Center, New York; Harvard Medical School, Boston; Newcastle University, Newcastle; Stanford University; University of Central Florida College of Medicine, Orlando). Four focus groups were completed during the annual conventions of both advocacy groups. Three of the 4 focus groups included caregivers and one also included patients. The participants volunteered to be part of these activities and signed a dedicated consent form. No compensation was provided for their participation.

Patients and caregivers were given a form describing the items of the HFMSE, in lay language, illustrating the activities included in the scale with some pictures. They were then asked to comment on the relevance of the individual items, whether each activity assessed in the items could be related to activities of daily living, and if and why this was relevant to them.

Each focus group was run by a psychologist and a member of our team (clinician or Physical therapist) who transcribed the responses immediately before moving to the next item.

The results of the various groups were analyzed by assigning a code to each response and by identifying consistencies across the various groups tabulating the frequency of individual responses in the various subgroups.

Part 2: Clinical meaningfulness of HFMSE changes

The aim for this part was to establish the view of the caregivers on the clinical relevance of HFMSE changes in relation to their children's functional level. This could only be performed in patients who had a recent clinical functional assessment. This study was part of an international effort.

From September 2015 to April 2016, we administered a questionnaire or conducted semi-structured telephone interviews with caregivers of type 2 and 3 SMA patients.

All consecutive patients attending our clinics, who routinely underwent functional assessments, were included. Telephone interviews were only conducted if patients had been seen within the previous 3 months and if the results of their functional assessments were available.

All centers shared the same training and had already performed inter-observer reliability for the HFMSE [10]. Study participants did not receive any form of compensation. Caregivers were first asked to provide general information regarding the patients' disease course over the last year and their expectations for the near future.

An innovative aspect of this questionnaire was the introduction of specific questions that were related to the subjects' motor performance as assessed by the standardized HFMSE functional scale. In the scale the items follow a hierarchical order with increasing difficulty, from top to bottom, built on the frequency distribution of findings observed in a large cohort of SMA patients The score on the scale provides a clear indication of the patient's functional level, and the subsequent activities represent activities likely to be achieved.

The advantage of this approach is that caregivers are asked questions about activities that are realistically close to their child's possible achievements, rather than generic questions on other activities, such as walking or running for non-ambulant type 2 SMA patients, that clearly would be highly desirable but difficult or impossible to achieve in a limited time frame.

The first two questions evaluated the caregiver's impression of the patient's overall function during the past year, and their expectations for the next two years (see appendix for details of the questionnaire).

The second set of questions included open-ended inquiries that were, according to the caregivers, the most important activities/functions of daily living that they hoped would be maintained or gained in their children.

Caregivers were finally asked to provide information on their expectations regarding clinical trials.

They were informed on the next three items that their child could not achieve on the HFMSE scale, asking more specifically, if achieving at least one of these abilities would justify their participation in a clinical trial.

The last question enquired whether the caregivers would consider having their child take part in a potential trial in the presence of mild side-effects. A trained clinician conducted the in-person interviews and telephone interviews using a semi-structured data collection sheet. The interviews lasted 15-20 min on average. The questions covered caregivers' views and expectations regarding a possible participation in a clinical trial.

Statistical Analysis: Responses of the non-ambulant and ambulant groups were compared for significant difference using the Wilcoxon-Mann-Whitney test. A p value of <0.05 was considered significant.

For the question assessing whether parents would consider entering in a study if their child could achive at least 1 (score0), two (score 1) or more than 2 activities on the HFMSE, a Chi-square analysis was used to was used to correlate the level of responses (0, 1, 2) with functional scores. A p value of <0.05 was considered significant.

Results
Part 1: Content validity
Sixty-three individuals participated in the focus groups. These included 30 caregivers and 25 patients. Eight professionals (psychologists, Physical Therapists or clinicians) conducted the interviews and facilitated the discussion by introducing the items without contributing to data collection in an effort to avoid bias.

Patient ages ranged from 14 to 35 years, 3 were ambulant and 22 non ambulant (20 type 2 and 2 type 3).

The caregivers were all parents (17 mothers and 13 fathers). The age of the patients represented by the caregivers ranged between 2 and 26 years, 5 were ambulant and 25 non ambulant (all type 2). Only one parent/caregiver was allowed to participate for each patient.

The caregivers commented on all the functional scale items and provided a comparison to activities of daily living for each of them. Table 1 shows the responses in the 4 focus groups illustrating whether some responses were reported in more than one focus group. Many activities (64.07%) were suggested by more than one group with only 37 of the 103 activities suggested by one group only. Of these 37, only 7 were suggested by the group including patients.

Part 2
One hundred-forty-nine of the 151 caregivers who were invited to participate agreed to complete the questionnaire (response rate 98.7%). The caregivers were all parents (Additional file 1).

The patient ages ranged from 17 months to 30 years. Thirty-three patients were ambulant and 116 non ambulant (109 type 2 and 7 type 3).

When asked to describe the patients' clinical course over the last year, 15% reported stability, 72% deterioration and 12% improvement.

When asked what to expect in the next 2 years, 21% anticipated a stable course, 70% a deterioration and 9% an improvement. Figure 1 summarizes the distribution of findings for both questions.

When asked to summarize their expectations regarding clinical trials, 72% of the caregivers would participate if the treatment slowed down deterioration, 88% if it

Table 1 Details of the caregivers and patients' responses in the 4 focus groups

HMFSE Item	HMFSE activities	Answers	Group 1	Group 2	Group 3	Group 4
1	Able to sit on chair or with legs off bed with or without hand support	Sitting on normal school chair or public spaces (stools in restaurant)	●	●	●	●
		Sitting on toilet	●	●		●
		Sitting in car			●	
		Independence out of the house	●			●
		Dress by herself/himself		●		
2	Able to sit on floor cross legged or legs stretched in front	Play on floor with siblings	●	●	●	●
		Sit on lounge chair, deck-chair		●		●
		Picnic			●	●
		Travel with less equipment	●			
		Inclusion in activities		●		
3	Able to bring hands to face at eye level	Wash face	●	●	●	●
		Brush and style	●	●	●	●
		Eat	●		●	
		Put on eye glasses	●	●		●
		Answer telephone			●	
		Blow nose	●			
4	Able to bring hands to head	Scratch head	●	●	●	●
		Wash, brush, style hair		●	●	●
		Put on hat	●	●		●
		Dress upper body	●		●	
5	Roll to side	Sleep by myself in my own room		●	●	
		Caregiver does not have to wake up to turn him/her	●	●		●
		Help during dressing lying down		●	●	
		Not having to turn head to see	●			
6-7-8-9	Roll	Play	●	●		
		Sleep well		●	●	
		Sunbathe		●	●	
		Experience space	●			●
		Reach for something at sides when lying down		●		●
10	Able to lye down from sitting	Independence: lye down and rest when tired	●	●	●	●
		Fun movement when falling	●	●		
		Rest on the back			●	
		Safety: Fall in a controlled way (avoid head trauma)	●			
11	Able to raise head when lying prone	Turn head react to stimulus, visual exploration of surroundings	●	●	●	
		Read a book	●		●	●
		Not be afraid of choking		●		
		Watch TV		●		●
		On beach not get sand in face	●			
12-13	Able to prop on forearms or extend arms	Read a book	●	●	●	

Table 1 Details of the caregivers and patients' responses in the 4 focus groups *(Continued)*

#	Item	Response	FG1	FG2	FG3	FG4
		Watch TV		•	•	•
		Stretch back	•			
		Sun bathe			•	
14	Able to sit up from lying	No need for assistant	•	•	•	
		Wake up and not have to wait for someone to sit me up	•	•	•	•
		Independence	•	•		
		Sit up and drink at night	•			•
15	Able to four-point kneel	Play like an animal in school	•		•	•
		Hiding				•
		Be able to fit under small spaces				•
16	Able to crawl	Move around	•	•	•	•
		Experience space		•	•	
		Go get objects	•	•		
		Play on floor			•	•
17	Lift head from supine	Change head position	•	•	•	
		Drink at night			•	•
		Read	•			
		Watch TV		•		
		Check the clock or alarm				•
18	Stand with support	Use toilet standing (boy)	•		•	•
		Use full length mirror, perceive body dimensions and proportions	•	•		
		Shower properly	•			
		Climb in car			•	
		Use kitchen burners, cook		•		
19	Stand without support	Public spaces: wait for bus, stand in cue		•		
		Cook			•	
		Use normal sink	•			
		Dress			•	
		Reach something on a shelf				•
20	Able to walk	Freedom	•	•	•	
		Go where and when you please	•	•	•	
		Get to places	•	•	•	
		Not to have to rely on wheelchair batteries			•	
21-22	Able to flex hip from supine	Dress (pants, socks)	•	•	•	•
		Scratch legs, kill mosquito	•	•		
		Change position			•	
23-24-25-26	Able to half kneel	Pick up object on floor		•	•	
		Tie shoe laces	•	•		
		Put away object on low surfaces	•			
		Pet a dog		•		
		Play			•	
		Make a proposal				•
		Kneel in church				•

Table 1 Details of the caregivers and patients' responses in the 4 focus groups *(Continued)*

		Talk with a kid				•
27	Able to go from standing to sitting	Not get hurt when falling or not fall in an embarrassing way	•		•	
		Sit on grass or sand	•	•		•
		Pet a dog			•	
		Sit beside a friend in same position/play on floor	•		•	
		Pick up something from floor		•		•
28	Able to squat	Sit when needed	•		•	
		Pick up objects on floor		•	•	•
		Pee	•			•
		Tie shoes			•	
		Pull up trousers	•			
29	Able to jump	Have fun, play	•	•	•	•
		Dance, gymnastics		•	•	
		Avoid obstacles	•	•		•
		Normality	•		•	
		Go to friends' home regardless of where they live	•		•	•
		Stay and live in my own home		•		
30-31-32-33	Go up and down stairs	Absence of barriers	•	•	•	•
		Normality	•	•		
		Go to friends' home regardless of where they live	•	•		•
		Stay and live in my own home			•	

would stop deterioration and 97% if the treatment produced an improvement.

When we correlated the responses to the functional status of the patients, the percentage of caregivers willing to take part in a clinical trial, if the treatment was expected to slow down deterioration, was higher in the non-ambulant group (76%) than in the ambulant group (61%) even though the difference was not significant ($p > 0.05$) (Figure 2 and 3).

When asked, after being informed of the next three items that their child could not achieve on the HFMSE

scale, if achieving at least one of these abilities completely (score 2) would justify their participation in a clinical trial, 75% would consider taking part if they could achieve at least one of these abilities, 89% if they could achieve 2 and 100% if they could achieve more than 2. The results were widely distributed across functional levels and age. The correlation between the responses and the functional scores was not significant ($p > 0.05$).

The percentage of caregivers considered participating in a clinical trial if their child might achieve one activity was not significantly different among the ambulant and

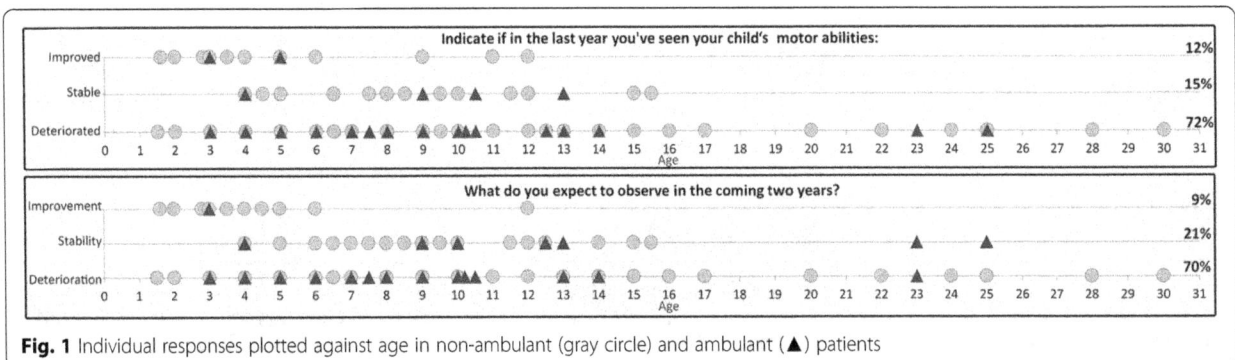

Fig. 1 Individual responses plotted against age in non-ambulant (gray circle) and ambulant (▲) patients

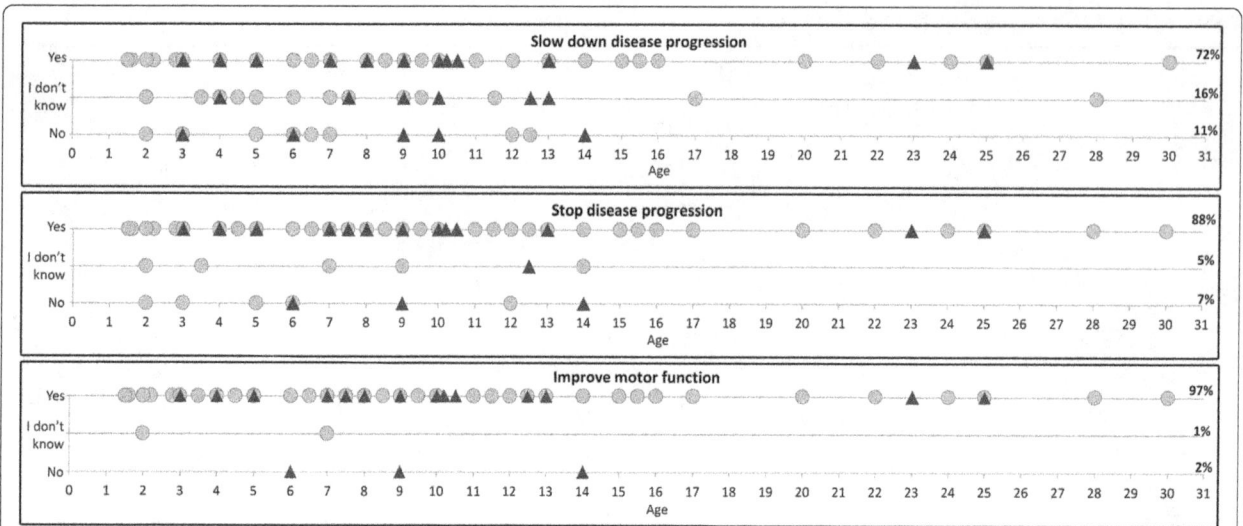

Fig. 2 Individual responses to the question: 'Would you agree to have your child take part in a potential trial if, in the absence of side-effects or with possible minimal side-effects, the prospect was to slow down a possible decline in motor function for at least two years?'

non ambulant groups ($p > 0.005$), a list of of the most frequent activities that caregivers hope will be achieved is provided in Table 2. The results were widely distributed across functional levels and age (Fig. 4).

Discussion

The results of our first study, assessing content validity, confirm that the activities of the HFMSE, known to be relevant both in clinical and research practice, are also clinically meaningful to patients and their caregivers. Following the FDA guidelines [18], we used a questionnaire exploring all items and a structured qualitative interview as part of focus groups, in a cohort of patients

and caregivers that included both genders, patients of different ages, and SMA patients who represent the full range of motor function captured on the HFMSE. The analysis of the transcripts of the focus groups demonstrated that each activity included in the HFMSE was related to activities of daily living that were relevant to patients and their caregivers, as often suggested by many participants in more than one focus group. The group including patients had similar responses to the other 3 groups, only including parents, for 101 of the 103 responses provided. Each of the items and the explored domains were thought to be appropriate for use in SMA.

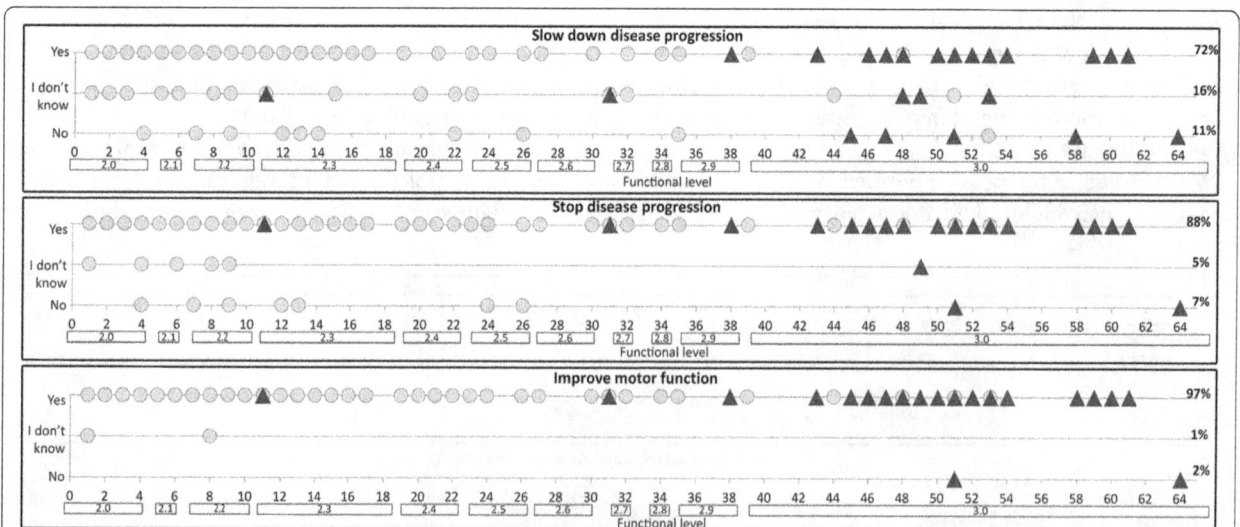

Fig. 3 Individual responses to the same question as in fig. 2. Responses are plotted against functional level for non ambulant (gray circle) and ambulant (▲) patients. Functional level is defined both using the raw HFMSE scores and the classification expressing severity in decimals, starting from 2.1, for patients who are just able to sit, to the strongest type 2, 2, who are able to stand but not to walk, to the type 3 [1]

Table 2 Details of the most frequent activities that caregivers hope will be achieved

Activities to achieve	%	Activities to achieve	%
Strength in the upper limbs	15,7%	Stand up from a chair	2,5%
Rolling	9,0%	Stand up from floor	2,5%
Walking	7,1%	Respiratory function	2,2%
Standing independently	6,2%	Writing skills	2,2%
Strength of the head	5,6%	Run	1,9%
Personal hygiene	4,9%	General autonomy	1,5%
Move independently	4,9%	Crawling	1,5%
Do stairs	4,6%	Hop/Jump	1,5%
Eat independently	3,1%	Strength of the hands	1,5%
Sit independently	3,1%	Use manual wheel-chair	1,2%
Strength in the lower limbs	2,8%	Balance	1,2%
Strength of the trunk	2,8%	Standing with support	1,2%

Not surprisingly, as also demonstrated in the second part of our study, the responses of patients and caregivers showed a degree of heterogeneity. This can be easily explained by the fact that the patients included in our study had a wide age range, from infants below age 2 years to adults in their thirties, and variable functional levels, from very weak patients with a HFMSE score of 0 who could only sit very briefly to strong ambulant patients who achieved the highest scores on the scale. It is, therefore, expected that the responses of individual patients/caregivers focused on the activities that were most challenging for them/their child, according to their respective functional levels.

In the second part of our study we also explored the perception of the families regarding their child's disease course with respect to motor function. The majority (72%) felt that over the last year their child had deterioration, whereas 15% reported a stabilization. The remaining 12% reported an improvement, and this occurred mainly in the younger end of the cohort. These results are in agreement with our recent collaborative study showing that a clinical improvement could be detected mainly in young children up to age 6 years as documented on the HFMSE. Clinical deterioration was more likely to occur around puberty [10].

As a result, over 70% of the caregivers felt that they would consider participating in a clinical trial if, in the absence of significant side effects, the intervention would slow down the rate of deterioration. Not surprisingly there were even higher percentages of caregivers considering participating in a trial if the prospect was stabilization (88%) or improvement (97%). These results should be interpreted with caution as considering participation in a clinical trial is complex and not all the studies have the same demands or the same possible outcomes. Nevertheless, these findings are already, in and of themselves, strongly indicative that caregivers would consider a trial even if the prospect was limited to influencing the rate of deterioration regardless of age or functional level.

In the second part of this study we tried to explore, in further detail, whether achieving or maintaining activities on the HFMSE had the same relevance regardless of HFMSE scores and, therefore, different functional levels.

The advantage of this approach is that the caregivers could relate the questions to the actual status of the child and were asked questions about activities that were realistically close to their child's possible achievements rather than generic questions on activities, such as walking or running that would be highly desirable but, at least in a limited time frame, difficult or impossible to achieve especially for the weakest patients. When asked if they would consider taking part in a trial if there was the possibility of achieving one, two, or more than two activities, 75% considered participation even if just one activity was achieved. These results were widely distributed across functional levels and age.

Conclusions

These findings suggest that even if the achievable activities are different, any improvement is considered to be meaningful, regardless as to whether the baseline score

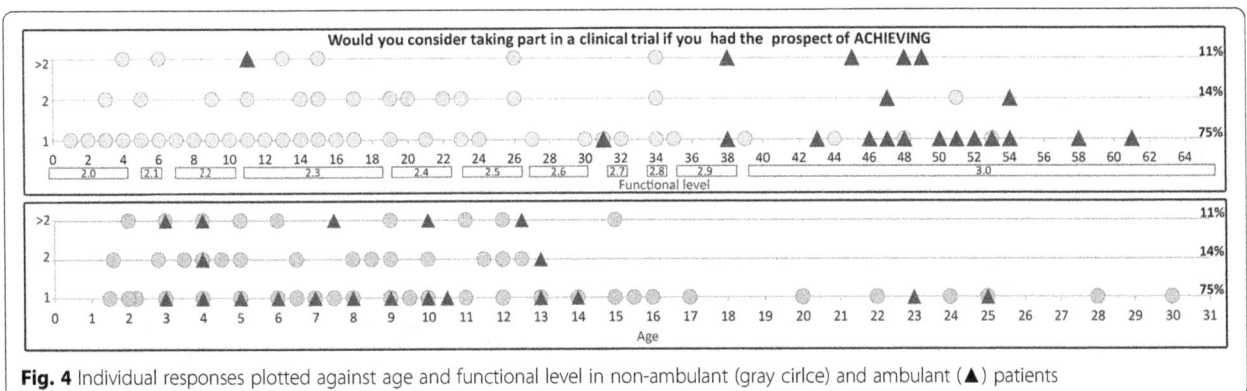

Fig. 4 Individual responses plotted against age and functional level in non-ambulant (gray cirlce) and ambulant (▲) patients

is very low, in the middle, or very high. This conclusion is particularly important considering the fact that the ordinal nature of the scale makes this comparison difficult.

This study has several limitations; first, the number of patients was relatively small but the range of age and functional level was quite wide and representative of the ambulant and non-ambulant SMA population. Since the Italian and English versions of the questionnaire's data collection sheet, and the forms used to illustrate the items with pictures from the scale manual, were piloted and validated before their use, these findings can justify another follow-on study with a larger cohort.

All the patients were followed in tertiary care centers or were part of advocacy groups and were unlikely to be representative of a more general population. While this is a potential bias, these patients are more likely to be representative of a trial population with appropriate standards of care and level of information and participation. Another apparent limitation is the fact that, in the second part of the study, we only involved caregivers. This was, however, necessary in order to include patients of all ages; very young patients would have not been able to complete the questionnaires. We acknowledge that the patient's perspective is however very important and further studies are in progress to collect data directly from patients who are older than age 12 years.

Despite these limitations, the study results support the use of the HFMSE as a robust outcome measure in clinical trials, not only because all the individual items appear to be meaningful to patients and caregivers, but also because even small changes detected on the scale appear to be relevant and to justify participation in a clinical trial. The great majority of the caregivers would already consider participation of their children in a clinical study even if the best outcome would be just to reduce deterioration. Of course, even more caregivers would agree to their child's participation if the prospect was to remain stable or improve; however, it is of interest that even when aiming for an improvement, a small improvement (just one activity) would already be sufficient in their mind to justify participation in a trial with an investigational drug.

Finally, these results are important as they provide the views of patients and caregivers and complement other studies currently being performed and designed to establish item response theory approach and the minimally important difference using statistical analysis.

Abbreviations
FDA: Food and Drug Administration.; HFMSE: Hammersmith Functional Motor Scale Expanded; SMA: Spinal muscular atrophy

Acknowledgments
None

Funding
In Italy, the study was supported by Famiglie SMA and Telethon (MC Pera and ES Mazzone; GUP: GSP13002). The authors are grateful to Famiglie SMA and ASAMSI Italy for their help in organizing the focus groups during their annual conferences. In UK, the SMA Trust financial provided support to M Scoto, D Ramsey and F Muntoni. The financial support of the Muscular Dystrophy UK Centre grant; of the MRC Translational Research Centre to UCL and Newcastle, and of the National Institute for Health Research Biomedical Research Centre at Great Ormond Street Hospital for Children NHS Foundation Trust and University College London is also gratefully acknowledged. In the US, the PNCR network is supported by SMA Foundation.

Author's contributions
MCP contributed to the study design, data collection and interpretation and manuscript review. GC conducted the statistical analysis, data collection and interpretation. NF contributed to data collection and manuscript review. ESM contributed to the design of the study, data collection and interpretation, and reviewed the manuscript. MS contributed to the design of the study, data collection and interpretation, and reviewed the manuscript. JM contributed to the design of the study, data collection and interpretation, and reviewed the manuscript. AP contributed to the design of the study, data collection and interpretation, and reviewed the manuscript. AM contributed to the design of the study, data collection and interpretation, and reviewed the manuscript. SM contributed to the design of the study, data collection and interpretation, and reviewed the manuscript. MS contributed to the design of the study, data collection and interpretation, and reviewed the manuscript. MM contributed to the design of the study, data collection and interpretation, and reviewed the manuscript. RML contributed to the design of the study, data collection and interpretation, and reviewed the manuscript. TD contributed to the design of the study, data collection and interpretation, and reviewed the manuscript. DR contributed to the design of the study, data collection and interpretation, and reviewed the manuscript. SD contributed to the design of the study, data collection and interpretation, and reviewed the manuscript. RS contributed to the design of the study, data collection and interpretation, and reviewed the manuscript. LF contributed to the study design, data collection and interpretation. MC contributed to the design of the study, data collection and interpretation, and reviewed the manuscript. RDS contributed to the study design, data collection and interpretation. LA contributed to the study design, data interpretation and manuscript review. LL contributed to the study design, data interpretation and manuscript review. SL contributed to the study design, data interpretation and analysis and manuscript review. MP contributed to the study design, data interpretation and manuscript review. JD contributed to the design of the study, data collection and interpretation, and reviewed the manuscript. BTD contributed to the study design, data interpretation and manuscript review. DCDV contributed to the study design, data interpretation and manuscript review and drafted the manuscript. FM contributed to the study design, data interpretation and manuscript review and drafted the manuscript. RF contributed to the study design, data interpretation and manuscript review and drafted the manuscript. EM contributed to the study design, data interpretation and manuscript review and drafted the manuscript. All authors read and approved the final manuscript.

Competing interests
The authors declare that they have no competing interests.

Author details
[1]Pediatric Neurology, Catholic University, Largo Gemelli 8, 00168 Rome, Italy. [2]Dubowitz Neuromuscular Centre, UCL Institute of Child Health & Great Ormond Street Hospital, London, UK. [3]Department of Neurology, Columbia University Medical Center, New York, NY, USA. [4]Department of Neurology, Boston Children's Hospital, Harvard Medical School, Boston, MA, USA. [5]John Walton Muscular Dystrophy Research Centre, Institute of Genetic Medicine, Newcastle University, Newcastle, UK. [6]Department of Clinical and Experimental Medicine and Nemo Sud Clinical Center, University of Messina, Messina, Italy. [7]Stanford University, Palo Alto, CA, USA. [8]Nemours Children's Hospital, University of Central Florida College of Medicine, Orlando, USA.

References

1. Main M, Kairon H, Mercuri E, Muntoni F. The Hammersmith functional motor scale for children with spinal muscular atrophy: a scale to test ability and monitor progress in children with limited ambulation. Eur J Paediatr Neurol. 2003;7(4):155-9.

2. O'Hagen JM, Glanzman AM, McDermott MP, Ryan PA, Flickinger J, Quigley J, Riley S, Sanborn E, Irvine C, Martens WB, et al. An expanded version of the Hammersmith Functional Motor Scale for SMA II and III patients. Neuromuscul Disord. 2007;17(9-10):693-7.

3. Mercuri E, Messina S, Battini R, Berardinelli A, Boffi P, Bono R, Bruno C, Carboni N, Cini C, Colitto F, et al. Reliability of the Hammersmith functional motor scale for spinal muscular atrophy in a multicentric study. Neuromuscul Disord. 2006;16(2):93-8.

4. Mercuri E, Mayhew A, Muntoni F, Messina S, Straub V, Van Ommen GJ, Voit T, Bertini E, Bushby K. Towards harmonisation of outcome measures for DMD and SMA within TREAT-NMD; report of three expert workshops: TREAT-NMD/ENMC workshop on outcome measures, 12th-13th May 2007, Naarden, The Netherlands; TREAT-NMD workshop on outcome measures in experimental trials for DMD, 30th June-1st July 2007, Naarden, The Netherlands; conjoint Institute of Myology TREAT-NMD meeting on physical activity monitoring in neuromuscular disorders, 11th July 2007, Paris, France. Neuromuscul Disord. 2008;18(11):894-903.

5. Finkel R, Bertini E, Muntoni F, Mercuri E, Group ESWS. 209th ENMC International Workshop: Outcome Measures and Clinical Trial Readiness in Spinal Muscular Atrophy 7-9 November 2014, Heemskerk. The Netherlands. Neuromuscul Disord. 2015;25(7):593-602.

6. Kayadjanian N, Burghes A, Finkel RS, Mercuri E, Rouault F, Schwersenz I, Talbot K. SMA-EUROPE workshop report: Opportunities and challenges in developing clinical trials for spinal muscular atrophy in Europe. Orphanet J Rare Dis. 2013;8:44.

7. Montes J, Glanzman AM, Mazzone ES, Martens WB, Dunaway S, Pasternak A, Riley SO, Quigley J, Pandya S, De Vivo DC, et al. Spinal muscular atrophy functional composite score: A functional measure in spinal muscular atrophy. Muscle Nerve. 2015;52(6):942-7.

8. Kaufmann P, McDermott MP, Darras BT, Finkel R, Kang P, Oskoui M, Constantinescu A, Sproule DM, Foley AR, Yang M, et al. Observational study of spinal muscular atrophy type 2 and 3: functional outcomes over 1 year. Arch Neurol. 2011;68(6):779-86.

9. Kaufmann P, McDermott MP, Darras BT, Finkel RS, Sproule DM, Kang PB, Oskoui M, Constantinescu A, Gooch CL, Foley AR, et al. Prospective cohort study of spinal muscular atrophy types 2 and 3. Neurology. 2012;79(18):1889-97.

10. Mercuri E, Finkel R, Montes J, Mazzone ES, Sormani MP, Main M, Ramsey D, Mayhew A, Glanzman AM, Dunaway S, et al. Patterns of disease progression in type 2 and 3 SMA: Implications for clinical trials. Neuromuscul Disord. 2016;26(2):126-31.

11. Kissel JT, Scott CB, Reyna SP, Crawford TO, Simard LR, Krosschell KJ, Acsadi G, Elsheik B, Schroth MK, D'Anjou G, et al. SMA CARNIVAL TRIAL PART II: a prospective, single-armed trial of L-carnitine and valproic acid in ambulatory children with spinal muscular atrophy. PLoS One. 2011;6(7):e21296.

12. Swoboda KJ, Scott CB, Crawford TO, Simard LR, Reyna SP, Krosschell KJ, Acsadi G, Elsheik B, Schroth MK, D'Anjou G, et al. SMA CARNI-VAL trial part I: double-blind, randomized, placebo-controlled trial of L-carnitine and valproic acid in spinal muscular atrophy. PLoS One. 2010;5(8):e12140.

13. Mercuri E, Bertini E, Messina S, Pelliccioni M, D'Amico A, Colitto F, Mirabella M, Tiziano FD, Vitali T, Angelozzi C, et al. Pilot trial of phenylbutyrate in spinal muscular atrophy. Neuromuscul Disord. 2004;14(2):130-5.

14. Mercuri E, Bertini E, Messina S, Solari A, D'Amico A, Angelozzi C, Battini R, Berardinelli A, Boffi P, Bruno C, et al. Randomized, double-blind, placebo-controlled trial of phenylbutyrate in spinal muscular atrophy. Neurology. 2007;68(1):51-5.

15. Chiriboga CA, Swoboda KJ, Darras BT, Iannaccone ST, Montes J, De Vivo DC, Norris DA, Bennett CF, Bishop KM. Results from a phase 1 study of nusinersen (ISIS-SMN (Rx)) in children with spinal muscular atrophy. Neurology. 2016;86(10):890-7.

16. U. S. Department of Health and Human Services. Guidance for Industry Use in Medical Product Development to Support Labeling Claims Guidance for Industry. 2009.

17. Qian Y, McGraw S, Henne J, Jarecki J, Hobby K, Yeh WS. Understanding the experiences and needs of individuals with Spinal Muscular Atrophy and their parents: a qualitative study. BMC Neurol. 2015;15:217.

18. R. USDoHaHSFaDfDa. Guidance for Industry Use in Medical Product Development to Support Labeling Claims Guidance for Industry. 2009.

24

Anti-N-methyl-D-aspartate receptor (NMDAR) antibody encephalitis presents in atypical types and coexists with neuromyelitis optica spectrum disorder or neurosyphilis

Kaiyu Qin, Wenqing Wu[*], Yuming Huang, Dongmei Xu, Lei Zhang, Bowen Zheng, Meijuan Jiang, Cheng Kou, Junhua Gao, Wurong Li, Jinglin Zhang, Sumei Wang, Yanfei Luan, Chaoling Yan, Dan Xu and Xinmei Zheng

Abstract

Background: Anti-N-methyl-D-aspartate receptor (NMDAR) encephalitis is a clinically heterogeneous disorder characterized by epileptic seizures, psychosis, dyskinesia, consciousness impairments, and autonomic instability. Symptoms are always various. Sometimes it presents in milder or incomplete forms. We report 4 cases of anti-NMDAR encephalitis with incomplete forms, 3 cases of which were accompanied by neuromyelitis optica spectrum disorder or neurosyphilis respectively.

Case presentation: A 33-year-old man presented with dysarthria, movement disorder and occasional seizures. He had 6 relapses in 28 years. When suffered from upper respiratory tract syndrome, he developed behavioral and consciousness impairment. Cranial MRI was normal. Viral PCR studies and oncologic work-up were negative. Anti-NMDAR antibody was detected in CSF and serum.

A 21-year-old female manifested dizziness and diplopia ten months and six months before, respectively. Both responded to steroid therapy and improved completely. This time she presented with progressive left limb and facial anesthesia, walking and holding unsteadily. Spinal cord MRI follow-up showed abnormality of medulla oblongata and cervical cord(C1). Anti-AQP4 and anti-NMDAR were positive in CSF. Steroid-pulse therapy ameliorated her symptoms.

A 37-year-old male experienced worsening vision. He was confirmed neurosyphilis since the CSF tests for syphilis were positive. Protein was elevated and the oligoclonal IgG bands(OB) and anti-NMDAR was positive in CSF. Anti-aquaporin 4(AQP4) antibodies and NMO-IgG were negative. Cranial MRI showed high FLAIR signal on frontal lobe and low T2 signal adjacent to the right cornu posterious ventriculi lateralis. Treatment for neurosyphlis was commenced with gradual improvement.

A 39-year-old male, developed serious behavioral and psychiatric symptoms. Examination showed abnormal pupils and unsteady gait. He was confirmed neurosyphilis according to the CSF tests for syphilis. Anti-NMDAR was positive in CSF and serum. Cranial MRI showed lateral ventricles and the third ventricle enlargement and signal abnormality involving bilateral temporal lobe, corona radiate and centrum semiovale. PenicillinG, pulsed methylprednisolone and intravenous immunoglobulin was administered. He was stable.

Conclusion: Anti-NMDAR encephalitis can present in atypical types. When relapsing, it may present with partial aspects or with isolated symptoms of the full-blown syndrome. Anti-NMDAR encephalitis may be related to neuromyelitis optica spectrum disorder or neurosyphilis.

Keywords: Anti-N-methyl-D-aspartate receptor(NMDAR), Atypical types, Neuromyelitis optica spectrum disorder, Neurosyphilis

* Correspondence: ruiyang56@aliyun.com
Department of neurology, Beijing Ditan Hospital, Capital Medical University, No.8 East Jing Shun Rd, Chaoyang District, Beijing, China

Background

Anti-NMDAR encephalitis is a severe but treatable auto-immune disorder. It can present with psychosis, memory deficits, seizures, dyskinesia, involuntary movements, decreased level of consciousness, and autonomic instability. Anti-NMDAR encephalitis usually evolves through several stages: flu-like prodromal syndromes, a psychotic stage, unresponsiveness with hypoventilation, autonomic instability and dyskinesia, and eventually death or recovery [1, 2]. The clinical phases of anti-NMDA receptor encephalitis may vary in sequence, presentation, and severity [3]. Milder or incomplete forms of the disorder can occur [4]. Here we report 4 cases presenting in atypical types.

Case presentation

Patient 1 was a 33-year-old male who was brought to our ward complaining of memory deficit, vision field with grids and stars background, and intermittent psychomotor agitation, following upper respiratory tract syndromes. His previous medical history indicated normal growth and development, except for epilepsy. He was diagnosed epilepsy during 9 years old because of paroxysmal formication responsive to antiepileptic drugs. There was no seizure until he manifested paroxysmal tongue rigidity and dysarthria for several days without any precipitating factor 16 years later. Thereafter, he developed episodes of "blank staring". Half a month later, he had paroxysmal head and eyes turning right, trismus, and rigidity of the left limbs. During having upper respiratory tract syndromes, that was accompanied by agitation, akathisia, hyperkinetic movements, disorientation to person and place, unresponsiveness, and consciousness impairment. Though antiepileptic drugs were prescribed, there were seizures every 3–5 years.

His reflexes were normal. There were no meningeal signs and no extensor plantar response. The CSF showed a lymphocyte pleocytosis, normal protein and glucose. Viral PCR studies for herpes simplex, cytomegalovirus, rubella, and toxoplasmosis were negative. Paraneoplastic tests such as Hu, Ri, Yo, CV_2, amphiphysin were negative, except for anti-NMDAR antibody positive in CSF and weakly positive in serum. Cranial MRI was normal.

He responded to steroid (dexamethasone 20 mg for 3 days and slow weaning of oral prednisolone) and anti-epileptic therapy. Relapse symptoms decreased after steroid received. Now he has weaned from anti-epileptic drugs for about 1 year, and there was no seizure. His blood test for anti-NMDAR-Ab became negative and CSF weakly positive when he recovered completely 1 year later. Despite an extensive oncologic work-up such as chest X-ray, pelvic and abdomen ultrasonic examination, there was no evidence of tumor, thus confirming the diagnosis of anti-NMDAR encephalitis.

Recently, he presented with paroxysmal choreiform movements of left hand, and slurring of speech (with delay of 3 years for the last relapse). His blood test for anti-NMDAR-Ab was reactive in 1:10 dilutions and CSF 1:100 dilutions. The movement disorder and dysarthria resolved after he was commenced on pulsed methylpre-dinisolone(500 mg). To prevent relapse, he received mycophenolate mofetil.

Patient 2, a 21-year-old female, suffered from progressive left limbs and facial anesthesia for a month, walking and holding unsteadily for 10 days. She also suffered from paroxysmal pain of facial and neck on the left side, and episodes of intractable vomiting, accompanied by anxiety. Ten months and six months before admission, she described dizziness, jittering vision, and diplopia on left gaze respectively, which responded to steroid therapy and improved completely. At her admission, examination noted fever(T:38.5 °C),facial dysesthesia on the left side,walking difficulties related to moderate superficial and deep sensory dysfunction and hemiparesis of the left limbs, difficulty in executing finger-to-nose and heel-to-knee maneuvers because of her ataxia. The left Babinski's sign, left Hoffmann's sign and Lhermitte's sign were positive.

Spinal cord MRI follow-up showed T2 hyperintensities and T1 hypointensities from the dorsal medulla to cervical cord(C1) (Fig. 1). Visual evoked potentials and EEG are normal. Analysis of the CSF showed almost acellular(1600/ml), normal protein and glucose concentration. OB(oligoclonal band) and MBP(myelin basic protein) are negative. Tests for paraneoplasia such as Hu, Ri, Yo, CV_2, amphiphysin were all negative. Anti-NMDAR-Ab was positive, and anti-aquaporin 4(AQP4) antibodies

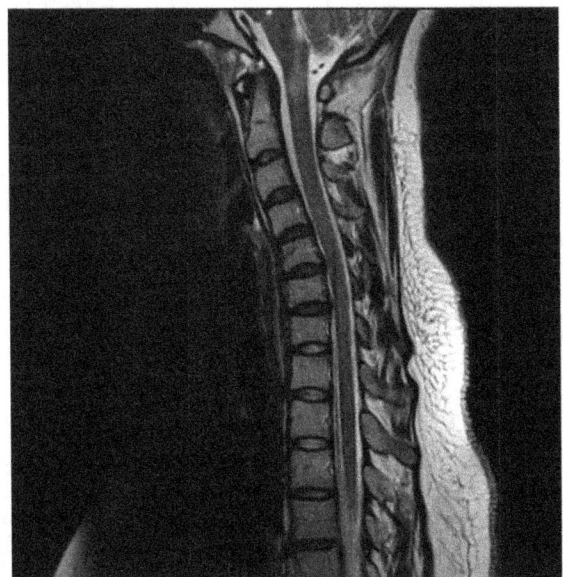

Fig. 1 T2-weighted MRI image showing high-signal intensity from the dorsal medulla to cervical cord(C1)

weakly positive in CSF, while anti-NMDAR-Ab negative and AQP4 antibodies weakly positive in serum. Oncologic tests, including chest X-ray, pelvic and abdomen ultrasonic examination, CA125, CEA(carcinoembryonic antigen), were all negative. Autoimmune tests such as ANA(antinuclear antibodies), ENA, and thyroid function were normal. She received pulsed methylpredinisolone(500 mg). Four days after the steroid therapy, unsteadiness of the left limbs was greatly improved. Considering anti-AQP4 and anti-NMDAR were positive in CSF, we gave her azathioprine to prevent relapse. No recrudescence developed throughout three months, and MRI showed improvement in the previously observed high T2 signal abnormalities.

Patient 3, a 37-year-old male, who was diagnosed syphilis 2 years before, presented with progressively reduced vision of both eyes to 0.02 for six months. Human immunodeficiency virus(HIV) testing was negative. The CSF was almost acellular(6/mm^3) with elevated protein 1.237 g/L, normal glucose, and tests for syphilis were positive for non-treponeal(Syphilis Toluidine Red Untreated Serum Test, TRUST reactive in 1:2 dilutions) and reactive in specific Treponema Pallidum particle agglutination and Treponema enzyme-linked immunosobent assays(IgG positive, IgM negative). The oligoclonal IgG bands(OB) and anti-NMDAR was positive in CSF. Anti-aquaporin 4(AQP4) antibodies and NMO-IgG were negative. Visual evoked potentials showed no P100 wave on the left side and delayed P100 latencies on the right side. Cranial MRI showed a focal slightly high FLAIR signal on frontal lobe (Fig. 2) and low T2 signal adjacent to the right cornu posterius ventriculi lateralis (Fig. 3). The patient was treated with intravenous penicillin G, followed by intramuscular injection of 2.4 million U of benzathine penicillin G weekly for 3 weeks. The vision was improved to 0.04 about 1 year later, and CSF tests for syphilis were negative for non-treponeal(TRUST).

Patient 4, a 39-year-old male, manifested progressive attention and memory impairments and episodes of anxiety and irritability reported by family members. Examination showed under illumination, his right and left pupils were 3 and 5 mm in diameter, respectively. Both pupils were insensitive to light. His gait was unsteady. He swayed a little from side to side when he stood erect with his eyes closed. HIV testing was negative. Blood tests for syphilis were positive for non-treponeal(TRUST reactive in 1:32 dilutions) and reactive in specific Treponema Pallidum particle agglutination and Treponema enzyme-linked immunosobent assays (IgG positive, IgM negative). The CSF was acellular with normal protein and glucose, and tests for syphilis were negative for non-treponeal(TRUST) and reactive in specific Treponema Pallidum particle agglutination and Treponema enzyme-linked immunosobent assays(IgG

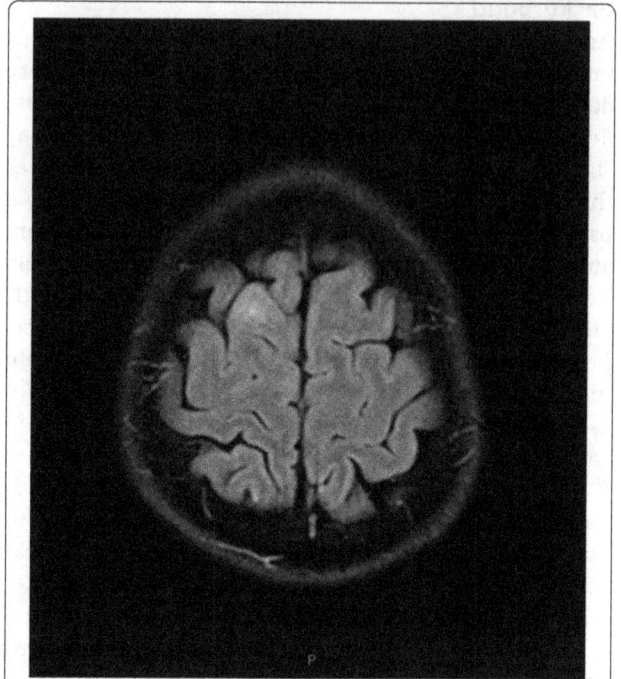

Fig. 2 FLAIR image showing high signal on right frontal lobe

positive, IgM negative). The oligoclonal IgG bands(OB) and anti-NMDAR was positive in CSF and serum. Cranial MRI showed lateral ventricles and the third ventricle enlargement (Fig. 4) and focal high T2/FLAIR signal abnormality involving bilateral temporal lobe, corona radiate and centrum semiovale (Figs. 5 and 6). We thought the patient may present 2 diseases: neurosyphilis and anti-NMDAR encephalitis. Besides penicillin G, pulsed methylprednisolone plus intravenous immunoglobulin was administered. He was stable afterwards.

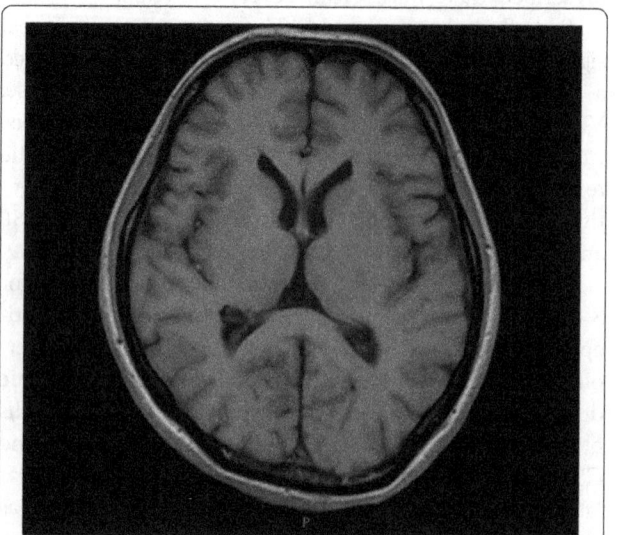

Fig. 3 T1-weighted Cranial MRI showing low-signal adjacent to the right cornu posterius ventriculi lateralis

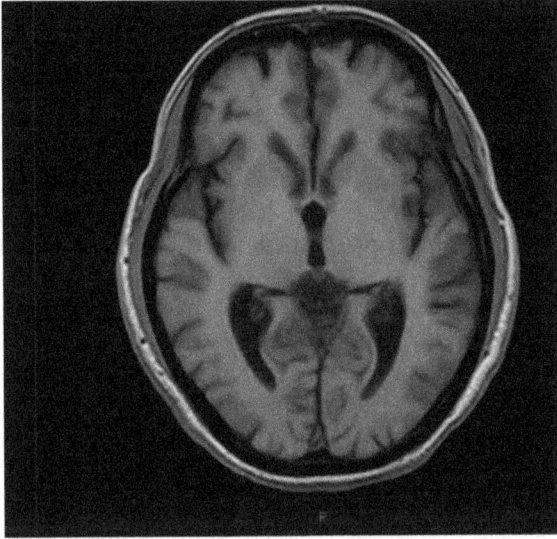

Fig. 4 T1-weighted head MRI showing lateral ventricles and the third ventricle enlargement

Conclusions

The NMDAR contributes to excitatory synaptic transmission across many brain regions. It plays a key role in neurodevelopment and synaptic plasticity. A highly active NMDAR is composed of glycine/D-serine-binding

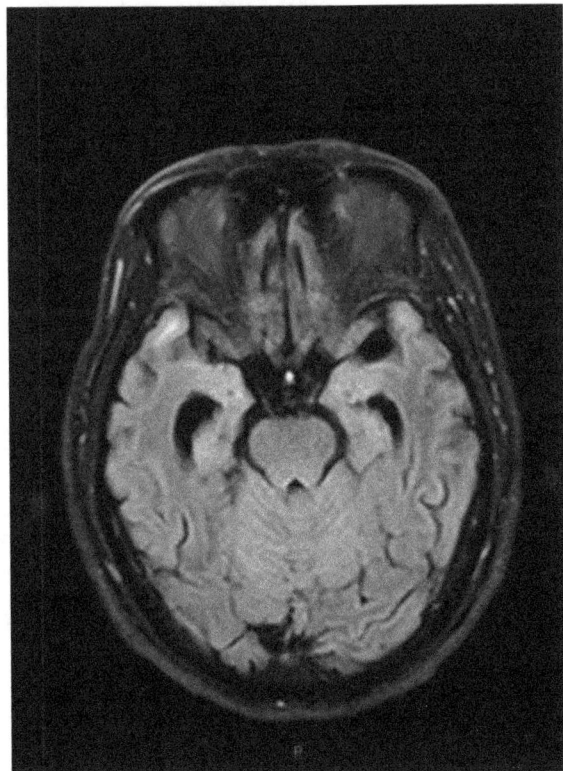

Fig. 6 T2-weighted head MRI showing high signal of bilateral corona radiate and centrum semiovale

NR1 subunit and multiple glutamate-binding NR2 subunits. The hyperactivation of NMDAR has been shown to induce acute neuronal death and chronic neurodegeneration, while the hypoactivation of NMDAR is related to the development of psychiatric state [5].

The NR1 subunit is considered obligatory for functional NMDAR assemblies. Recent advances in genetic, preclinical and clinical pharmacological, and brain studies have shown the role of disrupted NMDAR-NR1 subunit-mediated glutamatergic pathways in schizophrenia [6]. *Psychosis* is a canonical symptom of anti-NMDAR encephalitis. In our case, Patient 1, 2 and 4 all manifested episodes of agitation.

Approximately three-quarters of CNS disorders with antibodies to surface antigens manifest in epileptic seizures [7]. Some epileptics who are not sensitive to conventional anticonvulsants may have an immune-mediated etiology [8, 9], and that epilepsy with psychiatric symptoms may have anti-NMDAR encephalitis [10]. Patient 1 presented with occasional seizures accompanying with psychosis.

Anti-NMDAR encephalitis is proved to be antibody-mediated [11, 12]. The NMDA receptor antibodies are IgGs directed against *extracellular* epitopes of the GluN1 subunit [13]. The immunopathological findings of anti-

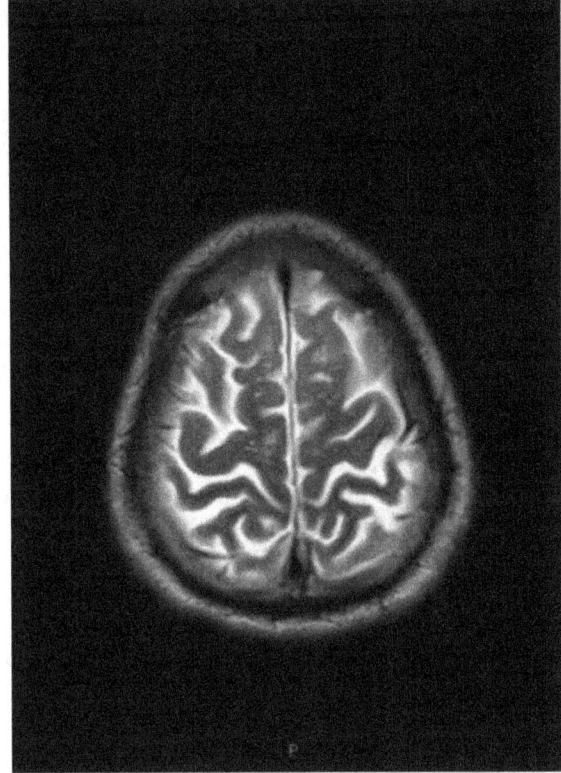

Fig. 5 FLAIR image showing high signal on bilateral temporal lobe

NMDAR encephalitis are increased deposits of immunoglobulin G and reactive microglial staining with anti-CD68 antibody, mainly in the basal forebrain, hippocampus, basal ganglion, and cervical spinal cord [2, 11, 13]. J.-P. Camdessanche thought perivascular inflammatory B-cell accumulation can appear in patients and play a positive role in brain T-cell infiltration, antibody secretion by plasmocytes, microglial and astro-glial proliferation [14].

Cui Li showed NMDAR played a critical role in regulation of oligodendrocyte precursor cells differentiation and remyelination [15]. Studies have indicated patients with anti-NMDAR encephalitis may develop episodes of demyelinating disorders, and conversely patients with NMO or demyelinating disorders in atypical types may have anti-NMDAR encephalitis [16, 17].

Patient 1 had 6 relapses in 28 years. He presented with seizures and dysarthria and movement disorder. We think the seizure of his 9-year-old is the first event. The delay range between relapses is 3–16 years. The level of anti-NMDAR antibodies in CSF and serum decreased when patient 1 show substantial clinical recovery. There are still different opinions on relationship between the level of anti-NMDAR and disease activity. Some researches indicate this relationship exists [13, 18, 19], while some show they are uncorrelated [20, 21].

Patient 2 had a relapsing disease course of CNS(central nervous system) demyelinating disorders. She presented with three subacute episodes of spinal cord and brainstem symptoms, which responded to steroid treatment. In view of MRI, cord spinal T2 lesions non-suggestive of MS, and tests for anti-aquaporin 4(AQP4) antibodies in serum and CSF were weakly positive, we diagnosed her neuromyelitis optica spectrum disorder(NMOSD). Although brainstem syndromes and short myelitis lesions [22] were reported in NMOSD [23, 24], we looked for other possible disorders involving auto-immune encephalitis and found anti-NMDAR-Ab in CSF and serum before steroid was applied.

Patient 1 and patient 2 both showed a relapsing disease course. In anti-NMDAR encephalitis, Relapse rate is reported to be 20-30%. [13, 25, 26]. At relapses, typical syndromes were usually lacking [27]. It can be separated by intervals of months or years. Between relapses is substantial recovery. Relapse rates may be higher in patients without immunotherapy during the first episode [18, 27] and in patients without detectable tumors [4, 18], suggesting importance of early immunotherapy. Differentiating from disorders with antibodies to intracellular antigens(Hu,Ri,Yo,Ma$_2$ and amphyphism antibodies), which is due to T-cell mediated cytotoxity, poorly responsive to immunotherapy, has a progressive course and its treatment is directed to the underlying malignancy [28], disorders with antibodies to cell surface antigens(VGKC-complex, NMDAR) may work by antibody-binding, internalization,

and loss of the target antigen [29], are often sensitive to treatment [4, 30], have a relapsing course, have a better prognosis, and are less commonly paraneoplastic [28, 31].

Patient 3 and Patient 4 were confirmed neurosyphilis, with anti-NMDAR antibody positive in CSF and serum. We have not found any reports about neurosyhilis accompanying with anti-NMDAR antibody so far.

We speculate the vision decrease of patient 3 may be caused by neurosyphilis. Patient 4 was diagnosed paralytic dementia. His MRI showed the lateral and third ventricles enlargement, which is associated with schizophrenia [32]. The oligoclonal IgG bands(OB) in CSF while not demonstrable in corresponding serum reflected a local B-cell response following central nervous system(CNS) inflammation. We cannot exclude that neurosyphilis has led to secondary immunological response of anti-NMDAR-Ab production. It's also possible that the patient may have presented 2 diseases concurrently: neurosyphilis and anti-NMDAR encephalitis. Such patients provide a compelling argument to pursue the possible relation of neurosyphilis and anti-NMDAR antibody.

This study has several limitations. The follow-up is relatively short. We cannot know if there are relapses of anti-NMDAR encephalitis in neurosyphilis. We recently gave patient 1 mycophenolate mofetil after 6 relapses, so we cannot know if that will prevent relapse. Since patient 1 had seizures every 3–5 years, it's a question whether anti-epileptic drugs are given initially.

Abbreviations

AQP4: Anti-aquaporin 4; CEA: Carcinoembryonic antigen; CSF: Cerebrospinal fluid; EEG: Electroencephalography; ENA: Extractable nuclear antigen antibody; FLAIR: Flow attenuated inversion recovery; MBP: Myelin basic protein; MRI: Magnetic resonance imaging; MS: Multiple sclerosis; NMDAR: N-methyl-D-aspartate receptor; NMO: Neuromyelitis optica; NMOSD: Neuromyelitis optica spectrum disorder; OB: Oligoclonal bands; PCR: Polymerase chain reaction; TRUST: Syphilis toluidine red untreated serum test; VGKC: Voltage-gated potassium channel-complex

Acknowledgements

We thank Professor Wenhui Lun who gave us instruction in treatment of neurosyphilis and other colleagues for the excellent care the patient received, and that made this report possible.

Funding

There's no funding available.

Authors' contributions

KQ was involved in the direct care of patients; she examined and assessed patients on admission, reviewed the literature, and wrote the case and the final draft. WW and YH were the treating neurologists involved in the care of patients; they helped in the design, made significant modifications in the manuscript and approved the final draft. DX was the treating neurologist involved in the care of the patients; she participated in obtaining the consent and designing. LZh, BZh, MJ, CK, WL, JG, JZh and XZh were involved in the direct care of patients; they examined and assessed patients. SW, ChY, DX and YL completed electrophysiological examinations and gave interpretention of data. All authors read and approved the final manuscript.

Competing interests

The authors declare that they have no competing interests.

References

1. Tuzune E, Dalmau J. Limbic encephalitis and variants: classification, diagnosis and treatment. Neurologist. 2007;13:261–71.
2. Dalmau J, Tuzune E, Wu H-Y, et al. Paraneoplastic anti-N-methyl-D-aspartate receptor encephalitis associated with ovarian teratoma. Ann Neurol. 2007;61:25–36.
3. Peery HE, Gregory S. Day, Anti-NMDA receptor encephalitis. The disorder, the diagnosis and the immunobiology. Autoimmun Rev. 2012;11:863–72.
4. Dalmau J, Lancaster E, Martinez-Hernandez E, et al. Clinical experience and laboratory investigations in patients with anti-NMDAR encephalitis. Lancet Neurol. 2011;10:63–74.
5. Miya K, Takahashi Y, Mori H, et al. Anti-NMDAR autoimmune encephalitis. Brain Dev. 2014;36:645–52.
6. Peijun J, Cui D. The involvement of N-methyl-D-aspartate receptor(NMDAR) subunit NR1 in the pathophysiology of schizophrenia. Acta Biochim Biophys Sin. 2016;48(3):209–19.
7. Irani SR, Bien CJ, Lang B. Autoimmune epilepsies. Curr Opin Neurol. 2011;24:146–53.
8. Rima N. Autoimmune and inflammatory epilepsies. Epilepsia. 2012; 53(Suppl4):58–62.
9. Quek AM, Britton JW, Mckeon A, et al. Autoimmune epilepsy: clinical characteristics and response to immunotherapy. Arch Neurol. 2012;69:582–93.
10. Kayser MS, Dalmau J. Anti-NMDA receptor encephalitis, autoimmunity, and psychosis. Schizophr Res. 2016;176(1):36–40.
11. Tuzun E, Zhou L, Baehring JM, et al. Evidence for antibody-mediated pathogenesis in anti-NMDAR encephalitis associated with ovarian teratoma. Acta Neuropathol. 2009;118:737–43.
12. Martinez-Hernandez E, Horvath J, Shiloh-Malawsky Y, et al. Analysis of complement and plasma cells in the brain of patients with anti-NMDAR encephalitis. Neurology. 2011;77(6):589–93.
13. Dalmau J, Gleichman AJ, Hughes EG, et al. Anti-NMDA-receptor encephalitis: case series and analysis of the effects of antibodies. Lancet Neurol. 2008;7:1091–8.
14. Camdessanche J-P, Streichenberger N, Cavillon G, et al. Brain immunohistopathological study in a patient with anti-NMDAR encephalitis. Eur J Neurol. 2011;18:929–31.
15. Li C, Xiao L, Liu X, et al. A functional role of NMDA receptor in regulating the differentiation of oligodendrocyte precursor cells and remyelination. Glia. 2013;61(5):732–49.
16. Titulaer MJ, Hoftberger R, Iizuka T, et al. Overlapping demyelinating syndromes and anti-N-methyl-D-aspartate receptor encephalitis. Ann Neurol. 2014;75:411–2.
17. Zoccarato M, Saddi MV, Serra G, et al. Aquaporin-4 antibody neuromyelitis optica following anti-NMDA receptor encephalitis. J Neurol. 2013;260:3185–87.
18. Irani SR, Bera K, Waters P, et al. N-methyl-D-aspartate antibody encephalitis: temporal progression of clinical and paraclinical observations in a predominantly non-paraneop lastic disorder of both sexes. Brain. 2010;133:1655–67.
19. Pruss H, Dalmau J, Harms L, et al. Retrospective analysis of NMDA receptor antibodies in encephalitis of unknown origin. Neurology. 2010;75:1735–9.
20. Alexopoulos H, Michalis L, Kosmidis ML, et al. Paraneoplastic anti-NMDAR encephalitis:long-term follow-up reveals persistent serum antibodies. J Neurol. 2011;258:1568–70.
21. Hansen C, Klingbeil C, Dalmau J, et al. Persistant intrathecal antibody synthesis 15 years after recovering from anti-N-methyl-D-aspartate receptor encephalitis. JAMA Neurol. 2013;70(1):117–9.
22. Flanagan EP, Weinshenker BG, Krecke KN. Short myelitis lesions in aquaporin-4-IgG-positive neurmyelitis optica spectrum. JAMA Neurol. 2015;72(1):81–7.
23. Lim BC, Chae JH, Kim S-K, et al. Aquaporin-4 auto immunity masquerading as a brainstem tumor. J Neurosurg Pediatrics. 2014;14:301–05.
24. Li Y, Jiang B, Chen B. Neuromyelitis optica spectrum disorders with multiple brainstem manifestations: a case report. Neurol Sci. 2016;37(2):309–13.
25. Titulaer MJ, McCracken L, Gabilondo I, et al. Traetment and prognostic factors for long-term outcome in patients with anti-NMDA receptor encephalitis: an observational cohort study. Lancet Neurol. 2013;12:157–65.
26. Florance NR, Davis RL, Lam C, et al. Anti-N-methyl-D- aspartate receptor(NMDAR) encephalitis in children and adolescents. Ann Neurol. 2009;66:11–8.
27. Gabilondo I, Saiz A, Galan L, et al. Analysis of relapses in anti-NMDAR encephalitis. Neurology. 2011;77(10):996–9.
28. Bien CG, Vincent A, Barnett MH, et al. Immunopathology of autoantibody-associated encephalitides: clues for pathogenesis. Brain. 2012;135:1622–38.
29 Hughes EG, Peng X, Gleichman AJ, et al. Cellular and synaptic mechanisms of anti-NMDA receptor encephalitis. J Neurosci. 2010;30:5866–75.
30 Malter MP, Frisch C, Schoene-Bake JC, et al. Outcome of limbic encephalitis with VGKC-complex antibodies: relation to antigenic specificity. J Neurol. 2014;261(9):1695–705.
31 Lancaster E, Martinez-Hernandez E, Dalmau J, et al. Encephalitis and antibodies to synaptic and neuronal cell surface proteins. Neurology. 2011;77:179–89.
32 Del Re EC, Konishi J, Bouix S, et al. Enlarged lateral ventricles inversely correlate with reduced corpus callosum central volume in first episode schizophrenia: association with functional measures. Brain Imaging and Behavior. 2015. Epub ahead of print.

25

Effects of acetyl-DL-leucine on cerebellar ataxia (ALCAT trial): study protocol for a multicenter, multinational, randomized, double-blind, placebo-controlled, crossover phase III trial

Katharina Feil[1,2,11]* , Christine Adrion[3], Julian Teufel[1,2], Sylvia Bösch[8], Jens Claassen[5], Ilaria Giordano[7], Holger Hengel[6], Heike Jacobi[7], Thomas Klockgether[7], Thomas Klopstock[1,4,12], Wolfgang Nachbauer[8], Ludger Schöls[6], Claudia Stendel[1,4], Ellen Uslar[5], Bart van de Warrenburg[9], Ingrid Berger[2], Ivonne Naumann[2], Otmar Bayer[2], Hans-Helge Müller[10], Ulrich Mansmann[3] and Michael Strupp[1,2]

Abstract

Background: Cerebellar ataxia (CA) is a frequent and often disabling condition that impairs motor functioning and impacts on quality of life (QoL). No medication has yet been proven effective for the symptomatic or even causative treatment of hereditary or non-hereditary, non-acquired CA. So far, the only treatment recommendation is physiotherapy. Therefore, new therapeutic options are needed. Based on three observational studies, the primary objective of the acetyl-DL-leucine on ataxia (ALCAT) trial is to examine the efficacy and tolerability of a symptomatic therapy with acetyl-DL-leucine compared to placebo on motor function measured by the Scale for the Assessment and Rating of Ataxia (SARA) in patients with CA.

Methods/Design: An investigator-initiated, multicenter, European, randomized, double-blind, placebo-controlled, 2-treatment 2-period crossover phase III trial will be carried out. In total, 108 adult patients who meet the clinical criteria of CA of different etiologies (hereditary or non-hereditary, non-acquired) presenting with a SARA total score of at least 3 points will be randomly assigned in a 1:1 ratio to one of two different treatment sequences, either acetyl-DL-leucine (up to 5 g per day) followed by placebo or vice versa. Each sequence consists of two 6-week treatment periods, separated by a 4-week wash-out period. A follow-up examination is scheduled 4 weeks after the end of treatment. The primary efficacy outcome is the absolute change in the SARA total score. Secondary objectives are to demonstrate that acetyl-DL-leucine is effective in improving (1) motor function measured by the Spinocerebellar Ataxia Functional Index (SCAFI) and SARA subscore items and (2) QoL (EuroQoL 5 dimensions and 5 level version, EQ-5D-5 L), depression (Beck Depression Inventory, BDI-II) and fatigue (Fatigue Severity Score, FSS). Furthermore, the incidence of adverse events will be investigated.

Discussion: The results of this trial will inform whether symptomatic treatment with the modified amino-acid acetyl-DL-leucine is a worthy candidate for a new drug therapy to relieve ataxia symptoms and to improve patient care. If superiority of the experimental drug to placebo can be established it will also be re-purposing of an agent that has been previously used for the symptomatic treatment of dizziness.

(Continued on next page)

* Correspondence: katharina.feil@med.uni-muenchen.de
[1]Department of Neurology with Friedrich-Baur-Institute, University Hospital, Munich, Germany
[2]German Center for Vertigo and Balance Disorders (DSGZ), University Hospital, Munich, Germany
Full list of author information is available at the end of the article

(Continued from previous page)

Keywords: Cerebellar ataxia, Amino acids, Acetyl-DL-leucine, Symptomatic therapy, Randomized controlled trial, Crossover design, Ataxia rating scales, Patient questionnaires, Quality of life

Background

Cerebellar ataxia (CA) is a frequent and often disabling syndrome which can severely impair motor functioning and quality of life (QoL) [1]. CAs are most often caused by neurodegenerative disorders of the cerebellum which are either hereditary or non-hereditary (sporadic); all in all, about 50% of the cases are sporadic. Studies suggest that the overall prevalence of CA in Europe is similar to that in Japan and may approach 20:100,000, i.e., 15,000 patients in Germany (www.ataxie.de) [2]. Due to the various etiologies and different courses of the diseases, there are no robust epidemiological data on CA-related mortality.

The leading clinical symptoms of CA are disturbances of stance or gait (>85%) with recurrent falls, limb ataxia with severe functional impairment of arm and hand movements, dysarthrophonia with impaired oral communication abilities, and ocular motor disturbances with impaired vision [1]. Further, most types of CA are progressive and therefore become more disabling in the course of the disease, severely impairing QoL and functioning [1]. In addition to functional impairment, CA also affects cognitive and psychosocial abilities and limits the ability to perform tasks of daily life. It is thus a severely disabling condition, progressively restricting autonomy and social participation. The care that is required is frequently provided by the family, thus further increasing the socioeconomic burden of disease [3]. Major cost components relevant for patients with CA are informal care, early retirement because of permanent disability, drugs, orthopedic devices, and rehabilitation. As the disease progresses, quality of life decreases and utilization of health resources increases [4].

No medication has yet been proven effective for the symptomatic or even causative treatment of degenerative CA [5]. Beneficial effects of Varenicline and Riluzole have been reported [6–8]. However, according to a consensus paper on management of degenerative CA, these findings need to be further confirmed in further placebo-controlled trials, in particular long-term and disease-specific studies [8, 9]. To date, the only treatment recommendation for CA is physiotherapy [10] and new therapeutic options are needed.

Acetyl-DL-leucine

Acetyl-DL-leucine (Tanganil; Pierre Fabre, Castres, France) is an acetylated derivative of a natural essential amino acid. Although it has been used for more than 50 years, mainly in France for the symptomatic treatment of acute vertigo and dizziness and improvement of central vestibular compensation [11], the therapeutic mode of action of acetyl-DL-leucine has so far not been very well examined. It may act due to its direct effect on neurons, as was shown in the vestibular nuclei [11]. In vitro studies in guinea pigs demonstrated that acetyl-DL-leucine acts mainly on abnormally hyperpolarized and/or depolarized vestibular neurons by normalizing the membrane potential and has only a minor effect on the membrane potential of vestibular neurons during normal resting potential [12]. In unilateral neurotomy and labyrinthectomy, the agent was described to normalize the vestibular asymmetry with showing an effect seen only in the subgroup of patients with residual vestibular function [11]. Due to the phylogenetical and electrophysiological similarities and close interactions between vestibular and deep cerebellar neurons [13], we had hypothesized that there may also be a positive effect on ataxic symptoms in cerebellar disorders. In an animal model on acute unilateral vestibulopathy, it was found that acetyl-DL-leucine improves compensation of postural symptoms most likely by activation of the vestibulocerebellum, since there was a significant increase of the regional cerebral metabolic rate for glucose in the paraflocculus/flocculus [14]. On cellular levels, it was demonstrated that acetyl-DL-leucine restores the membrane potential of hyperpolarized/depolarized vestibular neurons after unilateral labyrinthectomy in guinea pigs [12]. This mechanism may be mediated by its direct interactions with membrane phospholipids such as phosphatidylinositol 4,5-bisphosphate, which influences ion channel activity [15]. Thereby, acetyl-DL-leucine can stabilize the membrane potential. The input from cerebellar Purkinje cells and mossy/climbing fiber collaterals controls the action potential of the vestibular and the cerebellar nuclei [16], which in turn project to the brainstem, thalamus and spinal cord [13]. Therefore, acetyl-DL-leucine may act through afferent and efferent projections on upstream and downstream structures, thus influencing movement control.

Trial rationale

In a first case series on 13 patients with different types of hereditary and non-hereditary non-acquired CA, we reported positive effects of acetyl-DL-leucine (5 g per day for one week) on the motor function measured by the Scale for the Assessment and Rating of Ataxia (SARA) and the Spinocerebellar Ataxia Functional Index (SCAFI) [17]. The agent was well tolerated [17]. Mean total SARA decreased from 16.1 ± 7.1 (mean $\pm$ SD) at baseline to 12.8 ± 6.8 after one week on medication ($p = 0.002$), and patients showed better performance in the SCAFI consisting of the 8-m-walking-time (8 MW), 9-Hole-Peg-Test of the dominant hand (9HPTD) and the PATA rate task (timed speech task where the patient is asked to repeat "PATA" as quickly and distinctly as possible for 10 s two times). Preliminary FDG-PET-data in a case series of 18 patients suffering from degenerative CA with different etiologies showed central compensation processes in the group of responders mainly in the medulla (vestibular nuclei), midbrain (vestibular integration centers), thalami, basal ganglia and insular regions rather than neurons in the cerebellum, the primary site of dysfunction in CA syndromes [18]. In gait analysis, acetyl-DL-leucine improved the coefficient of variation of stride time in 14 out of 18 cerebellar patients. Acetyl-DL-leucine showed a reduction of gait variability during slow walking [19], whereas aminopyridines have been shown to improve gait variability mainly during fast walking [20, 21]. Subjective ambulatory gait scores and the SARA score also improved under treatment [19]. Further, in a case series on 12 patients with Niemann-Pick type C, a lysosomal storage disorder, there was also a significant improvement of symptoms of ataxia [22]. On the other side, the use of the liquid formula of acetyl-DL-leucine 5 g once daily for 7 days in 10 patients with degenerative CA failed to confirm a treatment benefit of the drug in combination with a short-term physio— and occupational therapy, although 7 out of 10 patients reported subjective improvement [23]. However, all these case studies provide limited evidence and have considerable methodological limitations. Efficacy outcomes were assessed unblinded, rendering objective evaluation of treatment response difficult. Large-scale double-blind randomized controlled trials are highly warranted. Based on these results, we designed the prospective ALCAT trial (Effects of Acetyl-DL-Leucine on Cerebellar ATaxia) to investigate the efficacy and safety of acetyl-DL-leucine with the aim of demonstrating superiority over placebo.

Methods/Design
Trial design and setting

The ALCAT trial is an investigator-initiated, multicenter, randomized, double-blind, placebo-controlled, 2-treatment 2-period crossover phase III trial. The study was initiated at the Department of Neurology and the German Center for Vertigo and Balance Disorders (University of Munich) and the Friedrich-Baur-Institute, and has been subsequently extended to other study sites located in Germany (University of Tuebingen, University of Essen, and DZNE Bonn), Austria (Innsbruck) and will be expanded to the Netherlands (Nijmegen). The study has been approved by the responsible ethics committees in Germany (project number 248–15 fed) as well as the ethics committee in Austria (project number AN2015–0252 355/2.1) and has been submitted to the ethics committee in the Netherlands. Furthermore, the study has been approved by the legal medical regulatory authorities (Federal Institute for Drugs and Medical Devices, in German: Bundesinstitut für Arzneimittelsicherheit und Medizinprodukte - BfArM in Germany, Austrian Agency for Health and Food Safety Ltd. AGES, in German: Österreichische Agentur für Gesundheit und Ernährungssicherheit GmbH in Austria, Central Committee on Research Involving Human Subjects, in Dutch: Centrale Commissie Mensgebonden Onderzoek – CCMO in the Netherlands). The first patient was randomized on January 25, 2016. The ALCAT trial is conducted in accordance with the International Conference for Harmonisation (of Technical Requirements for Pharmaceuticals for Human Use) - Good Clinical Practice Guideline (ICH-GCP) and the Declaration of Helsinki. The trial has been prospectively registered at www.clinicaltrialsregister.eu (EudraCT no. 2015–000460–34) and https://www.germanctr.de (DR KS-ID: DRKS00009733) on January 15, 2016. Patient insurance for the study has been arranged (policy number for Germany 39 130537 03026, for Austria 07208763–1, for Netherlands 081 50474–14005).

Patient population and eligibility criteria

Patients are screened for eligibility according to the inclusion and exclusion criteria. To be eligible for the study, patients aged 18 years or older must present with the clinical symptom of ataxia (hereditary or non-hereditary, non-acquired CA) with at least 3 points in the SARA total score and be able to understand and follow instructions and to give informed consent. All relevant medical and non-medical conditions should be taken into consideration when deciding whether this protocol is suitable for a particular subject. The exclusion criteria were chosen according to available data on acetyl-DL-leucine from the French Agence nationale de sécurité du médicament et des produits de santé (http://agence-prd.ansm.sante.fr/php/ecodex/notice/N0126720.htm, accessed on 24.04.2015, dated on 20.02.2007) and included, in particular, hypersensitivity to the agent. For a detailed description of inclusion and exclusion criteria see Table 1.

Table 1 Inclusion and exclusion criteria for patient selection

Inclusion criteria	Exclusion criteria

• Clinically confirmed CA with a SARA total score ≥ 3 (range 0-40) (CA (hereditary or non-hereditary, non-acquired)
• Patient did not receive any of the following prohibited medication within 4 weeks prior to randomization:
  o Aminopyridines
  o Acetyl-DL-leucine
  o Riluzole
  o Gabapentin
  o Varenicline
  o Chlorzoxazone
• The ability to follow study instructions and likely to attend and complete all required visits
• Written informed consent of the subject prior to any study-specific intervention
• Age ≥ 18 years
	• Subject is not able to give consent
	• Onset of ataxia in association with stroke, encephalitis, sepsis, hyperthermia or heat stroke
	• Toxic causes for ataxia of cerebellar type
	• Rapid progression of ataxia (development of severe ataxia in less than 12 weeks)
	• Subject suffers from any of the following:
	  o chronic diarrhea
	  o unexplained visual loss
	  o malignancies
	  o insulin-dependent diabetes mellitus
	• Ataxia due to multiple sclerosis, ischemia, hemorrhage or tumor of the posterior fossa as confirmed by imaging
	• Ataxia due to clinically likely multisystem atrophy type C (MSA-C)
	• Diagnosis of clinically likely Friedreich's ataxia
	• Known history of hypersensitivity to the investigational drug or derivatives
	• Liver failure defined as AST/ALT > 300 U/l
	• Simultaneous participation in another clinical trial or participation in any clinical trial involving administration of an investigational medical product within 30 days prior to the beginning of the clinical trial
	• Subjects with a physical or psychiatric condition which, in the opinion of the investigator, may put the subject at risk, may confound the trial results, or may interfere with the subject's participation in this clinical trial
	• Known or persistent abuse of medication, drugs or alcohol
	• Females of childbearing potential, who are not using and not willing to use medically reliable methods of contraception for the entire study duration as listed in the patient informed consent form
	• Current or planned pregnancy or nursing women
	• Patient has received any of the following prohibited medication within 4 weeks prior to randomization
	  o Aminopyridines (including sustained-release form)
	  o Acetyl-DL-leucine
	  o Riluzole
	  o Gabapentin
	  o Varenicline
	  o Chlorzoxazone

Recruitment and patient involvement

Patients will be recruited via personal correspondence and by routine care appointments at specialized tertiary referral centres (Neurological departments of University hospitals). In Germany, we also cooperate with the Deutsche Heredo-Ataxie Gesellschaft e.V. (DHAG), a self-help group of ataxia patients. All eligible CA patients who agree to participate in the study will be provided with a full verbal explanation of the trial and the Patient Information Sheet. This will include detailed information about the rationale, design and personal implications of the study. After information is provided to patients, they will have sufficient time to consider participation before they are asked whether they would be willing to take part in the trial. It is imperative that written consent be obtained before any trial-specific procedures commence.

Randomization, concealment, and blinding

Participants fulfilling the entry criteria at screening will be randomly assigned in a ratio of 1:1 to receive one of the two treatment sequences (active treatment followed by placebo, or vice versa). The randomization technique is based on permutated balanced blocks with random block length. The procedure considers stratification by study site and by genetic vs. sporadic CA to ensure balanced strata, maintaining allocation concealment. The allocation sequence will be generated by an independent person from the Institute of Medical Informatics, Biometry and Epidemiology (IBE) of the University of Munich who is not involved in assessing study outcomes. Neither the investigators nor other trial staff (data analysts, statisticians) or the patients will be informed about the treatment sequences to which a patient is allocated, and neither has access to the randomization list. Thus, randomisation will be conducted without any influence of the investigators or trial staff. The IBE will provide an internet-based, password-protected randomization tool ("Randoulette": https://wwwapp.ibe.med.uni-muenchen.de/randoulette), which chooses the treatment sequence for a new patient who fulfills the eligibility criteria and has signed the informed consent. Randoulette will register the patient by his or her screening number, gender, year of birth and strata before the allocated package number is provided. The current trial is subject— and investigator-blinded. Patients, clinicians, core laboratories, and trial staff (including data analysts and statisticians) will be unaware of the treatment that the participant will take during both double blind treatment periods.

Un-blinding will occur in the event of a clinical emergency in which the knowledge of the medication being taken is essential for the participant's clinical management. The investigator is supplied with an opaque sealed envelope for each participant that contains the corresponding treatment sequence for unblinding. Alternatively, the randomization code can be broken using Randoulette.

Trial procedures and interventions

Each treatment sequence consists of a first treatment period of 6 weeks (42 days), followed by a 4-week (28 days) wash-out period, and a second treatment period of 6 weeks (42 days). Finally, a post-treatment follow-up is scheduled 4 weeks (28 days) after the end of the second treatment period (see fig. 1). The 4-week wash-out period between consecutive treatments is assumed to be long enough to allow the effects of a treatment to wear off and prevent carry over from one treatment period to the next.

Patients will be screened and assessed for eligibility at visit 1. If within 4 weeks prior to visit 1 a patient has received any of the prohibited medications defined in the eligibility criteria, irrespective of the preceding treatment duration, a wash-out period of 4 weeks (screening period), prior to enrolment is required. Patients eligible for entry in the study will be randomized and assigned to one of the two sequence groups at visit 2. Visits 1 and 2 coincide if patients are not on prohibited medication

4 weeks prior to recruitment. At baseline, data on demographic and clinical characteristics including neurological assessment, ataxia rating scales, information about preceding physio– and speech therapy as well as patient questionnaires will be obtained. Figure 1 displays the crossover intervention scheme. Table 2 lists the schedule of enrolment and assessments together with pre-planned time points for clinic visits. Including the eligibility screening visit 1 and the post-treatment follow-up visit 8, a total of eight study visits (three in each treatment period) are scheduled.

Investigative drug and placebo

In the experimental treatment period, patients will receive tablets of acetyl-DL-leucine 500 mg (Tanganil®, manufactured by Pierre Fabre, Castres, France) (other ingredients: wheat starch, pregelatinized corn starch, calcium carbonate, and magnesium stearate as filling material). Tablets containing the active ingredient will be refilled from original packaging into blisters under sterile conditions and relabeled by the pharmacy of the university hospital of Heidelberg. An identically appearing tablet filled with wheat starch, pregelatinized corn starch, calcium carbonate, and magnesium stearate but not containing any active ingredient will be administered as placebo. Study medication blisters will be packed in boxes and study kits will be delivered to the participating centers.

Study medication will be delivered to the patient at the beginning of a 6-week treatment period (visits 2 and 5, respectively). Patients are instructed to apply a 2-week up-titration scheme and will be provided with written

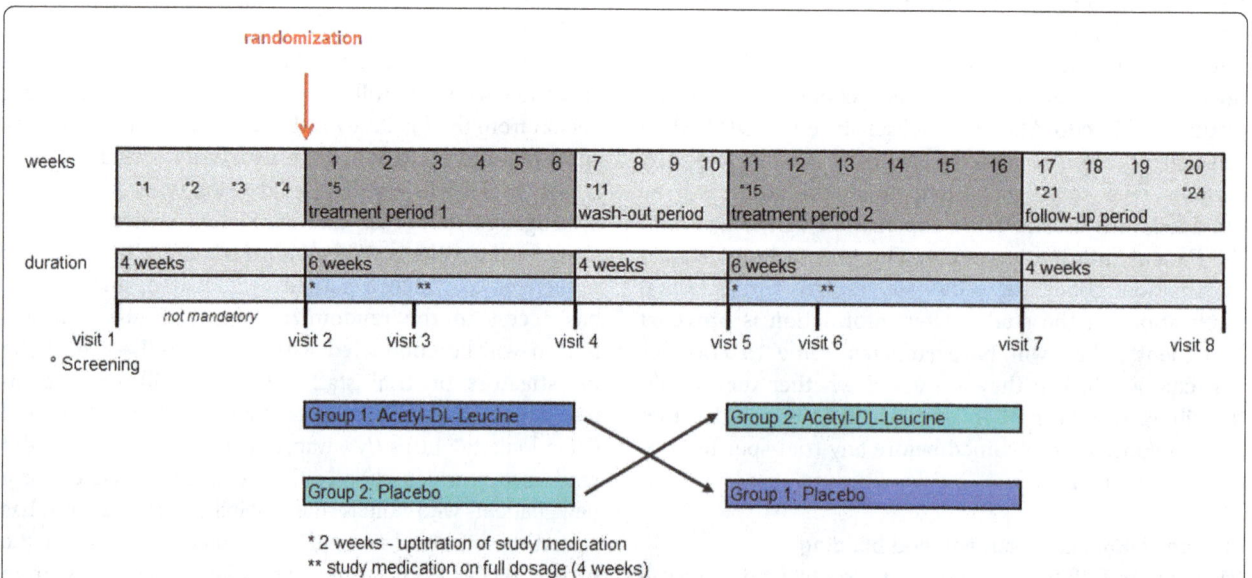

Fig. 1 ALCAT trial: crossover intervention scheme. Screening (visit 1) and visit 2 can take place on the same date, if patients are not on prohibited medication within 4 weeks prior to enrolment. If patients have received any of the prohibited medications 4 weeks prior to enrolment, a wash-out period of 4 weeks prior to visit 2 (randomization) is required to rule out a carryover effect

Table 2 Schedule of enrolment, interventions, and assessments

	Enrollment		Treatment period 1			Wash-out 4 weeks	Treatment period 2			Close-out
	Before	Eligibility Screening Visit 1[c]	Visit 2 (Baseline)	Visit 3 2 weeks after V2	Visit 4 6 weeks after V2		Visit 5	Visit 6 2 weeks after V5	Visit 7 6 weeks after V5	Follow-up Visit 8 4 weeks after V7
Timeline (days)		0/-28	0	14	42	70	70	84	112	140
Informed consent[a]	X									
Inclusion/exclusion criteria		X								
Medical history, including demographics & medications		X								
Documentation of physiotherapy/ speech therapy		X	X[b]	X	X		X	X	X	X
Neurological examination		X								
Blood tests		X[d]			X[d]		X[d]		X[d]	
Randomization			X							
Dispensing of trial drug			X				X			
Return of trial drug					X				X	
Compliance check				X	X			X	X	
Patient questionnaires (EQ-5D-5 L, BDI-II, FSS)			X	X	X		X	X	X	X
Ataxia rating scale: SARA		X	X[b]	X	X		X	X	X	X
Ataxia rating scale: SCAFI			X	X	X		X	X	X	X
Documentation of (S)AEs		X	X[b]	X	X		X	X	X	X
Documentation of concomitant medication (drug history)			X	X	X		X	X	X	X

A delay of -3 and +5 days is acceptable for visits 2 and 5, for all other visits a delay of ± 5 days is acceptable

[a] prior to first study-specific intervention and allocation

[b] If visit 1 and visit 2 take place at the same time, the ataxia rating scale (SARA), documentation of physiotherapy/speech therapy and documentation of (S)AE are assessed only once

[c] If patients are on medication due to cerebellar symptoms at visit 1, a 4-week wash-out (screening period) prior to randomization at visit 2 is required (adherence will again be checked before randomization at V2). Otherwise, visit 1 and visit 2 coincide

[d] incl. negative pregnancy test for women of childbearing potential

information. The up-titration scheme is as follows: in the first week an initial dosage of 1.5 g per day (500 mg t.i.d.), followed by 3 g per day (500 mg 2 tablets t.i.d.) in the second week. After that (and another study visit), the full dosage of 5 g per day (500 mg 3–3–4) will be administered for another 4 weeks. If adverse events (AEs) are noted, patients are permitted to down-titrate to a minimum dosage of 1.5 g per day (in the maintaining phase from week 3 to 6) within the current treatment period, which is then considered to be their maximal dose. The patients are instructed that the study medication has to be taken at least 30 min before and at least 2 h after a meal. Treatment adherence will be assessed by counting tablets at the end of the treatment period, and by recording the number of skipped intakes.

Study objectives and outcomes

The primary objective of the ALCAT trial is to demonstrate that acetyl-DL-leucine is effective at improving motor function measured by the SARA total score. The primary efficacy endpoint is the absolute change in the SARA total score from period-level baseline to the end of the 6-week treatment period, i.e. the difference between post-treatment values at the end of each treatment period and the corresponding period-level baseline values:

$$\text{Delta (SARAtotal)} = \text{SARAtotal (post-treatment)} - \text{SARAtotal (period baseline)}$$

We presume a minimum clinically relevant difference in the SARA total score of 1.5 points. The secondary objectives are to determine whether Acetyl-DL-Leucine is effective at:

a) improving motor function measured by the Spinocerebellar Ataxia Functional Index (SCAFI) and SARA subscore items
b) improving QoL, as well as the common comorbidities depression and fatigue.

The secondary efficacy outcome measures will be absolute changes in the subscores of SARA as well as the

SCAFI total score and subscores of SCAFI (8 MW testing gait, 9HPT testing limb ataxia and the PATA rate task for speech). Furthermore, patient-reported outcomes using the EuroQoL 5 dimensions and 5 level version (EQ-5D-5 L), Beck's Depression Inventory (BDI-II) as well as the Fatigue Severity Scale (FSS) will be recorded.

For all these scores, the treatment effect will be assessed at the end of each treatment period and at the post-treatment follow-up visit.

During the whole study period any AE (any untoward medical occurrence, including an abnormal laboratory finding, regardless of its causal relation to the study treatment) will be recorded.

Ataxia rating scales

The clinical severity of ataxia will be assessed by two different clinical ataxia rating scales — namely SARA [24] and SCAFI [25, 26]. The scores will be assessed by the investigators. Both scales assess ataxia and dysarthria, and are widely used in clinical practice [26] and clinical trials covering the whole range of impaired motor function in ataxic patients. The scales are measured at each clinic visit.

The SARA total score serves as a key inclusion criterion measuring the severity of ataxia prior to enrollment. The SARA total score has eight categories reflecting neurologic manifestations of CA. Each category represents a crucialmovement feature in CA rated by an examiner (gait, stance, sitting, speech disturbance, finger chase, nose-finger test, fast alternating hand movements, heel-shin slide) resulting in a score ranging from 0 (no ataxia) to 40 points (most severe ataxia). It is a reliable and valid clinical scale with a high internal consistency that measures the severity of ataxia and increases with disease stage [25, 27, 28].

The SCAFI includes the 8 MW testing gait, the 9HPT testing limb ataxia and the PATA rate task for speech and therefore represents vital movement features. In contrast to the SARA, the SCAFI uses a timed approach rated by an examiner. After the assessment, raw scores are transformed into reciprocals and converted into subtest Z-scores. The resulting SCAFI is defined as the arithmetic mean of all three Z-scores.

Patient questionnaires for quality of life, depression and fatigue

A self-administered questionnaire to evaluate QoL, namely the EQ-5D-5 L [29] (multiple choice questionnaire and a visual analogue scale) will be used. The EQ-5D-5 L is a standardized measure of health status that provides a simple, generic measure of health for clinical and economic appraisal and consists of 2 parts — the EQ-5D descriptive system and the EQ visual analogue scale (EQ-VAS). The EQ-5D-5 L descriptive system comprises the following 5 dimensions: mobility, self-care, usual activities, pain/discomfort and anxiety/depression. Each dimension has 5 levels: no problems, slight problems, moderate problems, severe problems, and extreme problems.

As depression and fatigue are known common comorbidities in patients with CA, trial participants are instructed to complete the BDI-II [30–32] and FSS [32] questionnaires at each clinic visit. The BDI-II is a multiple choice self-report inventory for measuring the severity of depression and is composed of items related to symptoms of depression such as hopelessness and irritability, emotions such as guilt or feelings of being punished, as well as physical symptoms such as fatigue, weight loss and lack of interest in sex. The FSS captures the patient's experience of mental or psychological fatigue and how it interferes with performing certain activities (exercise, work and family life). It is a self-reporting scale of 9 items. The mean of all answered items represents the fatigue severity.

Laboratory examinations

A routine blood sample will be taken to exclude liver or kidney failure, and a pregnancy test for women of childbearing potential will be performed. A pregnancy test is not required for postmenopausal (amenorrhea >12 months), surgically sterilized or hysterectomized women. The following laboratory parameters will be assessed (but not routinely documented in the CRF): sodium, potassium, creatinine, serum bilirubin level, AST, ALT, urea, ALP, TSH, hemoglobin, erythrocytes, hematocrit, thrombocytes, leukocytes, pregnancy test for women of childbearing potential. In a case of an AE, laboratory parameters will be documented. The total amount of blood taken per subject during the entire trial will be approximately 20 ml. Laboratory examinations are carried out at visit 1, visit 4, visit 5 and visit 7.

Concomitant drug and non-drug therapies

Trial participants should not begin physiotherapy or speech therapy while they are enrolled in the trial. If they are already under therapy, the amount of sessions of physiotherapy and speech therapy (measured in hours of therapy per week) will be documented in the patient's medical record and in the case report form (CRF) during the trial and for 6 months prior to randomization. To adhere to the protocol, the non-pharmacological concomitant therapy should be continued with the same intensity while the patient is enrolled in the trial.

Guided by the eligibility criteria, the administration of 4-aminopyridine, Riluzole, Varenicline, Gabapentin or Chlorzoxazone is not allowed during the trial because of a possible beneficial effect in CA.

Participation discontinuation and follow-up of participants 'off protocol'

If a participant withdraws from the study, the reason will be documented. 'Off protocol' is defined as those study participants who cease trial medications on clinical grounds. Regardless of the decision to continue with study medication, these participants will be asked to participate in all scheduled follow-up appointments, as if they were maintaining full participation, in order to prevent further missing data. Those who are unwilling or unable to do this will be asked to agree to a phone or mail follow-up, and/or permission for study staff to continue ascertainment of outcomes.

Statistical planning and analyses
Power considerations and sample size calculation

The sample size was calculated on the basis of the primary hypothesis, using our own preliminary case series data (13 patients [17]) and a similar placebo-controlled trial (20 patients [7]) investigating the efficacy of varenicline on the change in SARA total score in patients with SCA 3. Hence, assuming a minimum clinically relevant difference in the SARA total score of 1.5 points [25] to be detected (i.e. the absolute change on acetyl-DL-leucine is 1.5 score points better than the change on placebo) and a standard deviation of the individual SARA change of 4.2, a sample size of 86 (85 is calculated but 2 sequences are needed) in total is will have 90% power to detect a difference in means of 1.5, using a paired t-test with a 0.05 two-sided significance level [Software used: nQuery Advisor 7.0]. On the basis of our experience with patient compliance in previous studies, we expect a dropout rate of about 20%. Thus, a total of 108 patients have to be enrolled. With a proportion of about 50–55% recruited patients out of the number to be screened, about 200 patients have to be assessed for eligibility. There is no interim analysis planned for this study.

Statistical analyses for primary and secondary endpoints

Efficacy analyses are based on the intention to treat (ITT) principle in that all participants randomized will be analyzed according to the treatment sequences to which they were allocated and irrespective of the extent of intervention received. In this study, the term 'full analysis set' is used to describe the analysis set, which is as complete as possible and as close as possible to the ITT ideal of including all randomised participants (i.e, the ITT population). All statistical tests are two-sided, and the significance level alpha is set to 5%.

For the primary efficacy outcome change in SARA total score (DeltaSARA), the null hypothesis will be tested that there is no difference in mean change between placebo and acetyl-DL-leucine.

Absolute change, calculated as the difference between the period-level baseline score and the score measured at the 2-week and 6-week visits of the acetyl-DL-leucine/placebo period, will be considered for a model-based primary efficacy analysis. If not revised in the statistical analysis plan (SAP), a linear mixed effects model for DeltaSARA will be performed (fixed effects: factor for treatment, visit, treatment-by-visit interaction, and mean of both period-level baseline SARA total scores as covariate; normally distributed patient-specific random intercepts and slopes) in order to deal with repeated measurements within periods and measurements not made at equivalent times in each subject due to unscheduled or missed clinic visits. This subject-specific modelling approach allows individual change scores over time to be calculated. To analyse the differences between both interventions at the end of the 6-week treatment period, 95% confidence intervals will be provided to quantitatively describe treatment effects.

Sensitivity analyses will be performed on a per protocol approach which takes into account treatment adherence and compliance with the trial protocol. Additional efficacy analyses adjusting for genetic vs. sporadic CA, gender, age, or trial site, will be performed. In addition, the robustness of the overall efficacy result will be investigated by analyses adjusting for the amount of physiotherapy the patient received when he or she was enrolled in the trial (which should be comparable to the amount received before randomization), as considered appropriate during the blinded data review and depending on the data quality. Since this analysis will also be based on variables measured after randomization, the susceptibility for bias will be given consideration and will be discussed.

In case of a statistically significant primary efficacy result, confirmatory testing will be extended to the EQ-5D-5 L (VAS and descriptive scale). SCAFI (total score and 3 subscores), SARA subscale items, as well as patient-reported outcomes BDI-II and FSS are not considered in the hierarchical multiple testing procedures. Descriptive comparisons between treatment groups at the end of the 6-week acetyl-DL-leucine/placebo period will be performed using a two-sided Wilcoxon signed rank test, and additionally, Hodges-Lehmann estimation of the location shift between the two groups will be provided, as considered appropriate based on the blinded data. The same non-parametrical tests will be employed to estimate treatment differences at the follow-up visit 8 (close-out visit). Further methodological details will be provided in the SAP.

Safety assessment

Outcome assessors will judge the severity (mild, moderate, or severe), seriousness, and causality (definitely related, probably related, possibly related, possibly not related, definitely not related to the intervention, or not assessable).

All adverse events will be listed by trial site and patient and displayed in summary tables. The incidence of adverse events and their relationship to the study drug will be analyzed descriptively, guided by the Medical Dictionary for Regulatory Activities (MedDRA) classification.

Data collection
Results from the trial assessments will be recorded in an electronic CRF (e-CRF) via a validated open-source electronic data capture (EDC) system based on the OpenClinica® Community Edition. At each clinical site, study personnel will enter data directly into the EDC system. Data will be transferred on a regular basis to the official study database stored in SAS (Version 9.2 for Linux, SAS Institute, Cary, NC) for quality checks and query management. Statistical analyses will be performed using SAS, as well as the software package R version 3.3.0 or higher [33].

Data safety and monitoring board (DSMB)
An independent DSMB has been established. The function of the DSMB is to monitor the course of the study and if necessary to give a recommendation to the coordinating investigator and sponsor of the trial for discontinuation, modification or continuation of the study. Furthermore, the DSMB will periodically review the safety data of Development Safety Update Reports.

Discussion
Because there is no approved causal or symptomatic drug therapy yet, there is an urgent need for effective and well-tolerated drug treatment. Based on different case series in hereditary or non-hereditary non-acquired CA of different etiologies [17, 19, 22] and its good safety profile (since 1957 on the market in France for symptomatic dizziness and vertigo treatment) the modified amino-acid acetyl-DL-leucine is a good candidate.

In this multicenter, multinational, randomized, double-blind, placebo-controlled, phase III trial, short-term treatment efficacy and safety are evaluated with a 2-treatment 2-period crossover design comprised of 6-week treatment periods. The primary inclusion criterion SARA total score of at least 3 points ensures that patients are at least moderately affected by the disease and allows CA patients with a wide spectrum of clinical severity to be included. Except for the blood tests, all examinations and assessments applied are non-invasive and also performed in clinical routine. If superiority of acetyl-DL-leucine compared to placebo intervention can be established, this medication could offer a complete new therapeutic approach for the target population. Due to the high prevalence and the participation of many centers in three European countries, recruitment to reach the target sample size of 108 participants seems achievable within the planned time frame of 32 months. Due to the pragmatic nature of the trial

design, the primary question of interest relates to intervention effectiveness, i.e. whether the intervention works under real-life conditions. In particular, trial participants are allowed to maintain physio- or speech therapy during the trial provided that they have already started this therapy before recruitment.

Of course, this trial has some limitations: first, so far we do not know what the optimal dosage is. The dose of 5 g per day used in this trial is based on case series. Second, we do not know what the optimal dosage interval is. Third, since the plasma levels are not measured, we cannot correlate them with the clinical effect and we cannot exclude patients taking acetyl-DL-leucine in addition to the study medication. Fourth, as we include multiple types of CA (hereditary or non-hereditary non-acquired) we will not know if the agent is more effective with one CA than with another due to small numbers of the different CA types. Last, but not least, the observational period is quite short, so we cannot evaluate the effect of the drug on the long-term progression of the disease compared to placebo intervention. This, however, could easily be done as soon as its efficacy and safety in symptomatic treatment is demonstrated.

Trial status
At the time of manuscript submission, the study design had been evaluated by independent international reviewers and has been approved by the responsible ethics committee of the University of Munich and the ethics committee in Austria as well as the authorities in Germany (BfArM) and Austria (AGES). The study is being prepared for submission in the Netherlands. The first study participant was randomized on January 25, 2016 with the opening of the trial site of the coordinating investigator. As of October, 1st, we have included a total of 92 patients.

Abbreviations
(S)AE(s): (serious) adverse event(s); (S)CA: (spino-) cerebellar ataxia; 8 MW: 8-m-walking-time; 9HPTD: 9-Hole-Peg-Test of the dominant hand; AGES: Österreichische Agentur für Gesundheit und Ernährungssicherheit GmbH in Austria (Austrian agency for health and food safety Ltd.); BDI-II: Beck's depression inventory; BfArM: Bundesinstitut für Arzneimittelsicherheit und Medizinprodukte (Federal institute for drugs and medical devices); CCMO: Centrale Commissie Mensgebonden Onderzoek (Central committee on research involving human subjects); CRF: Case report form; DHAG: Deutsche Heredo-Ataxie Gesellschaft e.V.; DSMB: Data safety and monitoring board; e-CRF: Electronic CRF; EDC: Electronic data capture; EQ-5D-5L: EuroQol 5 dimensions and 5 level version; EQ-VAS: EuroQol Visual analogue scale; FSS: Fatigue severity scale; ICH-GCP: International conference for harmonisation (of technical requirements for pharmaceuticals for human use) - good clinical practice guideline; ITT: Intention to treat; MedDRA: Medical dictionary for regulatory activities; MSA-C: Multisystem atrophy type C; QoL: Quality of Life; SAP: Statistical analysis plan; SARA: Scale for the assessment and rating of ataxia; SCAFI: Spinocerebellar ataxia functional index; SD: Standard deviation; SDP: Sponsor's delegated person

Acknowledgment
The authors thank Katie Ogston for copy-editing the manuscript. Further, we are very grateful to all the patients who decided to participate in this study.

Funding
This investigator-initiated trial is funded by the German Federal Ministry of Education and Research (BMBF, No. 01KG1422). The funder had no influence on the design of protocol, and will not have any impact on patient recruitment, data generation, statistical analyses or writing of the final manuscript.

Authors' contributions
MS, KF and JT initiated the initial case series pre-study, leading to the study concept and design of the ALCAT trial. MS is the sponsor delegated person (SDP) and coordinating investigator. MS and KF are responsible for the implementation of the study.

MS, KF, OB, JT, CA and HHM made substantial contributions to the conception and the trial design, and wrote the study protocol or preceding research proposals for funding.

SB, JC, IG, HH, HJ, TK, TK, WN, LS, CS, EU, BW made contributions to the study protocol or research proposals and revised the final manuscript for medical content.

KF and CA drafted the manuscript. HHM and CA developed the statistical concept and performed the sample size calculation. UM has the main responsibility for statistical analyses and supervised parts of the protocol development. IB and IN contributed decisively to approval to ethics and regulatory authorities and made substantial contribution to the study protocol. All authors read and approved the final manuscript.

Competing interests
Michael Strupp, is Joint Chief Editor of the Journal of Neurology, Editor in Chief of Frontiers of Neuro-otology and Section Editor of F1000. He has received speaker's honoraria from Abbott, Actelion, Biogen, Eisai, GSK, Hennig Pharma, Pierre Fabre, MSD Sharp & Dohme, TEVA, and UCB and works as a consultant for Abbott, Heel, IntraBio, Sensorion and Synthon.
Bart van de Warrenburg reports research funding from the Radboud University Medical Center and ZonMW.
The other co-authors declare no competing interests.
All authors provided feedback on drafts of this paper and read and approved the final manuscript.

Author details
[1]Department of Neurology with Friedrich-Baur-Institute, University Hospital, Munich, Germany. [2]German Center for Vertigo and Balance Disorders (DSGZ), University Hospital, Munich, Germany. [3]Institute for Medical Informatics, Biometry and Epidemiology (IBE), University Hospital, Munich, Germany. [4]German Center for Neurodegenerative Diseases (DZNE), Munich 80336, Germany. [5]Department of Neurology, University Hospital Essen, University of Duisburg-Essen, Essen, Germany. [6]Department of Neurology and Hertie Institute for Clinical Brain Research, University Hospital Tübingen, Tübingen, Germany. [7]German Center for Neurodegenerative Diseases (DZNE), Center for Clinical Research, Bonn, Germany. [8]Department of Neurology, Medical University Innsbruck, Innsbruck, Austria. [9]Department of Neurology, Donders Institute for Brain, Cognition, and Behaviour, Radboud University Medical Centre, Nijmegen, Netherlands. [10]Institute for Medical Biometry and Epidemiology, Philipps University Marburg, Marburg, Germany. [11]Department of Neurology and German Center for Vertigo and Balance Disorders, University Hospital, Campus Grosshadern, Marchioninistrasse 15, Munich 81377, Germany. [12]Munich Cluster for Systems Neurology (SyNergy), Munich 80336, Germany.

References
1. Jacobi H, et al. The natural history of spinocerebellar ataxia type 1, 2, 3, and 6: a 2-year follow-up study. Neurology. 2011;77(11):1035–41.
2. Klockgether T. Sporadic adult-onset ataxia of unknown etiology. Handb Clin Neurol. 2012;103:253–62.
3. Perlman SL. Symptomatic and disease-modifying therapy for the progressive ataxias. Neurologist. 2004;10(5):275–89.
4. Lopez-Bastida J, et al. Social economic costs and health-related quality of life in patients with degenerative cerebellar ataxia in Spain. Mov Disord. 2008;23(2):212–7.
5. Ilg W, Bastian AJ, Boesch S, Burciu RG, Celnik P, Claaßen J, Feil K, Kalla R, Miyai I, Nachbauer W, Schöls L, Strupp M, Synofzik M, Teufel J, Timmann D. Consensus paper: management of degenerative cerebellar disorders. Cerebellum. 2014;13(2):248-68. doi:10.1007/s12311-013-0531-6.
6. Ristori G, et al. Riluzole in cerebellar ataxia: a randomized, double-blind, placebo-controlled pilot trial. Neurology. 2010;74(10):839–45.
7. Zesiewicz TA, et al. A randomized trial of varenicline (Chantix) for the treatment of spinocerebellar ataxia type 3. Neurology. 2012;78(8):545–50.
8. Romano S, et al. Riluzole in patients with hereditary cerebellar ataxia: a randomised, double-blind, placebo-controlled trial. Lancet Neurol. 2015; 14(10):985–91.
9. Ilg W, et al. Consensus paper: management of degenerative cerebellar disorders. Cerebellum. 2014;13(2):248–68.
10. Ilg W, et al. Intensive coordinative training improves motor performance in degenerative cerebellar disease. Neurology. 2009;73(22):1823–30.
11. Ferber-Viart C, Dubreuil C, Vidal PP. Effects of acetyl-DL-leucine in vestibular patients: a clinical study following neurotomy and labyrinthectomy. Audiol Neurootol. 2009;14(1):17–25.
12. Vibert N, Vidal PP. In vitro effects of acetyl-DL-leucine (tanganil) on central vestibular neurons and vestibulo-ocular networks of the guinea-pig. Eur J Neurosci. 2001;13(4):735–48.
13. Highstein SM, Holstein GR. The anatomy of the vestibular nuclei. Prog Brain Res. 2006;151:157–203.
14. Gunther L, et al. N-acetyl-L-leucine accelerates vestibular compensation after unilateral labyrinthectomy by action in the cerebellum and thalamus. PLoS One. 2015;10(3):e0120891.
15. Suh BC, Hille B. PIP2 is a necessary cofactor for ion channel function: how and why? Annu Rev Biophys. 2008;37:175–95.
16. Witter L, et al. The cerebellar nuclei take center stage. Cerebellum. 2011; 10(4):633–6.
17. Strupp M, et al. Effects of acetyl-DL-leucine in patients with cerebellar ataxia: a case series. J Neurol. 2013;260(10):2556–61.
18. Becker-Bense S, Feuerecker R, Xiong G, Feil K, Bartenstein P, Strupp M, Dieterich M. Effects of acetyl-DL-leucine on the cerebral activation pattern in cerebellar ataxia (FDG-PET study) - Oral Sessions No. O1201. Eur J Neurol. 2015;22:21–117.
19. Schniepp R, et al. Acetyl-DL-leucine improves gait variability in patients with cerebellar ataxia-a case series. Cerebellum Ataxias. 2016;3:8.
20. Schniepp R, et al. 4-aminopyridine and cerebellar gait: a retrospective case series. J Neurol. 2012;259(11):2491–3.
21. Schniepp R, et al. 4-Aminopyridine improves gait variability in cerebellar ataxia due to CACNA 1A mutation. J Neurol. 2011;258(9):1708–11.
22. Bremova T, M.V., Amraoui Y, Mengel E, Reinke J, Kolníková M, Strupp M Acetyl-DL-leucine in Niemann-Pick type C: a case series. Neurology. Neurology, 2015. In press.
23. Pelz JO, et al. Failure to confirm benefit of acetyl-DL-leucine in degenerative cerebellar ataxia: a case series. J Neurol. 2015;262(5):1373–5.
24. Subramony SH. SARA–a new clinical scale for the assessment and rating of ataxia. Nat Clin Pract Neurol. 2007;3(3):136–7.
25. Schmitz-Hubsch T, et al. Scale for the assessment and rating of ataxia: development of a new clinical scale. Neurology. 2006;66(11):1717–20.
26. Schmitz-Hubsch T, et al. SCA Functional Index: a useful compound performance measure for spinocerebellar ataxia. Neurology. 2008;71(7):486–92.
27. Weyer A, et al. Reliability and validity of the scale for the assessment and rating of ataxia: a study in 64 ataxia patients. Mov Disord. 2007;22(11):1633–7.
28. Yabe I, et al. Usefulness of the scale for assessment and rating of ataxia (SARA). J Neurol Sci. 2008;266(1-2):164–6.
29. Rabin R, de Charro F. EQ-5D: a measure of health status from the EuroQol Group. Ann Med. 2001;33(5):337–43.
30. Schmitz-Hubsch T, et al. Self-rated health status in spinocerebellar ataxia– results from a European multicenter study. Mov Disord. 2010;25(5):587–95.
31. Schmitz-Hubsch T, et al. Depression comorbidity in spinocerebellar ataxia. Mov Disord. 2011;26(5):870–6.
32. Brusse E, et al. Fatigue in spinocerebellar ataxia: patient self-assessment of an early and disabling symptom. Neurology. 2011;76(11):953–9.
33. R Core Team, R: A language and environment for statistical computing. R Foundation for Statistical Computing,. Vienna, Austria 2016. http://www.R-project.org/.

26

Screening for onconeural antibodies in neuromyelitis optica spectrum disorders

Benjamin Berger*(iD), Tilman Hottenrott, Sebastian Rauer and Oliver Stich

Abstract

Background: Some so-called "non-classical" paraneoplastic neurological syndromes (PNS), namely optic neuritis and myelitis, clinically overlap with neuromyelitis optica spectrum disorders (NMOSD), and conversely, in cancer-associated NMOSD, a paraneoplastic etiology has been suggested in rare cases. Therefore, we retrospectively investigated the prevalence of onconeural antibodies, which are highly predictive for a paraneoplastic etiology, and the prevalence of malignancies in NMOSD patients.

Methods: We retrospectively screened 23 consecutive patients from our clinic with NMOSD (13 were anti-aquaporin-4 [AQP4] antibody positive, 10 were AQP4 negative) for onconeural antibodies using an immunoblot.

Results: All patients were negative for a broad spectrum of antibodies targeting intracellular onconeural antigens (Hu, Yo, Ri, CV2/CRMP5, Ma1, Ma2, Zic4, SOX1, Tr, and amphiphysin). Notably, only two patients had a malignancy. However, neoplastic entities (astrocytic brain tumor and acute myeloid leukemia) were not typical for PNS.

Conclusions: Our data suggest that there is no need to routinely screen anti-AQP4 antibody positive NMOSD patients with a typical presentation for onconeural antibodies. Furthermore, absence of these antibodies in NMOSD, which is typically non-paraneoplastic, confirms their high specificity for PNS.

Keywords: Aquaporin-4, Neuromyelitis optica spectrum disorders, NMOSD, Onconeural antibodies, Paraneoplastic

Background

Neuromyelitis optica (NMO) is a rare, immune-mediated, demyelinating disorder of the central nervous system (CNS), typically presenting with relapsing optic neuritis (ON) and/or ≥ three vertebral segment longitudinally extensive transverse myelitis (LETM) [1, 2]. Pathogenetic antibodies targeting the water channel protein aquaporin-4 (AQP4) are found in the majority of patients with NMO [3]. Since their discovery, the spectrum of clinical manifestations within the CNS associated with AQP4 antibodies has expanded [4]. Therefore, diagnostic criteria have recently been revised, introducing the term "neuromyelitis optica spectrum disorders (NMOSD)" [5]. According to these revised criteria, an NMOSD diagnosis can also be established in absence of anti-AQP4 antibodies. For simplicity, in the following, the term "NMOSD" is consistently used for both NMO and NMOSD.

Paraneoplastic neurological syndromes (PNS) are remote effects of cancer and often are associated with high concentrations of so-called well-characterized onconeural antibodies (anti-Hu, Yo, Ri, CV2/CRMP5, Ma1, Ma2, and amphiphysin) that help to establish the diagnosis [6]. Notably, some "non-classical" PNS (ON, myelitis) have a clinical presentation similar to NMOSD [6–10]. Conversely, previous studies of cancer-associated NMOSD, comprising mainly case reports, postulated a paraneoplastic etiology [11–17], particularly if the tumor expresses AQP4 [18–22]. However, onconeural antibodies were not systematically investigated in NMOSD.

Regarding a previously suggested paraneoplastic etiology in rare cases, we retrospectively investigated the prevalence of onconeural antibodies and malignancies in NMOSD patients.

Methods

Consecutive patients were identified by an electronic database search. Based on clinical records, NMOSD diagnosis was verified according to recently revised

* Correspondence: benjamin.berger@uniklinik-freiburg.de
Department of Neurology and Neurophysiology, Medical Center—University of Freiburg, Faculty of Medicine, Breisacher Strasse 64, D-79106 Freiburg, Germany

criteria [5]. This approach identified 35 patients with NMOSD who were treated in our clinic (Department of Neurology and Neurophysiology, Medical Center—University of Freiburg, Germany) between 2003 and 2015. Stored serum samples kept at −80 °C from 25 therapy naïve patients were available for analysis. Of these patients, two declined analysis. Finally, 23 patients entered the study. Demographic and clinical data, including anti-AQP4 antibody status, were obtained from patients' records.

Screening for antibodies targeting intracellular onconeural antigens (Hu, Yo, Ri, CV2/CRMP5, Ma1, Ma2, Zic4, SOX1, Tr, and amphiphysin) was performed on serum samples using a commercial immunoblot with highly purified recombinant antigens according to the manufacturer's instructions (kindly provided by ravo Diagnostika, Freiburg, Germany).

Dichotomized variables are presented using numbers and percentages; continuous variables are presented using means or medians, range, and standard deviation (SD). The local ethics committee approved the study, and all patients gave written informed consent to the study protocol.

Results

Table 1 summarizes clinical data of 23 patients fulfilling revised criteria for NMOSD diagnosis and entering the study. Mean age was 44 years (range 19–75, SD 17.2) at disease manifestation, and 49 years (range 20–75, SD 15.8) at diagnosis. Eighteen (78.3%) were female, and 13 (56.5%) were anti-AQP4 antibody positive. Two patients (Table 1: patients #5 and #15) had a malignoma: one had an anaplastic astrocytoma that occurred 7 years after NMOSD manifestation and that progressed to secondary glioblastoma; the other had acute myeloid leukemia (AML) that was treated with stem cell transplantation 4 years before the NMOSD manifestation. Follow-up information was available in all patients with a median duration of 5.0 years (range 0.5–10.0 years, SD 2.7). Remarkably, none had antibodies targeting intracellular onconeural antigens (Hu, Yo, Ri, CV2/CRMP5, Ma1, Ma2, Zic4, SOX1, Tr, and amphiphysin).

Discussion

Inspired by previous reports suggesting a paraneoplastic etiology in rare cases of cancer-associated NMOSD

Table 1 Demographic and clinical characteristics of 23 patients with NMOSD

Patient	Anti-AQP4	Clinical characteristics	Malignoma	Associated autoimmune disease	Duration of follow-up (years)
#1	+	ON and LETM	-	Sjögren's syndrome	4
#2	-	ON and LETM	-	-	3
#3	-	ON and LETM	-	Hashimoto's thyroiditis	6
#4	+	LETM	-	-	5,5
#5	-	ON and LETM	Astrocytoma[a]	-	10
#6	+	LETM	-	-	2
#7	-	ON and LETM	-	-	5
#8	-	ON and LETM	-	Hashimoto's thyroiditis	5
#9	-	ON and LETM	-	-	5
#10	-	ON and LETM	-	Hashimoto's thyroiditis	9
#11	+	ON and LETM	-	-	0.5
#12	+	LETM	-	Systemic lupus erythematosus	5
#13	+	ON and LETM	-	-	6
#14	-	ON and LETM	-	-	5.5
#15	-	ON and LETM	AML	-	6
#16	+	ON and LETM	-	Sjögren's syndrome	1
#17	-	ON and LETM	-	-	2
#18	+	ON and LETM	-	-	8
#19	+	ON and LETM	-	Non-differentiated collagenosis	3.5
#20	+	ON and LETM	-	-	8
#21	+	LETM	-	-	0.5
#22	+	LETM	-	Hashimoto's thyroiditis	7
#23	+	ON and LETM	-	-	1

Abbreviations: NMOSD neuromyelitis optica spectrum disorders, *AQP4* aquaporin-4, *ON* optic neuritis, *LETM* longitudinal extensive transverse myelitis, *AML* acute myeloid leukemia
[a]Anaplastic astrocytoma that progressed to secondary glioblastoma

[11–22], this is the first study systematically investigating the seroprevalence of onconeural antibodies (anti-Hu, Yo, Ri, CV2/CRMP5, Ma1, Ma2, Zic4, SOX1, Tr, and amphiphysin) in NMOSD patients.

The principal finding was that all 23 patients' samples were antibody-negative. However, we acknowledge that the absence of onconeural antibodies does not exclude PNS [6]. In addition, only two patients in our study had a malignancy; yet neoplastic entities (astrocytic brain tumor and AML) are not typically associated with PNS [6]. By contrast, previous reports on putative paraneoplastic NMOSD described associated malignancies that typically occur in PNS patients, predominantly lung and breast cancer [11–22]. Unfortunately, these reports did not systematically investigate onconeural antibodies for comparison with our data. In this regard, there is currently only one case report describing anti-Hu antibodies in a patient with anti-AQP4 positive NMOSD and recurrent thymoma [23].

Limitations of our study were the retrospective design and therefore patients were not systematically screened for occult malignomas. Furthermore, the case number was limited, since serum was available for only 25 of 35 patients (71.4%) previously identified by an electronic database search for those with an NMOSD diagnosis.

Conclusions

According to our data, the routine screening for onconeural antibodies in NMOSD patients is not mandatory. However, clinicians should pay particular attention in anti-AQP4 negative patients, in patients with a known malignancy or cancer risk factors (e.g. smoking), and/or if clinical presentation is atypical, since paraneoplastic myelitis and/or ON in association with anti-CV2/CRMP5, –Hu or –amphiphysin antibodies might clinically mimic NMOSD [7–10]. Finally, the absence of onconeural antibodies in a typically non-paraneoplastic disorder corresponds to their high specificity for PNS [6]. Finally, larger retrospective trials are necessary to verify these results and to determine the proportion of anti-AQP4 negative NMOSD patients with onconeural antibodies.

Abbreviations

AML: Acute myeloid leukemia; AQP4: Aquaporin-4; CNS: Central nervous system; LETM: Longitudinally extensive transverse myelitis; NMO: Neuromyelitis optica; NMOSD: Neuromyelitis optica spectrum disorders; ON: Optic neuritis; PNS: Paraneoplastic neurological syndromes; SD: Standard deviation

Acknowledgements
Not applicable.

Funding
Not applicable.

Authors' contributions
BB conceived the study, drafted the manuscript, performed antibody testing, and collected patients' data. TH collected patients' data. SR and OS helped to draft the manuscript. All authors read and approved the final manuscript.

Competing interests
BB received travel grants from Bayer Vital GmbH, Ipsen Pharma GmbH, and Genzyme. TH received travel grants from Bayer Vital GmbH and Novartis. OS and SR report receiving consulting and lecture fees, and grant and research support from Baxter, Bayer Vital GmbH, Biogen Idec, Genzyme, Merck Serono, Novartis, Sanofi-Aventis, and Teva. Furthermore, SR is a founding executive board member of ravo Diagnostika GmbH, which sells in-vitro diagnostic medical devices for the detection of infectious diseases and paraneoplastic autoantibodies. None of the authors have any financial or personal relationships with individuals or organizations that could inappropriately influence this publication.

References
1. Wingerchuk DM, Lennon VA, Pittock SJ, Lucchinetti CF, Weinshenker BG. Revised diagnostic criteria for neuromyelitis optica. Neurology. 2006;66(10): 1485–9.
2. Wingerchuk DM, Hogancamp WF, O'Brien PC, Weinshenker BG. The clinical course of neuromyelitis optica (Devic's syndrome). Neurology. 1999;53(5): 1107–14.
3. Paul F, Jarius S, Aktas O, et al. Antibody to aquaporin 4 in the diagnosis of neuromyelitis optica. PLoS One. 2007;4(4), e133.
4. Jarius S, Wildemann B, Paul F. Neuromyelitis optica: clinical features, immunopathogenesis and treatment. Clin Exp Immunol. 2014;176(2):149–64.
5. Wingerchuk DM, Banwell B, Bennett JL, et al. International consensus diagnostic criteria for neuromyelitis optica spectrum disorders. Neurology. 2015;85(2):177–89.
6. Graus F, Delattre J, Antoine J, et al. Recommended diagnostic criteria for paraneoplastic neurological syndromes. J Neurol Neurosurg Psychiatry. 2004;75:1135–41.
7. Cross SA, Salomao DR, Parisi JE, et al. Paraneoplastic autoimmune optic neuritis with retinitis defined by CRMP-5-IgG. Ann Neurol. 2003;54(1):38–50.
8. Ducray F, Roos-Weil R, Garcia P, et al. Devic's syndrome-like phenotype associated with thymoma and anti-CV2/CRMP5 antibodies. J Neurol Neurosurg Psychiatry. 2007;78(3):325–7.
9. Jarius S, Wandinger KP, Borowski K, Stoecker W, Wildemann B. Antibodies to CV2/CRMP5 in neuromyelitis optica-like disease: case report and review of the literature. Clin Neurol Neurosurg. 2012;114(4):331–5.
10. Keegan BM, Pittock SJ, Lennon VA. Autoimmune myelopathy associated with collapsin response-mediator protein-5 immunoglobulin G. Ann Neurol. 2008;63(4):531–4.
11. Al-Harbi T, Al-Sarawi A, Binfalah M, Dermime S. Paraneoplastic neuromyelitis optica spectrum disorder associated with stomach carcinoid tumor. Hematol Oncol Stem Cell Ther. 2014;7(3):116–9.
12. Cai G, He D, Chu L, Dai Q, Xu Z, Zhang Y. Paraneoplastic neuromyelitis optica spectrum disorders: three new cases and a review of the literature. Int J Neurosci. 2016;126(7):660–8.
13. De Santis G, Caniatti L, De Vito A, De Gennaro R, Granieri E, Tola MR. A possible paraneoplastic neuromyelitis optica associated with lung cancer. Neurol Sci. 2009;30(5):397–400.
14. Moussawi K, Lin DJ, Matiello M, Chew S, Morganstern D, Vaitkevicius H. Brainstem and limbic encephalitis with paraneoplastic neuromyelitis optica. J Clin Neurosci. 2016;23:159–61.
15. Mueller S, Dubal DB, Josephson SA. A case of paraneoplastic myelopathy associated with the neuromyelitis optica antibody. Nat Clin Pract Neurol. 2008;4(5):284–8.
16. Ontaneda D, Fox R. Is neuromyelitis optica with advanced age of onset a paraneoplastic disorder? Int J Neurosci. 2014;124(7):509–11.
17. Pittock SJ, Lennon VA. Aquaporin-4 autoantibodies in a paraneoplastic context. Arch Neurol. 2008;65(5):629–32.
18. Armagan H, Tüzün E, Icöz O, et al. Long extensive transverse myelitis associated with aquaporin-4 antibody and breast cancer: favorable response to cancer treatment. J Spinal Cord Med. 2012;35(4):267–9.
19. Figueroa M, Guo Y, Tselis A, et al. Paraneoplastic neuromyelitis optica spectrum disorder associated with metastatic carcinoid expressing aquaporin-4. JAMA Neurol. 2014;71(4):495–8.

Permissions

All chapters in this book were first published in NEUROLOGY, by BioMed Central; hereby published with permission under the Creative Commons Attribution License or equivalent. Every chapter published in this book has been scrutinized by our experts. Their significance has been extensively debated. The topics covered herein carry significant findings which will fuel the growth of the discipline. They may even be implemented as practical applications or may be referred to as a beginning point for another development.

The contributors of this book come from diverse backgrounds, making this book a truly international effort. This book will bring forth new frontiers with its revolutionizing research information and detailed analysis of the nascent developments around the world.

We would like to thank all the contributing authors for lending their expertise to make the book truly unique. They have played a crucial role in the development of this book. Without their invaluable contributions this book wouldn't have been possible. They have made vital efforts to compile up to date information on the varied aspects of this subject to make this book a valuable addition to the collection of many professionals and students.

This book was conceptualized with the vision of imparting up-to-date information and advanced data in this field. To ensure the same, a matchless editorial board was set up. Every individual on the board went through rigorous rounds of assessment to prove their worth. After which they invested a large part of their time researching and compiling the most relevant data for our readers.

The editorial board has been involved in producing this book since its inception. They have spent rigorous hours researching and exploring the diverse topics which have resulted in the successful publishing of this book. They have passed on their knowledge of decades through this book. To expedite this challenging task, the publisher supported the team at every step. A small team of assistant editors was also appointed to further simplify the editing procedure and attain best results for the readers.

Apart from the editorial board, the designing team has also invested a significant amount of their time in understanding the subject and creating the most relevant covers. They scrutinized every image to scout for the most suitable representation of the subject and create an appropriate cover for the book.

The publishing team has been an ardent support to the editorial, designing and production team. Their endless efforts to recruit the best for this project, has resulted in the accomplishment of this book. They are a veteran in the field of academics and their pool of knowledge is as vast as their experience in printing. Their expertise and guidance has proved useful at every step. Their uncompromising quality standards have made this book an exceptional effort. Their encouragement from time to time has been an inspiration for everyone.

The publisher and the editorial board hope that this book will prove to be a valuable piece of knowledge for researchers, students, practitioners and scholars across the globe.

List of Contributors

Deborah Cristina Gonçalves Luiz Fernani and Maria Tereza Artero Prado
University of West Paulista, Presidente Prudente, SP, Brazil
Laboratory Design and Scientific Writing Department of Basic Sciences, ABC Faculty of Medicine, Av. Príncipe de Gales, 821, Vila Principe de Gales, Santo André, SP 09060-650, Brazil

Luiz Carlos de Abreu
Laboratory Design and Scientific Writing Department of Basic Sciences, ABC Faculty of Medicine, Av. Príncipe de Gales, 821, Vila Principe de Gales, Santo André, SP 09060-650, Brazil

Fernando Henrique Magalhães and Talita Dias da Silva
School of Arts, Sciences and Humanities, University of São Paulo, São Paulo, SP, Brazil

Thais Massetti
Post-graduate Program in Rehabilitation Sciences, Faculty of Medicine, University of São Paulo, São Paulo, SP, Brazil

Carlos Bandeira de Mello Monteiro
Laboratory Design and Scientific Writing Department of Basic Sciences, ABC Faculty of Medicine, Av. Príncipe de Gales, 821, Vila Principe de Gales, Santo André, SP 09060-650, Brazil
School of Arts, Sciences and Humanities, University of São Paulo, São Paulo, SP, Brazil
Post-graduate Program in Rehabilitation Sciences, Faculty of Medicine, University of São Paulo, São Paulo, SP, Brazil

Helen Dawes
Oxford Institute of Nursing and Allied Health Research, Oxford Brookes University, Oxford, UK
Department of Clinical Neurology, University of Oxford, Oxford, UK

Han-Jui Lee and Chui-Mei Tiu
Department of Radiology, Taipei Veterans General Hospital, Taipei, Taiwan
School of Medicine, National Yang-Ming University, Taipei, Taiwan

Tzu-Hung Chu and Chia-Feng Yang
School of Medicine, National Yang-Ming University, Taipei, Taiwan
Department of Pediatrics, Taipei Veterans General Hospital, Taipei, Taiwan

Ting-Rong Hsu and Dau-Ming Niu
Institute of Clinical Medicine, National Yang-Ming University, Taipei, Taiwan
Department of Pediatrics, Taipei Veterans General Hospital, Taipei, Taiwan

Sheng-Che Hung
Department of Radiology, Taipei Veterans General Hospital, Taipei, Taiwan
School of Medicine, National Yang-Ming University, Taipei, Taiwan
Department of Biomedical Imaging and Radiological Sciences, National Yang-Ming University, Taipei, Taiwan

Wen-Chung Yu
School of Medicine, National Yang-Ming University, Taipei, Taiwan
Division of Cardiology, Department of Medicine, Taipei Veterans General Hospital, Taipei, Taiwan

Svetlana Bizjajeva
Shire, Zug, Switzerland

Lijun Zuo
Department of Neurology, Beijing Tiantan Hospital, Capital Medical University, Beijing, China

Wei Zhang
Department of Neurology, Beijing Tiantan Hospital, Capital Medical University, Beijing, China
Epilepsy Center, Guangdong Sanjiu Brain Hospital, Jinan University, No. 578, Sha Tai Nan Lu, Guangzhou 510510, China

Xingzhou Liu and Qiang Guo
Epilepsy Center, Guangdong Sanjiu Brain Hospital, Jinan University, No. 578, Sha Tai Nan Lu, Guangzhou 510510, China

Qi chen
School of Psychology, South China Normal University, Guangzhou, China

Yongjun Wang
China National Clinical Research Center for Neurological Diseases, Beijing, China
Department of Neurology, Tiantan Clinical Trial and Research Center for Stroke, Beijing Tiantan Hospital, Capital Medical University, Beijing, China
Vascular Neurology, Department of Neurology, Beijing Tiantan Hospital, Capital Medical University, Beijing, China

Chaohua Yang, Baoqing Yu, Jianmin Huang, Bin Yu and Jianjun Feng
Department of Orthopaedics, Shanghai Pudong Hospital, Fudan University Pudong Medical Center, Shanghai 201399, China

Fenfen Ma and Huiping Lu
Department of Pharmacy, Shanghai Pudong Hospital, Fudan University, Shanghai 201399, China

Qinghua You
Department of Pathology, Shanghai Pudong Hospital, Fudan University Pudong Medical Center, Shanghai 201399, China

Jianlan Qiao
Department of Radiology, Shanghai Pudong Hospital, Fudan University Pudong Medical Center, Shanghai 201399, China

Paolo Solla, Antonino Cannas, Gianluca Floris, Davide Fonti and Gianni Orofino
Department of Neurology, Movement Disorders Center, Institute of Neurology, University of Cagliari, SS 554 Bivio per Sestu, Monserrato 09042, Cagliari, Italy

Francesco Marrosu
Department of Neurology, Movement Disorders Center, Institute of Neurology, University of Cagliari, SS 554 Bivio per Sestu, Monserrato 09042, Cagliari, Italy
Department of Medical Sciences and Public Health, University of Cagliari, Cagliari, Italy

Gioia Mura
Department of Medical Sciences and Public Health, University of Cagliari, Cagliari, Italy

Mauro Giovanni Carta
Chair of Quality of Care and Applied Medical Technologies, Department of Public Health, Clinical and Molecular Medicine, University of Cagliari, Monserrato, Italy

Jinfeng Wu
Department of Dermatology, Huashan Hospital, Fudan University, #12 Middle Wurumuqi Road, Shanghai 200040, People's Republic of China

Haibo Zhang, Yang Xu, Wei Zhu, Yi Zhang, Liang Chen and Wei Hua
Department of Neurosurgery, Huashan Hospital, Fudan University, #12 Middle Wurumuqi Road, Shanghai 200040, People's Republic of China

Jingwen Zhang
Department of Neurosurgery, Huashan Hospital, Fudan University, #12 Middle Wurumuqi Road, Shanghai 200040, People's Republic of China
Department of Ultrasound, Hebei General Hospital, #348 West Heping Road, Shijiazhuang, Hebei Province 050000, People's Republic of China

Ying Mao
Department of Neurosurgery, Huashan Hospital, Fudan University, #12 Middle Wurumuqi Road, Shanghai 200040, People's Republic of China
Institutes of Biomedical Sciences, Fudan University, #131 Dong'an Road, Shanghai 200040, People's Republic of China
State Key Laboratory of Medical Neurobiology, School of Basic Medical Sciences and Institutes of Brain Science, Fudan University, Shanghai 200040, People's Republic of China
The Collaborative Innovation Center for Brain Science, Fudan University, Shanghai 200040, People's Republic of China

Junliang Yuan, Shuna Yang, Wei Qin, Lei Yang and Wenli Hu
Department of Neurology, Beijing Chaoyang Hospital, Capital Medical University, Chaoyang District, Beijing, China

Shuangkun Wang
Department of Radiology, Beijing Chaoyang Hospital, Capital Medical University, Beijing, China

Liang Shen, Sheng Qiu, Zhongzhou Su and Xudong Ma
Department of Neurosurgery, Huzhou Central Hospital, 198 Hongqi Road, Huzhou, Zhejiang 313000, China

Teiji Tominaga
Department of Neurosurgery, Tohoku University Graduate School of Medicine, Sendai, Japan

Renfu Yan
Department of Neurosurgery, Huzhou Central Hospital, 198 Hongqi Road, Huzhou, Zhejiang 313000, China
School of Medicine, Huzhou University, 759 East Second Ring Road, Huzhou, Zhejiang 313000, China

Satoru Ohtomo and Hiroaki Arai
Department of Neurosurgery, South Miyagi Medical Center, 38-1 Azanishi, Ogawara-machi, Shibata-gun, Miyagi 989-1253, Japan

Yoshiteru Shimoda
Department of Neurosurgery, South Miyagi Medical Center, 38-1 Azanishi, Ogawara-machi, Shibata-gun, Miyagi 989-1253, Japan
Department of Neurosurgery, Tohoku University Graduate School of Medicine, Sendai, Japan

Takashi Ohtoh
Department of Pathology, South Miyagi Medical Center, Shibata-gun, Miyagi, Japan

Gun-Ha Kim
Department of Pediatrics, College of Medicine, Korea University, Seoul, South Korea
Comprehensive Epilepsy Center, Florida Hospital for Children and Florida Hospital, 615 E. Rollins Street, Orlando, FL 32803, USA

Joo Hee Seo, James E. Baumgartner, Fatima Ajmal and Ki Hyeong Lee
Comprehensive Epilepsy Center, Florida Hospital for Children and Florida Hospital, 615 E. Rollins Street, Orlando, FL 32803, USA

Salvatore Monaco and Sergio Ferrari
Department of Neuroscience, Biomedicine and Movement Sciences, Section of Neurology, University of Verona, Verona, Italy

Sara Mariotto
Department of Neuroscience, Biomedicine and Movement Sciences, Section of Neurology, University of Verona, Verona, Italy
Clinical Department of Neurology, Medical University of Innsbruck, Innsbruck, Austria

Patrick Peschl and Markus Reindl
Clinical Department of Neurology, Medical University of Innsbruck, Innsbruck, Austria

Ilaria Coledan and Romualdo Mazzi
Department of Diagnostics and Public Health, Section of Infectious Diseases, University of Verona, Verona, Italy

Romana Höftberger
Institute of Neurology, Medical University of Vienna, Vienna, Austria

Wen Li Hu and Jun Liang Yuan
Department of Neurology, Beijing Chaoyang Hospital, Capital Medical University, Beijing 100020, China

Shuang Kun Wang and Tao Jiang
Department of Radiology, Beijing Chaoyang Hospital, Capital Medical University, Beijing 100020, China

Fanfan Chen, Yongfu Cao, Yongjun Yi, Jingwen Zhuang, Wuhua Le, Wei Xie, Lanbo Tu and Peng Li
Neurosurgery Department, Guangzhou First People's Hospital, Guangzhou Medical University, 1# Panfu Road, Guangzhou, Guangdong 510180, China

Lei Chen
Neurosurgery Department, Shenzhen Second People's Hospital, Shenzhen University, 3002# Sungang Road, Shenzhen 518037, China

Yimin Fang
Tuberculosis Department, Guangzhou Chest Hospital, 62# Hengzhi Gang Road, Guangzhou, Guangdong 510095, China

Ling Li
Record Department, Guangzhou First People's Hospital, Guangzhou Medical University, 1# Panfu Road, Guangzhou, Guangdong 510180, China

Yuqing Kou and Kaikai Fu
Department of Navy Medicine, The Second Military Medical University, 800# Xiangyin Road, Shanghai 200433, China

Hua He
Neurosurgery Department, Changzheng Hospital, The Second Military Medical University;State key Laboratory of Drug Research, Shanghai Institute of Material Medical, Chinese Academy of Sciences, 415# Fengyang Road, Shanghai 200003, China

Hongbin Ju
Spinal Surgery Department, Guangzhou First People's Hospital, Guangzhou Medical University, 1# Panfu Road, Guangzhou, Guangdong 510180, China

Daisuke Taniguchi, Hideki Shimura, Masao Watanabe and Takao Urabe
Department of Neurology, Juntendo University Urayasu Hospital, 2-1-1 Tomioka, Urayasu, Chiba 279-0021, Japan

Nobutaka Hattori
Department of Neurology, Juntendo University School of Medicine, 2-1-1 Hongo, Bunkyo-ku, Tokyo 113-8421, Japan

Vanesa Bochkezanian
Department of Exercise and Health Sciences, School of Health, Medical and Applied Sciences, Central Queensland University, Building 34.1.02, Bruce Highway, North Rockhampton, Qld 4702, Australia
Exercise Medicine Research Clinic, Edith Cowan University, Perth, Australia
Centre for Sports and Exercise Science, School of Medical and Health Sciences, Edith Cowan University, Joondalup, Australia

Robert U. Newton
Exercise Medicine Research Clinic, Edith Cowan University, Perth, Australia
Centre for Sports and Exercise Science, School of Medical and Health Sciences, Edith Cowan University, Joondalup, Australia
UQ Centre for Clinical Research, The University of Queensland, Brisbane, Australia

Timothy S. Pulverenti and Anthony J. Blazevich
Centre for Sports and Exercise Science, School of Medical and Health Sciences, Edith Cowan University, Joondalup, Australia

Gabriel S. Trajano
School of Exercise and Nutrition Sciences, Institute of Health and Biomedical Innovation, Queensland University of Technology (QUT), Brisbane, Australia

Amilton Vieira
UDF-University Centre, Brasilia, Brazil

Kanitpong Phabphal and Suparat Chisurajinda
Neurology Unit, Department of Medicine, Faculty of Medicine, Prince of Songkla University, Hat Yai, Songkhla 90110, Thailand

Thapanee Somboon and Kanjana Unwongse
Prasat Neurological Institute, Bangkok 10400, Thailand

Alan Geater
Epidemiology Unit, Department of Epidemiology, Faculty of Medicine, Prince of Songkla University, Hat Yai, Songkhla 90110, Thailand

Rui-li Li, Jun Sun and Hong-jun Li
Department of Radiology, Beijing YouAn Hospital, Capital Medical University, No.8, Xi Tou Tiao, Youanmen Wai, Feng Tai District, Beijing 100069, China

Zhen-chao Tang
School of Mechanical, Electrical & Information Engineering, Shandong University, No.180, West Wenhua Road, Weihai 264209, Shandong Province, China

Jing-ji Zhang
STD and AIDS clinical treatment center, Beijing YouAn Hospital, Capital Medical University, No.8, Xi Tou Tiao, Youanmen Wai, Feng Tai District, Beijing 100069, China

Anna Misyail Abdul Rashid
Department of Medicine, Faculty of Medicine and Health Sciences, Universiti Putra Malaysia, Serdang, Malaysia

Mohamad Syafeeq Faeez Md Noh
Department of Imaging, Faculty of Medicine and Health Sciences, Universiti Putra Malaysia, Serdang, Malaysia

Hong Qiao
Department of General Affairs Section, Second Affiliated Hospital of Mudanjiang Medical University, Mudanjiang, Heilongjiang 157009, People's Republic of China

Yong-Bo Wang and Yu-Mei Gao
Department of Respiratory Medicine, Second Affiliated Hospital of Mudanjiang Medical University, Mudanjiang, Heilongjiang 157009, People's Republic of China

Li-Li Bi
Department of Medical Instruments, Second Affiliated Hospital of Mudanjiang Medical University, Mudanjiang, Heilongjiang 157009, People's Republic of China

Tian Song, Xindi Li and Xinghu Zhang
Neuroinfection and Neuroimmunology Center, Department of Neurology, Beijing Tiantan Hospital, Capital Medical University, 6 TiantanXili, Dongcheng District, Beijing 100050, People's Republic of China
China National Clinical Research Center for Neurological Diseases, Beijing Tiantan Hospital, Capital Medical University, 6 TiantanXili, Dongcheng District, Beijing 100050, People's Republic of China

Yonghong Liu
Department of Neurology, Beijing Rehabilitation Hospital, Capital Medical University,Xixiazhuang, Shijingshan District, Beijing 100050, People's Republic of China

Yuzhi Gao, Qiang Li, Chunshuang Wu, Shaoyun Liu and Mao Zhang
Department of Emergency Medicine, Second Affiliated Hospital, Zhejiang University School of Medicine, No. 88, Jiefang Road, Hangzhou City 310009, Zhejiang Province, China

Malek Chouchi
Department of Genetic, Tunis El Manar University, Faculty of Medicine of Tunis, 15 Jebel Lakhdhar street, La Rabta, 1007 Tunis, Tunisia
Department of Child Neurology, National Institute Mongi Ben Hmida of Neurology, UR12SP24 Abnormal Movements of Neurologic Diseases, Jebel Lakhdhar street, La Rabta, 1007 Tunis, Tunisia

Hedia Klaa and Ilhem Ben-Youssef Turki
Department of Child Neurology, National Institute Mongi Ben Hmida of Neurology, UR12SP24 Abnormal Movements of Neurologic Diseases, Jebel Lakhdhar street, La Rabta, 1007 Tunis, Tunisia

Wajih Kaabachi and Kalthoum Tizaoui
Division of Histology and Immunology Division, Department of Basic Sciences, Faculty of Medicine of Tunis, 15 Jebel Lakhdhar street, La Rabta, 1007 Tunis, Tunisia

Lamia Hila
Department of Genetic, Faculty of Medicine of Tunis, 15 Jebel Lakhdhar street, La Rabta, 1007 Tunis,Tunisia

Richard Finkel and Matthew Civitello
Nemours Children's Hospital, University of Central Florida College of Medicine, Orlando, USA

Maria C. Pera, Giorgia Coratti, Nicola Forcina, Elena S. Mazzone, Lavinia Fanelli, Roberto de Sanctis, Laura Antonaci, Leonardo Lapenta, Simona Lucibello, Marika Pane and Eugenio Mercuri
Pediatric Neurology, Catholic University, Largo Gemelli 8, 00168 Rome, Italy

Mariacristina Scoto, Marion Main, Danielle Ramsey and Francesco Muntoni
Dubowitz Neuromuscular Centre, UCL Institute of Child Health & Great Ormond Street Hospital, London, UK

Jacqueline Montes, Sally Dunaway, Rachel Salazar and Darryl C. De Vivo
Department of Neurology, Columbia University Medical Center, New York, NY, USA

Amy Pasternak and Basil T. Darras
Department of Neurology, Boston Children's Hospital, Harvard Medical School, Boston, MA, USA

Anna Mayhew and Robert Muni Lofra
John Walton Muscular Dystrophy Research Centre, Institute of Genetic Medicine, Newcastle University, Newcastle, UK

Sonia Messina and Maria Sframeli
Department of Clinical and Experimental Medicine and Nemo Sud Clinical Center, University of Messina, Messina, Italy

Tina Duong and John Day
Stanford University, Palo Alto, CA, USA

Kaiyu Qin, Wenqing Wu, Yuming Huang, Dongmei Xu, Lei Zhang, Bowen Zheng, Meijuan Jiang, Cheng Kou, Junhua Gao, Wurong Li, Jinglin Zhang, Sumei Wang, Yanfei Luan, Chaoling Yan, Dan Xu and Xinmei Zheng
Department of neurology, Beijing Ditan Hospital, Capital Medical University, No.8 East Jing Shun Rd, Chaoyang District, Beijing, China

Michael Strupp and Julian Teufel
Department of Neurology with Friedrich-Baur-Institute, University Hospital, Munich, Germany
German Center for Vertigo and Balance Disorders (DSGZ), University Hospital, Munich, Germany

Ingrid Berger, Ivonne Naumann and Otmar Bayer
German Center for Vertigo and Balance Disorders (DSGZ), University Hospital, Munich, Germany

Christine Adrion and Ulrich Mansmann
Institute for Medical Informatics, Biometry and Epidemiology (IBE), University Hospital, Munich, Germany

Claudia Stendel
Department of Neurology with Friedrich-Baur-Institute, University Hospital, Munich, Germany German Center for Neurodegenerative Diseases (DZNE), Munich 80336, Germany

Jens Claassen and Ellen Uslar
Department of Neurology, University Hospital Essen, University of Duisburg-Essen, Essen, Germany

Ludger Schöls and Holger Hengel
Department of Neurology and Hertie Institute for Clinical Brain Research, University Hospital Tübingen, Tübingen, Germany

Ilaria Giordano, Heike Jacobi and Thomas Klockgether
German Center for Neurodegenerative Diseases (DZNE), Center for Clinical Research, Bonn, Germany

Sylvia Bösch and Wolfgang Nachbauer
Department of Neurology, Medical University Innsbruck, Innsbruck, Austria

Bart van de Warrenburg
Department of Neurology, Donders Institute for Brain, Cognition, and Behaviour, Radboud University Medical Centre, Nijmegen, Netherlands

Hans-Helge Müller
Institute for Medical Biometry and Epidemiology, Philipps University Marburg, Marburg, Germany

Katharina Feil
Department of Neurology with Friedrich-Baur-Institute, University Hospital, Munich, Germany German Center for Vertigo and Balance Disorders (DSGZ), University Hospital, Munich, Germany Department of Neurology and German Center for Vertigo and Balance Disorders, University Hospital, Campus Grosshadern, Marchioninistrasse 15, Munich 81377, Germany

Thomas Klopstock
Department of Neurology with Friedrich-Baur-Institute, University Hospital, Munich, Germany German Center for Neurodegenerative Diseases (DZNE), Munich 80336, Germany Munich Cluster for Systems Neurology (SyNergy), Munich 80336, Germany

Benjamin Berger, Tilman Hottenrott, Sebastian Rauer and Oliver Stich
Department of Neurology and Neurophysiology, Medical Center—University of Freiburg, Faculty of Medicine, Breisacher Strasse 64, D-79106 Freiburg, Germany

Index

www.ingramcontent.com/pod-product-compliance
Lightning Source LLC
Chambersburg PA
CBHW082016190326
41458CB00010B/3202